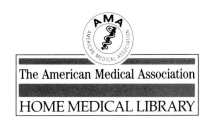

The American Medical Association

HOME MEDICAL LIBRARY

MEDICAL DICTIONARY AND INDEX

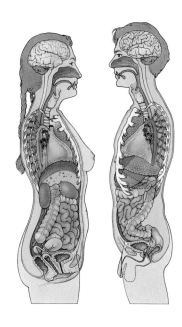

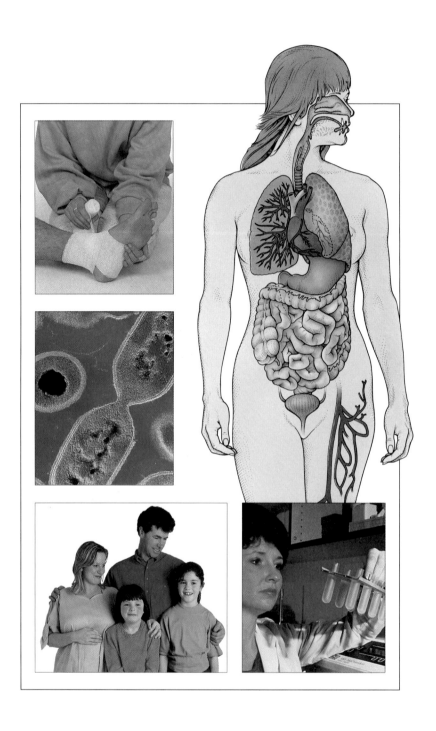

THE AMERICAN
MEDICAL ASSOCIATION

MEDICAL DICTIONARY AND INDEX

Medical Editor
CHARLES B. CLAYMAN, MD

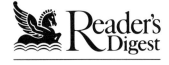

THE READER'S DIGEST ASSOCIATION, INC.
Pleasantville, New York/Montreal

The AMA Home Medical Library was created and produced
by Dorling Kindersley, Ltd., in association with the
American Medical Association.

The information in this book reflects current medical knowledge. The
recommendations and information are appropriate in most cases;
however, they are not a substitute for medical diagnosis. For specific
information concerning your personal medical condition, the AMA
suggests that you consult a physician.

The names of organizations, products, or alternative therapies appearing
in this book are given for informational purposes only. Their inclusion
does not imply AMA endorsement, nor does the omission of any
organization, product, or alternative therapy indicate AMA disapproval.

The AMA Home Medical Library is distinct from and unrelated to the
series of health books published by Random House, Inc., in conjunction
with the American Medical Association under the names ''The AMA Home
Reference Library'' and ''The AMA Home Health Library.''

Library of Congress Cataloging in Publication Data

Medical dictionary and index / medical editor, Charles B. Clayman.
    p.   cm. — (The American Medical Association home medical
library)
  Includes index.
  ISBN 0-89577-540-9
  1. Medicine—Dictionaries.   2. American Medical Association home
medical library—Indexes.   I. Clayman, Charles B.   II. American
Medical Association.   III. Series.
R121.M493 1993
610'.3—dc20   93-1729

FOREWORD

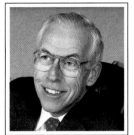 With health care a top priority for Americans, it is more important now than ever before for you to work with your doctor in a partnership to protect your health and the health of family members. The surest path to a successful relationship between you and your doctor is communication – your ability to communicate your concerns and his or her ability to answer your questions in clear language that you can understand.

We at the American Medical Association want to help you become better prepared for and more confident about discussing your health care concerns with your doctor. We have developed the AMA Home Medical Library, a 19-volume series, to introduce you to many aspects of health and medicine. Each book is extensively illustrated, full of facts, and written in concise, easy-to-understand language.

This final volume will guide you through the enormous amount of useful medical information contained in the AMA Home Medical Library. It serves both as an illustrated medical dictionary and an index to the series.

At one time, much of the content of this series of books would have been accessible only to medical professionals. But we believe that there is no such thing as having too much information because it allows you to make intelligent health care decisions. The series, with topics ranging from first aid to the latest discoveries in genetics, provides you with basic facts that make you a more knowledgeable consumer of health care.

We at the AMA wish you and your loved ones good health and, through our series of books, a better understanding of how to preserve it.

James S. Todd MD

JAMES S. TODD, MD
Executive Vice President
American Medical Association

CONTENTS

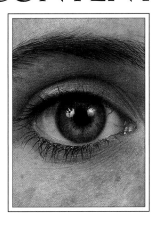

Foreword   *5*

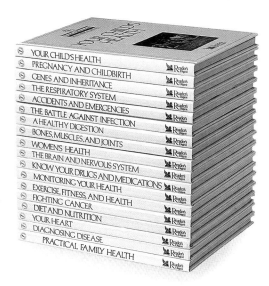

HOW TO USE THE AMA HOME MEDICAL LIBRARY

The AMA Home Medical Library is a valuable reference source covering all aspects of medicine and health. The series is extensively illustrated to make the information more usable for you and members of your family. The Library consists of 18 volumes in addition to the book you are holding in your hand – which contains an illustrated MEDICAL DICTIONARY and an index to direct you to information anywhere in the series. In the AMA HOME MEDICAL LIBRARY INDEX on pages 104 to 144, each book in the series has an assigned code letter that identifies it. The individual volumes and their code letters are shown on these pages.

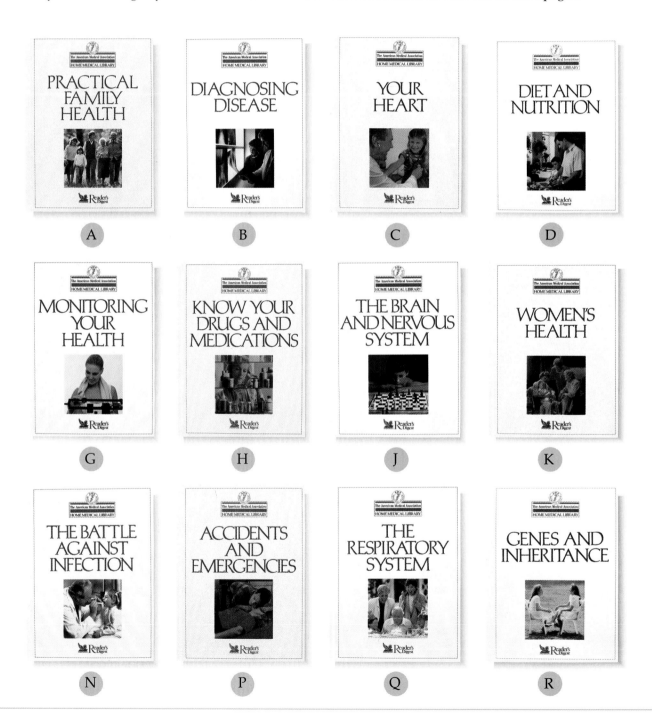

There are many ways to find the information you need in the AMA Home Medical Library.

◆ Usually it will be obvious which volume of the AMA Home Medical Library contains the information you are looking for. For example, you are most likely to find information about heart function and disease in the volume **Your Heart** and information about nutrition in the **Diet and Nutrition** volume. Consult the index at the back of the individual volume to find the specific information you are seeking.

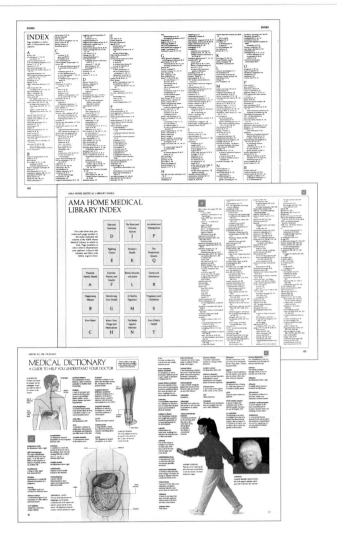

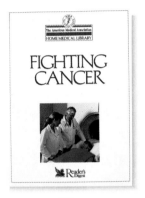

 E

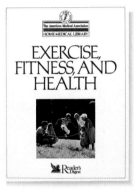

 F

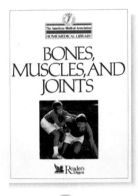

 L

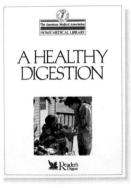

 M

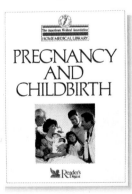

 S

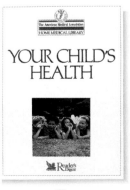

 T

◆ For a more extensive listing of places to find information about a particular subject, consult the AMA HOME MEDICAL LIBRARY INDEX on pages 104 to 144 of this volume. It will direct you to the pages in the various volumes on which you will find references to the subject you are interested in.

◆ If you want to know the meaning of a medical phrase or term, consult the illustrated MEDICAL DICTIONARY on pages 20 to 103 of this volume.

◆ If you are interested in learning about a particular symptom, disorder, surgical procedure, or drug, you will want to read the relevant instructive section (HOW TO ANSWER QUESTIONS ABOUT SYMPTOMS, HOW TO LEARN ABOUT DISEASES AND DISORDERS, ... SURGICAL PROCEDURES, and .... DRUGS) on pages 10 to 16.

◆ You can learn how to find information in an emergency by reading the section HOW TO USE THE AMA HOME MEDICAL LIBRARY IN AN EMERGENCY on pages 18 and 19.

HOW TO ANSWER QUESTIONS ABOUT SYMPTOMS

The AMA HOME MEDICAL LIBRARY INDEX on pages 104 to 144 will help direct you to places throughout the series where particular symptoms are discussed.

On pages 134 to 141 of the volume **Accidents and Emergencies**, you will find a section called EMERGENCY SYMPTOMS that can help you recognize those symptoms requiring immediate medical attention.

In addition, a total of 38 MONITOR YOUR SYMPTOMS charts, describing the symptoms that occur most often in both adults and children, can be found throughout the AMA Home Medical Library. The question-and-answer format of the charts makes it easy for you to learn about the possible causes of common symptoms and to find out what action you can take.

At right is a list of the symptoms described in the 38 charts; each is accompanied by a code letter indicating the volume of the AMA Home Medical Library containing the chart and the page on which it appears. A key to the code letters is on pages 8 and 9.

Questions
Each question requires a "yes" or "no" answer. Follow the arrows directing you to the next question and continue until you reach the information that applies to your condition.

CONSULT YOUR DOCTOR WITHOUT DELAY!

This instruction is used for a serious condition requiring immediate medical assessment but for which a delay of a few hours is unlikely to be harmful. Seek your doctor's advice within 24 hours. That usually means calling to make an appointment for the same day.

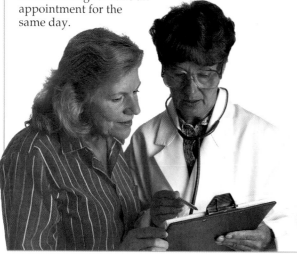

Introduction
The introductory section of each symptom chart describes the symptom, gives its most common causes, and provides useful information such as the degree of severity of the symptom or the combination of symptoms that would indicate you should consult your doctor.

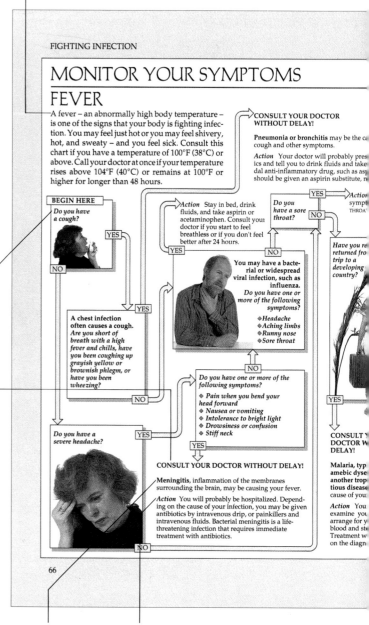

FIGHTING INFECTION

MONITOR YOUR SYMPTOMS
FEVER

A fever – an abnormally high body temperature – is one of the signs that your body is fighting infection. You may feel just hot or you may feel shivery, hot, and sweaty – and you feel sick. Consult this chart if you have a temperature of 100°F (38°C) or above. Call your doctor at once if your temperature rises above 104°F (40°C) or remains at 100°F or higher for longer than 48 hours.

CONSULT YOUR DOCTOR WITHOUT DELAY!

Pneumonia or bronchitis may be the ca cough and other symptoms.

Action Your doctor will probably pres ics and tell you to drink fluids and take dal anti-inflammatory drug, such as asp should be given an aspirin substitute, r

BEGIN HERE
Do you have a cough?
YES / NO

Action Stay in bed, drink fluids, and take aspirin or acetaminophen. Consult your doctor if you start to feel breathless or if you don't feel better after 24 hours.

Do you have a sore throat?
YES / NO

Action sympt THROA'

You may have a bacterial or widespread viral infection, such as influenza.
Do you have one or more of the following symptoms?
◆ Headache
◆ Aching limbs
◆ Runny nose
◆ Sore throat

Have you re returned fro trip to a developing country?

A chest infection often causes a cough. *Are you short of breath with a high fever and chills, have you been coughing up grayish yellow or brownish phlegm, or have you been wheezing?*
NO

Do you have one or more of the following symptoms?
◆ Pain when you bend your head forward
◆ Nausea or vomiting
◆ Intolerance to bright light
◆ Drowsiness or confusion
◆ Stiff neck

Do you have a severe headache?
YES / NO

CONSULT YOUR DOCTOR WITHOUT DELAY!

Meningitis, inflammation of the membranes surrounding the brain, may be causing your fever.

Action You will probably be hospitalized. Depending on the cause of your infection, you may be given antibiotics by intravenous drip, or painkillers and intravenous fluids. Bacterial meningitis is a life-threatening infection that requires immediate treatment with antibiotics.

CONSULT DOCTOR W DELAY!

Malaria, typ amebic dyse another trop tious disease cause of you

Action You examine you arrange for y blood and te Treatment w on the diagn

66

The diagnosis
In most cases, the series of questions leads to a probable diagnosis.

Action
If you need to consult a doctor, we tell you whether you are likely to be hospitalized and what types of tests and treatments you might have. When appropriate, we offer you tips about things you can do at home to treat your illness.

EMERGENCY CALL YOUR DOCTOR NOW!

This instruction is used for potentially life-threatening conditions. Call your doctor immediately for advice. If you cannot get hold of your doctor, proceed as for EMERGENCY CALL FOR MEDICAL HELP NOW!

EMERGENCY CALL FOR MEDICAL HELP NOW!

This advice is given for life-threatening situations. Call 911 or your local emergency number. If the person can be moved safely, you may have to drive him or her to the nearest hospital emergency room.

MONITOR YOUR SYMPTOMS CHARTS

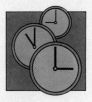

The charts are listed by symptom rather than by title.

YOUR BODY'S DEFENSES

A kidney or bladder infection may cause a fever and other symptoms. *Do you have one or more of the following symptoms?*
- Pain in the middle portion or small of your back
- Abnormally frequent urination
- Pain when urinating
- Pink or cloudy urine

YES → **CONSULT YOUR DOCTOR WITHOUT DELAY!**

A kidney or bladder infection is a possibility.

Action Your doctor will examine you and take a urine specimen and may prescribe an antibiotic. Your doctor may also arrange for you to have a kidney X-ray or ultrasound examination. Further treatment depends on the results of the tests.

NO

Do you have a rash on your trunk or on your arms and legs?

YES → **CONSULT YOUR DOCTOR WITHOUT DELAY!**

An infectious disease such as chickenpox, measles, rubella, or Rocky Mountain spotted fever may be causing your rash. These infectious diseases can be very serious in adults.

Action Your doctor will probably advise you to rest, drink plenty of fluids, and take a nonsteroidal anti-inflammatory drug such as aspirin.

WARNING
Consult your doctor without delay if you have had recurrent bouts of elevated temperature for no apparent reason or if you have been sweating profusely at night, especially if you also feel sick. Some chronic infections and disorders of the lymphatic system cause such symptoms.

NO

Has your urine changed to a brownish color and/or have the whites of your eyes or your skin turned yellow?

NO → *Do you have diarrhea?* → NO → *Are you a woman?* → YES → *Do you have pain in the lower part of your abdomen or have you had a heavy or unpleasant-smelling vaginal discharge?*

YES (diarrhea) → **Viral gastroenteritis** (inflammation of the stomach and intestines) may be the cause of your diarrhea.

Action If your symptoms are severe, or they continue longer than 24 to 48 hours, consult your doctor immediately.

NO (woman)

YES (urine) → **CONSULT YOUR DOCTOR WITHOUT DELAY!**

Viral hepatitis may be causing your dark urine or yellow skin or eyes, which are signs of jaundice.

Action Treatment, which includes rest, depends on the type of virus causing the jaundice.

Action Consult your doctor if you are unable to make a diagnosis from this chart and your temperature has not returned to normal within 48 hours, or if it rises again.

NO / YES → **CONSULT YOUR DOCTOR NOW!**

A fallopian tube infection (salpingitis) or pelvic inflammatory disease may be causing your symptoms.

Action Your doctor will probably perform a vaginal examination and take a sample of vaginal discharge for analysis. If tests confirm the diagnosis, antibiotics will be prescribed.

67

CONSULT YOUR DOCTOR NOW!

In this case, you might have a serious condition that requires prompt treatment. Call your doctor immediately for instructions. If you cannot reach your doctor within an hour, proceed as for EMERGENCY CALL FOR MEDICAL HELP NOW!

Warning boxes
Warning boxes draw your attention to potentially serious symptoms and advise you about what action to take.

HOW TO LEARN ABOUT DISEASES AND DISORDERS

The AMA HOME MEDICAL LIBRARY INDEX at the back of this volume will help direct you to places in the series where particular disorders are discussed. In addition, the AMA Home Medical Library contains more than 100 CASE HISTORIES describing the usual symptoms, diagnosis, treatment, and outcome of a number of common disorders, diseases, and injuries. Below, and at right, is an alphabetical listing of the topics covered in the CASE HISTORIES. Each case history is accompanied by a code letter indicating the volume that contains it and the page on which it appears. A key to the code letters can be found on pages 8 and 9.

The person
A photograph of the person discussed in the case history is accompanied by his or her name, age, and occupation along with information about the health of family members.

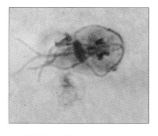

Additional information
Illustrations and captions help to explain the detailed medical information presented in every case history.

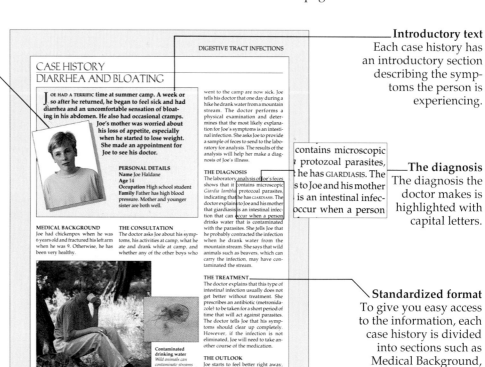

Introductory text
Each case history has an introductory section describing the symptoms the person is experiencing.

The diagnosis
The diagnosis the doctor makes is highlighted with capital letters.

Standardized format
To give you easy access to the information, each case history is divided into sections such as Medical Background, The Consultation, The Diagnosis, The Treatment, and The Outlook.

CASE HISTORY SUBJECTS

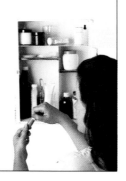

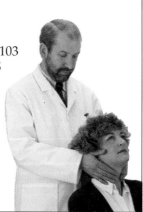

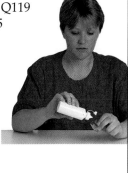

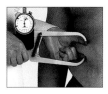

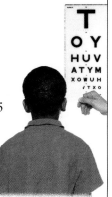

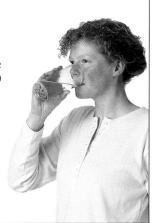

HOW TO LEARN ABOUT SURGICAL PROCEDURES

The AMA HOME MEDICAL LIBRARY INDEX at the back of this volume will help direct you to places in the series where particular surgical procedures are explained. Many of the most frequently performed operations are highlighted in SURGICAL PROCEDURES features – scattered throughout the series – that describe and illustrate the stages of the operation step-by-step.

On the opposite page is an alphabetical listing of the 28 SURGICAL PROCEDURES boxes that appear in various books in the series. Each listing is accompanied by a code letter indicating the volume of the AMA Home Medical Library in which the procedure is featured, and the page number on which it appears. A key to the code letters can be found on pages 8 and 9.

Background information
For each surgical procedure, an introductory section provides background information, such as the reasons for the operation, the chances for a successful outcome, and the probable recovery time.

The problem
Illustrations and X-rays or other medical images show the diseased or injured area to be operated on.

Incision sites
Solid or dotted lines drawn on anatomical illustrations show the position and shape of the surgeon's incision.

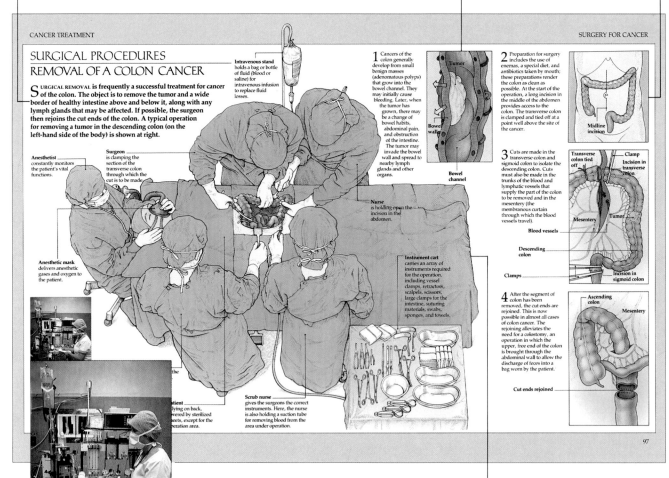

The equipment
Illustrations draw your attention to specialized equipment used during the operation, such as the mobile anesthetic cart shown at left.

The procedure
For some surgical procedures, illustrations depict the operating-room setting and show the roles played by the medical specialists involved.

The patient
Illustrations show the position of the patient on the operating table and highlight the preparations carried out before the operation, such as application of a tourniquet.

Step-by-step text and illustrations
Explanatory text and detailed illustrations take you through the stages of the surgical procedure.

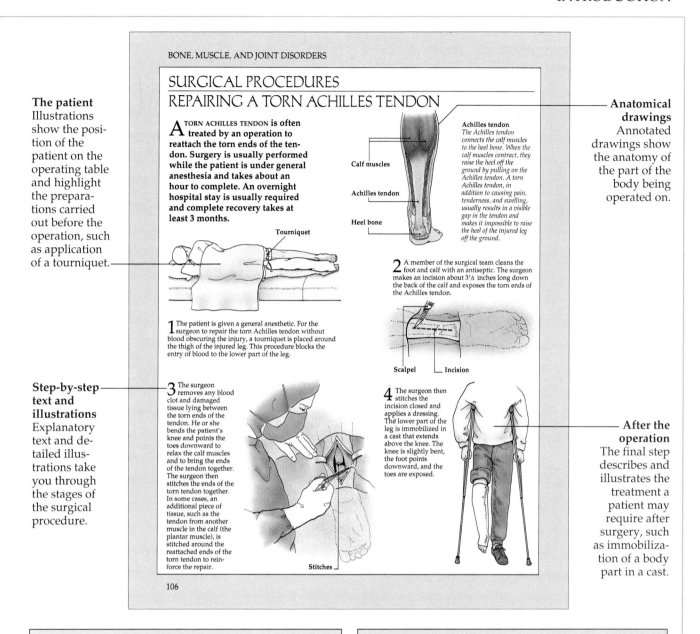

BONE, MUSCLE, AND JOINT DISORDERS

SURGICAL PROCEDURES
REPAIRING A TORN ACHILLES TENDON

A TORN ACHILLES TENDON is often treated by an operation to reattach the torn ends of the tendon. Surgery is usually performed while the patient is under general anesthesia and takes about an hour to complete. An overnight hospital stay is usually required and complete recovery takes at least 3 months.

Calf muscles

Achilles tendon

Heel bone

Tourniquet

Achilles tendon
The Achilles tendon connects the calf muscles to the heel bone. When the calf muscles contract, they raise the heel off the ground by pulling on the Achilles tendon. A torn Achilles tendon, in addition to causing pain, tenderness, and swelling, usually results in a visible gap in the tendon and makes it impossible to raise the heel of the injured leg off the ground.

1 The patient is given a general anesthetic. For the surgeon to repair the torn Achilles tendon without blood obscuring the injury, a tourniquet is placed around the thigh of the injured leg. This procedure blocks the entry of blood to the lower part of the leg.

2 A member of the surgical team cleans the foot and calf with an antiseptic. The surgeon makes an incision about 3 1/2 inches long down the back of the calf and exposes the torn ends of the Achilles tendon.

Scalpel   Incision

3 The surgeon removes any blood clot and damaged tissue lying between the torn ends of the tendon. He or she bends the patient's knee and points the toes downward to relax the calf muscles and to bring the ends of the tendon together. The surgeon then stitches the ends of the torn tendon together. In some cases, an additional piece of tissue, such as the tendon from another muscle in the calf (the plantar muscle), is stitched around the reattached ends of the torn tendon to reinforce the repair.

Stitches

4 The surgeon then stitches the incision closed and applies a dressing. The lower part of the leg is immobilized in a cast that extends above the knee. The knee is slightly bent, the foot points downward, and the toes are exposed.

106

Anatomical drawings
Annotated drawings show the anatomy of the part of the body being operated on.

After the operation
The final step describes and illustrates the treatment a patient may require after surgery, such as immobilization of a body part in a cast.

SURGICAL PROCEDURES BOXES

Achilles tendon repair L106
Aneurysm repair J112
Appendectomy M124
Arthroscopic repair of a shoulder injury L99
Balloon angioplasty C118
Breast cancer surgery E92
Bypass surgery, coronary artery C78
Cesarean section S114
Cholecystectomy M109
Colon cancer surgery E96
Colostomy M121
Dilatation and curettage K101
Drainage of a pancreatic pseudocyst M113
Gallbladder removal M109
Heart transplant C96
Heart valve replacement C89

Hip joint replacement L82
Hole-in-the-heart repair C71
Hysterectomy K106
Internal fixation of fractured femur L72
Laparoscopic cholecystectomy M109
Liver transplant M104
Lobectomy for lung cancer Q127
Lumpectomy E92
Mastectomy
    Partial E92
    Modified radical E93
    Subcutaneous E93
Meniscectomy F111
Microdiscectomy L120
Nerve repair J35
Prostate cancer surgery E94
Resection of the rectum M132
Spinal fusion L127
Stereotaxic surgery J99

HOW TO LEARN ABOUT DRUGS

The AMA HOME MEDICAL LIBRARY INDEX at the back of this volume will help direct you to places throughout the series where you can find information about particular drug groups (for example, antihistamines, beta blockers, or analgesic drugs) and a number of the most widely used generic drugs.

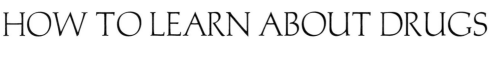

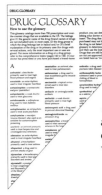

In addition, the DRUG GLOSSARY on pages 134 to 141 of **Know Your Drugs and Medications** catalogs, by generic name, about 700 prescription and over-the-counter drugs and provides a brief description of each drug's uses and/or the drug group to which it belongs.

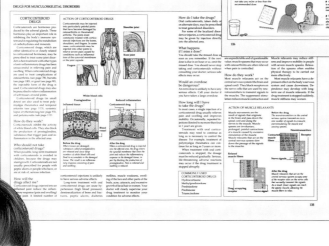

There are also special sections on DRUGS FOR THE HEART AND CIRCULATION on pages 126 to 139 of **Your Heart** and on DRUGS FOR MUSCULOSKELETAL DISORDERS on pages 128 to 139 of **Bones, Muscles, and Joints.**

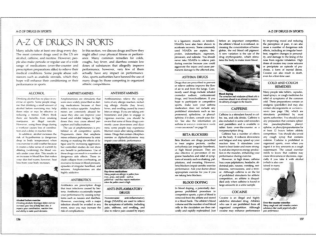

On pages 136 to 139 of **Exercise, Fitness, and Health**, you will find a reference section called A-Z OF DRUGS IN SPORTS.

MORE SOURCES OF INFORMATION

The AMA Home Medical Library provides many other useful and informative reference sections.

A–Z OF
MEDICAL TESTS
**Diagnosing
Disease** pages
128 to 141

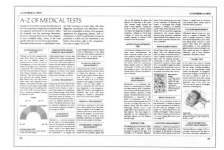

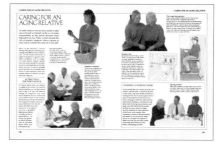

CARING FOR AN AGING RELATIVE ▶
Women's Health pages 138 to 139

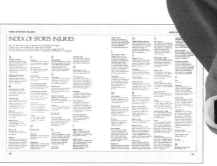

◀ CANCER FACT FILE
Fighting Cancer
pages 122 to 141

INDEX OF SPORTS INJURIES ▶
Exercise, Fitness, and Health
pages 140 to 141

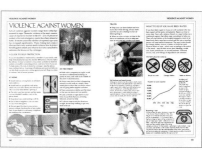

VIOLENCE AGAINST WOMEN ▶
Women's Health pages 140 to 141

▲
FACT FILE OF SINGLE-GENE DISORDERS
Genes and Inheritance
pages 136 to 139

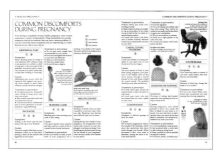

◀
COMMON DISCOMFORTS OF PREGNANCY
Pregnancy and Childbirth
pages 40 to 45

HOW TO USE THE AMA HOME MEDICAL LIBRARY IN AN EMERGENCY

Knowing what to do in the event of an accident or when severe symptoms begin suddenly can make the difference between life and death. In the AMA Home Medical Library, you will find information about how to handle almost any emergency, with illustrated, step-by-step instructions for first aid and clear guidelines on when to seek medical help.

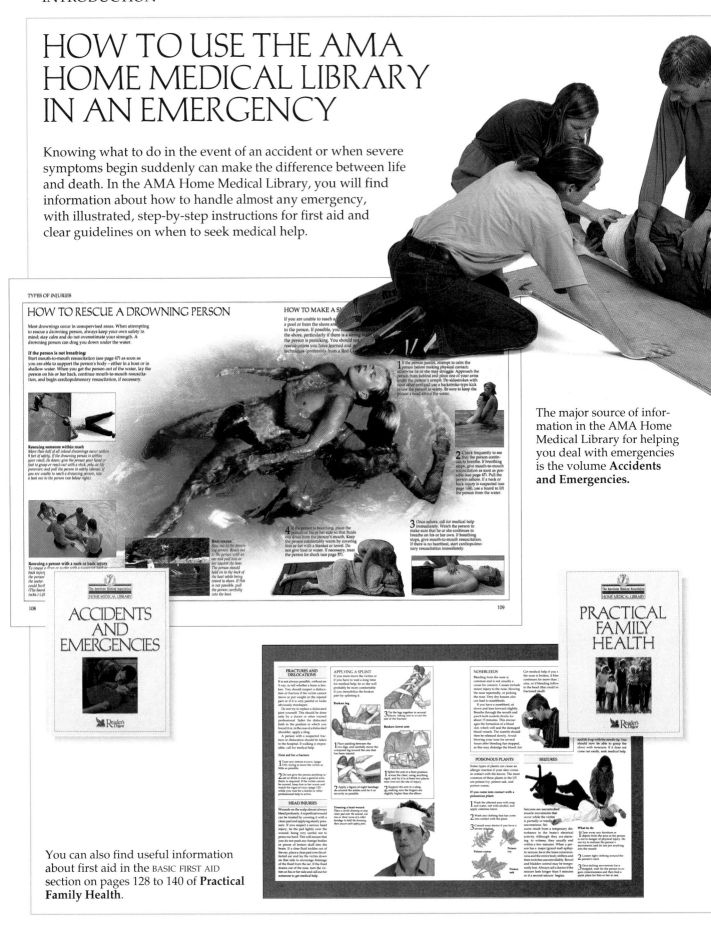

The major source of information in the AMA Home Medical Library for helping you deal with emergencies is the volume **Accidents and Emergencies.**

You can also find useful information about first aid in the BASIC FIRST AID section on pages 128 to 140 of **Practical Family Health**.

If you experience serious symptoms related to the digestive system – such as severe abdominal pain, vomiting blood, or passing dark or bloody feces – consult the section ABDOMINAL EMERGENCIES on pages 134 to 139 of **A Healthy Digestion**.

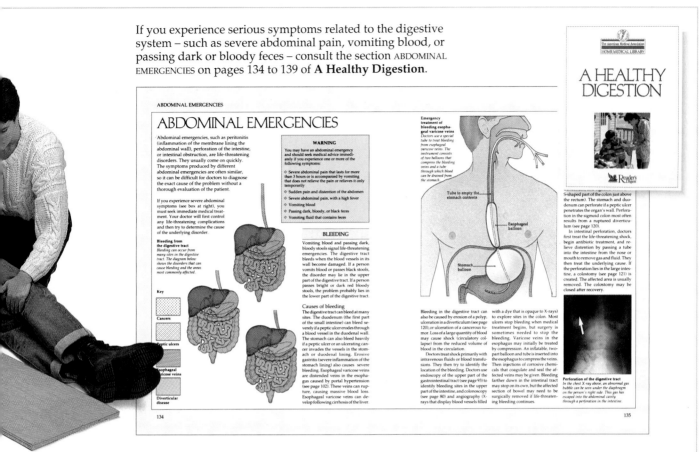

If the emergency results from a drug overdose, consult the DEALING WITH DRUG POISONING EMERGENCIES section on pages 132 to 133 of **Know Your Drugs and Medications.**

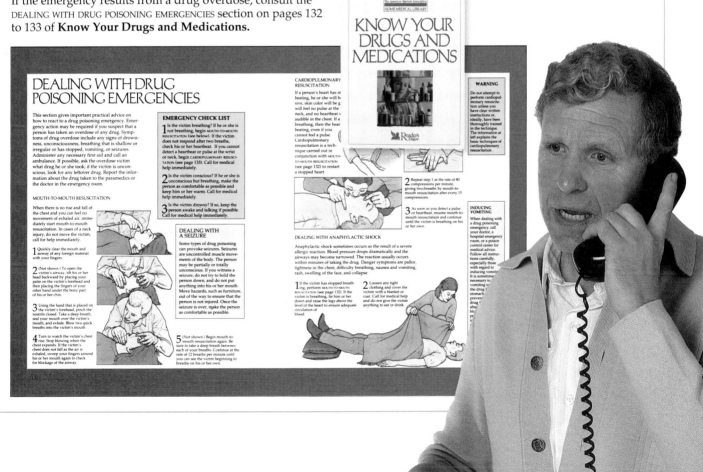

MEDICAL DICTIONARY
A GUIDE TO HELP YOU UNDERSTAND YOUR DOCTOR

Terms in *italics* in the main entries and terms in **boldface** in the captions refer to other entries in the dictionary.

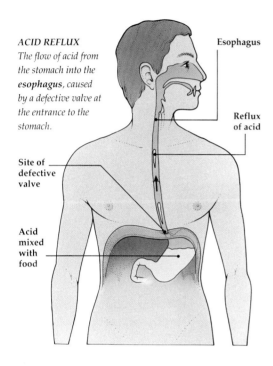

ACID REFLUX
The flow of acid from the stomach into the **esophagus**, *caused by a defective valve at the entrance to the stomach.*

Esophagus

Reflux of acid

Site of defective valve

Acid mixed with food

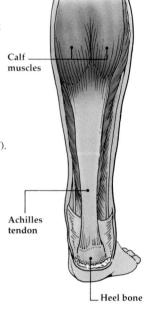

Calf muscles

Achilles tendon

Heel bone

ACHILLES TENDON
The strong **tendon** *connecting the muscles of the calf to the heel; it raises the heel and extends the ankle.*

a

Abdominal cavity
See illustration below right.

ABO blood groups
The major classification of human blood into four types – A, B, AB, and O – based on the presence or absence of specific *proteins* on *red blood cells.*

Abortifacient
A drug or other agent that causes *abortion.*

Abortion
Spontaneous or medically induced termination of a pregnancy.

Abscess
A pus-filled cavity surrounded by inflamed tissue.

Absence seizure
A momentary lapse of consciousness; it is also called a petit mal seizure.

ACE inhibitor
Angiotensin-converting enzyme inhibitor.

Acetylcholine
An important chemical transmitter of *nerve* impulses between cells.

Achalasia
A condition in which the muscle at the lower end of the *esophagus* does not relax, causing difficulty swallowing and regurgitation of recently eaten food.

Achilles tendon
See illustration above right.

Achlorhydria
Absence of acid usually formed in the stomach.

Achondroplasia
A *genetic disorder* characterized by short stature and disproportionately short limbs.

ABDOMINAL CAVITY
The area of the body between the **diaphragm** *and the* **pelvis**, *containing most of the organs of the digestive system and the urinary system. The abdominal cavity also contains internal reproductive organs.*

Acid-base balance
The maintenance of body fluids in a state of chemical neutrality for healthy body functioning.

Acidosis
A state of increased acid content in the blood that occurs in uncontrolled *diabetes mellitus*, severe kidney disease, and some lung diseases.

Acid phosphatase
An *enzyme* found mainly in the *prostate gland*; its level is elevated in cases of advanced prostate cancer.

Acid reflux
See illustration at left.

Acne
A condition, common in adolescents, characterized by *blackheads* and inflamed, pus-filled areas on the skin.

Acoustic neuroma
A noncancerous tumor of the *auditory nerve.*

Acquired
Describes a disease or condition that develops during life, compared with one present at birth.

Acquired immune deficiency syndrome
A disease resulting from a deficiency of the body's *immune system*, caused by infection with the *human immunodeficiency virus* (HIV).

Acquired immunity
Resistance to infection developed as a result of a previous infection or *immunization.*

ACTH
Adrenocorticotropic hormone.

Actinomycosis
A lung infection caused by a bacterium that forms colonies resembling those of fungi.

Acuity
The sharpness of sensory perception, as of vision.

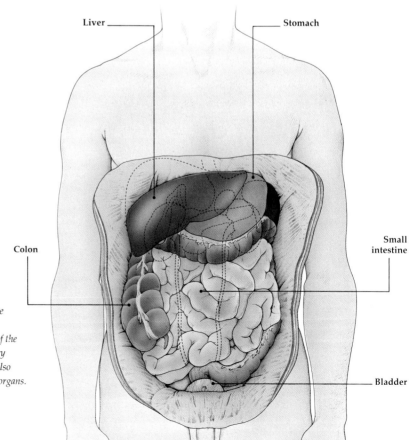

Liver

Stomach

Colon

Small intestine

Bladder

Acute
Describes an illness that is short-lived and usually relatively severe.

Acute respiratory distress syndrome
An emergency in which breathing is difficult and the oxygen supply in the blood is dangerously low.

Adams-Stokes syndrome
Recurrent episodes of temporary loss of consciousness caused by insufficient blood flow from the heart to the brain, resulting from an abnormally slow heartbeat.

Addiction
Uncontrollable dependence on a substance or activity to such an extent that cessation causes severe mental or physical reactions.

Addison's disease
Life-threatening weakness and weight loss caused by insufficient production of *corticosteroid hormones* by the *adrenal glands*.

Adenitis
Inflammation of a *lymph node,* resulting from infection; the node becomes swollen and tender.

Adenoid
One of the masses of *lymphoid tissue* that lie on either side of the back wall of the nose and the upper part of the throat.

Adenomatous polyp
A noncancerous *tumor* in which the cells form microscopic glandlike structures.

Adenosine triphosphate
A chemical compound that stores energy in muscles; the energy is released when the compound breaks down.

Adenoviruses
A group of *viruses* that cause respiratory and gastro-intestinal *infections* and a severe form of *conjunctivitis.*

Adhesion
A band of scar tissue that joins normally separated internal parts of the body and may cause disease.

Adipose tissue
Fatty tissue.

Adjuvant therapy
Treatment for cancer using drugs or *radiation therapy* along with surgery.

Adrenal failure
A life-threatening condition that occurs when the *adrenal glands* stop producing their hormones, causing low blood pressure and *shock.*

Adrenal glands
A pair of small, triangular glands that secrete several *hormones*; they are located on top of the kidneys.

Adrenaline
Epinephrine.

Adrenergic
Describes nerve pathways that secrete or are activated by *epinephrine* or similar substances.

Adrenocorticotropic hormone
A hormone produced by the *pituitary gland* that acts on the outer layer of the *adrenal glands* to stimulate the release of *corticosteroid hormones.*

Adverse reaction
A harmful, unintended reaction to a drug or other treatment.

Aerobic exercise
See illustration below left.

Affective disorders
A group of mental disorders dominated by mood disturbances and inappropriate emotional responses.

Afferent nerve
A nerve that carries signals to the *central nervous system.*

AFP
Alpha-fetoprotein.

Afterbirth
The *placenta* and membranes that are expelled from the *uterus* after childbirth.

Afterpains
Normal contractions of the *uterus* that occur during the first few days after a woman has given birth.

Agonist
A drug or natural substance that can interact with specific sites on certain cells to produce a known response.

Agoraphobia
An abnormal fear of being in a wide open space or in crowded or public places.

AIDS
Acquired immune deficiency syndrome.

AIDS-related complex
A group of signs and symptoms seen in *HIV-*infected people who have not yet developed *AIDS.*

Air embolism
The blockage of an *artery* by bubbles of air that have entered the blood during surgery, after an injury, or in a pressure accident, such as when a diver comes too quickly to the surface.

Airway obstruction
Any impediment to the free movement of air through the airways into the *lungs.*

Airways
The tubular passages through which air moves into and out of the *lungs.*

Albinism
See illustration below right.

Albumin
A soluble *protein* found in the blood and all tissues.

Albuminuria
The presence of *albumin* in the urine, which is an indication of *kidney* disease.

Alcoholic cardiomyopathy
A severe disorder of the heart muscle caused by excessive alcohol intake and resulting in heart failure.

Aldosterone
A *corticosteroid hormone* secreted by the *adrenal glands* that indirectly controls blood pressure by regulating *sodium* and *potassium* balance in the blood.

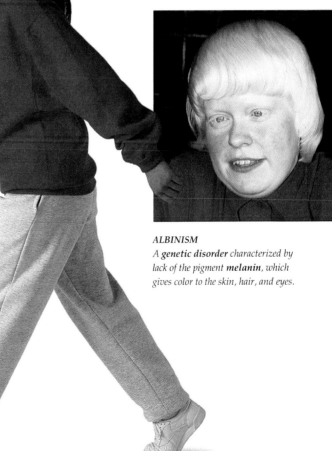

AEROBIC EXERCISE
Physical exercise requiring the heart and lungs to work harder to meet the muscles' increased demand for oxygen.

ALBINISM
*A **genetic disorder** characterized by lack of the pigment **melanin**, which gives color to the skin, hair, and eyes.*

Alexia
Loss of the ability to understand written language, usually resulting from brain damage.

Alimentary canal
The *digestive tract*.

Alkali
A compound that will neutralize an acid.

Alkaline phosphatase
An *enzyme* found in many body tissues; a raised level in the blood is found in some liver and bone diseases and in some other illnesses.

Alkaloids
A group of plant-derived substances (including morphine and caffeine), some of which are used as drugs.

Alkalosis
An abnormal and dangerous state of reduced acidity of blood and body fluids that may be caused by excessive vomiting, *hyperventilation*, or exposure to high altitudes.

Alkylating agents
Substances that interfere with cell division, which makes them especially useful in the treatment of cancer.

Allele
One of two or more forms of a *gene* that occupy corresponding positions on *chromosome* pairs.

Allergen
A substance – such as house dust, animal dander, or molds – that can produce *hypersensitivity* or an *allergic reaction* in some people.

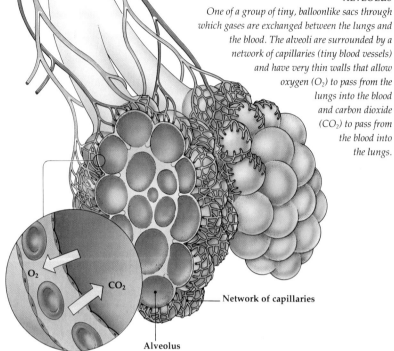

ALVEOLUS
One of a group of tiny, balloonlike sacs through which gases are exchanged between the lungs and the blood. The alveoli are surrounded by a network of capillaries (tiny blood vessels) and have very thin walls that allow oxygen (O_2) to pass from the lungs into the blood and carbon dioxide (CO_2) to pass from the blood into the lungs.

Network of capillaries

Alveolus

Allergic reaction
The body's response to a particular substance (such as a food) that a person has developed *antibodies* against.

Allergic rhinitis
Inflammation of the nasal passages and membrane covering the white of the eye as the result of an *allergic reaction*; symptoms include sneezing, a runny nose, and itchy, tearing eyes.

Allergy
Symptoms caused by a person's reaction to a particular substance that in most people causes no reaction.

Alopecia areata
See illustration below left.

Alpha₁-antitrypsin deficiency
A *genetic disorder* in which, as the result of a lack of a substance in the blood called alpha₁-antitrypsin, *enzymes* released from *white blood cells* cause tissue damage, especially in the lungs.

Alpha-fetoprotein
A *protein* excreted by a *fetus* into the *amniotic fluid* that can be passed to the pregnant woman's blood; abnormal levels in these fluids may be a sign of abnormality in the fetus.

ALS
Amyotrophic lateral sclerosis.

Altitude sickness
An illness with symptoms such as headache, nausea, and dizziness caused by reduced oxygen in the atmosphere at heights of 8,000 feet or above.

Alveolus
See illustration above.

Alzheimer's disease
A condition in which nerve cells in the brain degenerate, producing gradual memory loss, confusion, and physical debilitation.

Ambulatory
Able to walk.

Ameba
A microscopic single-celled organism.

Amebiasis
An infection, often involving the *colon* and liver, acquired by ingesting food or water contaminated with a disease-causing *ameba*.

Amebic dysentery
Inflammation of the *colon* caused by infection with an *ameba*, producing watery, bloody diarrhea.

Amenorrhea
Absence or cessation of menstrual periods.

Amino acids
A group of chemical compounds that are the building blocks of *proteins*.

Aminoglycosides
A group of *antibiotics* that act by interfering with the production of harmful bacterial proteins.

Amnesia
Loss of memory or the ability to recall information stored in memory.

Amniocentesis
See illustration at right.

Amniotic fluid
A clear fluid that surrounds the *fetus* during pregnancy.

Amniotic sac
A thin-walled bag that contains the *fetus* and *amniotic fluid* during pregnancy.

Amphetamine
A type of drug, often abused, that stimulates the nervous system.

Amyotrophic lateral sclerosis
The most common *motor neuron disease*, characterized by progressive loss of muscle function; its cause is unknown.

Anabolic steroid
A drug similar in action to the male hormone *testosterone* that builds up tissue, promotes muscle growth and repair, and strengthens bones.

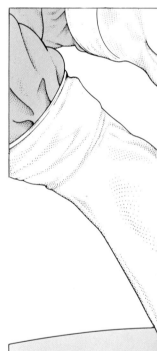

AMNIOCENTESIS
*A prenatal diagnostic procedure in which a small amount of **amniotic fluid** is withdrawn for laboratory analysis. The procedure is guided by **ultrasound scanning.***

ALOPECIA AREATA

A disorder of unknown cause characterized by defined patches of baldness on the head or other hair-bearing areas of the body.

Anabolism
Processes in cells in which simple substances are converted into more complex chemicals.

Anaerobic exercise
Strenuous exercise of limited duration (such as weight lifting) during which muscles generate energy without using oxygen.

Anal fissure
An elongated ulceration of the skin of the anus.

Anal fistula
An abnormal channel connecting the *anus* with the surface of the skin surrounding it.

Analgesic
A drug used for pain relief.

Anal sphincter
A ring of muscle fibers at the outlet of the *anus* that maintains control of the outlet.

Anaphylactic shock
A severe, life-threatening *allergic reaction* causing difficulty breathing and dangerously low blood pressure.

Anastomosis
A natural or artificial connection of two tubular channels, such as blood vessels, that may or may not normally be joined.

Androgen
A *hormone* that stimulates the development of the male sex organs and other male characteristics.

Anemia
A disorder in which the blood contains too little of the oxygen-carrying compound *hemoglobin*.

Anencephaly
A fatal birth defect in which the brain and *spinal cord* have failed to develop.

Anesthesia
Lack of sensation, either in a localized part of the body or throughout the body.

Anesthetic
A drug used to relieve pain.

Aneurysm
Abnormal ballooning of a weakened area in the wall of an artery.

Angina pectoris
A tight, gripping pain in the chest caused by an insufficient supply of oxygen to the heart muscle.

Angioedema
An *allergic reaction* that causes swelling in the skin, throat, or other areas.

Angiography
An X-ray procedure that is used to visualize the inside of blood vessels after they have been injected with a *contrast medium*.

Angioma
A noncancerous tumor consisting of blood vessels or lymph vessels.

Angioplasty
Surgical reconstruction or widening of blood vessels.

Angiotensin-converting enzyme inhibitor
A drug that widens narrowed blood vessels and improves blood flow; it is used to control high blood pressure and to prevent or treat *heart failure*.

Ankylosing spondylitis
An inflammatory disease affecting joints in the spine and adjacent structures.

Anorexia nervosa
An eating disorder (most frequent in young women) characterized by an abnormal fear of looking fat, prolonged avoidance of food, and severe weight loss.

Anovulation
Absence of *ovulation*.

Anoxia
A deficiency of oxygen in a body tissue.

Antacid
A drug that relieves the symptoms of indigestion by neutralizing stomach acid.

Anterior
Relating to or located in the front of the body.

Antiangina drugs
Drugs that relieve the symptoms of *angina pectoris* by increasing blood flow to the heart muscle and reducing the work load on the heart.

Antiarrhythmics
Drugs that are used to prevent or correct an abnormal heart rhythm.

Antibacterials
Synthetic drugs used to treat bacterial infections.

Antibiotic resistance
Immunity developed by a class of bacteria to a particular antibiotic, making the bacteria difficult to eradicate.

Antibiotics
See illustration below.

Antibiotic sensitivity test
A laboratory test used to determine whether a particular bacterial infection is susceptible to treatment with a particular *antibiotic*.

Antibody
A *protein* manufactured by the *immune system* to neutralize a specific *antigen* in the body.

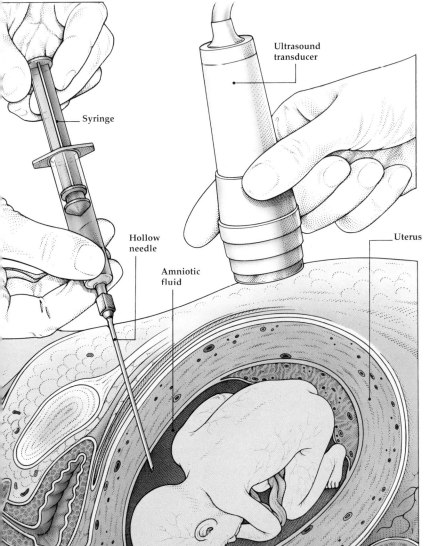

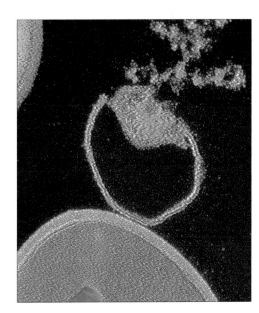

ANTIBIOTICS
Drugs used to treat bacterial infections; originally derived from a mold or fungus, they are now made synthetically. In the photograph above, a bacterium is disintegrating as a result of antibiotic action.

Anticholinergics
Drugs that help to control muscle spasms; they are used to treat *Parkinson's disease, irritable bowel syndrome*, and some respiratory disorders.

Anticoagulants
Drugs used to prevent abnormal blood clotting.

Anticonvulsants
Drugs used to prevent or minimize the frequency and severity of *seizures*.

Antidepressants
Drugs used to prevent or relieve *depression*.

Antidiarrheals
Drugs used to relieve the symptoms of diarrhea.

Antidiuretic hormones
Hormones that act on the kidneys to increase the reabsorption of water.

Antidote
A substance that neutralizes the effects of a poison.

Antiemetics
Drugs used to prevent or relieve nausea and vomiting.

Antifungals
Drugs used to treat infections caused by fungi.

Antigen
A *protein* recognized as foreign by the *immune system*, which produces an *antibody* to fight it.

Antihistamines
Drugs that block the effects of *histamine*.

Antihypertensives
Drugs used to reduce high blood pressure.

Anti-inflammatories
Drugs, such as aspirin, that reduce inflammation.

Antimalarials
Drugs used to prevent or treat *malaria*.

Antimetabolites
Drugs that interfere with cell division, used to treat cancer.

Antimicrobials
Drugs used to treat infection by any type of disease-causing organism.

Antinuclear antibodies test
A test used to detect a class of *antibodies* that develop in people who have certain *autoimmune diseases*.

Antioncogene
A *gene* that acts to prevent uncontrolled cell division such as that in cancer.

Antioxidants
Compounds that protect against cell damage caused by *oxygen free radicals*, which are considered a major cause of aging and cancer.

Antiparasitics
Drugs used to treat infections caused by parasites such as lice.

Antipsychotics
Drugs used to treat major mental disorders.

Antirenins
Drugs that reduce high blood pressure by blocking the action of renin, an *enzyme* that causes some types of high blood pressure.

Antiseptic
A chemical that kills bacteria and other *microorganisms*.

Antispasmodics
Drugs used to prevent spasms in the walls of blood vessels, the uterus, the intestine, or any muscle in the body.

Antithyroid drugs
Drugs used to treat an overactive *thyroid gland*.

Antitoxin
A substance, usually injected, that neutralizes the effects of a *toxin* produced by a bacterium.

Antitussives
Drugs that suppress or relieve coughing.

Antivirals
Drugs used to treat an infection caused by a virus; few effective ones exist.

Anuria
Failure of the kidneys to produce urine.

Anus
The opening at the end of the digestive tract through which feces are passed.

Aorta
The body's main artery, which carries blood away from the heart.

Aortic aneurysm
A localized ballooning in the wall of the *aorta*.

Aortic insufficiency
Leaking of the *aortic valve*, which reduces the heart's pumping efficiency.

Aortic stenosis
Narrowing of the *aortic valve*, causing *angina pectoris* and *heart failure*; it is the most common heart valve disorder.

Aortic valve
See illustration at left.

Apgar score
A system used to evaluate the physical condition of a newborn.

Aphasia
A deficiency of previously acquired language skills, usually following an injury to the brain.

Apheresis
A procedure in which blood is withdrawn from a person, then reinfused after selected components have been removed.

Aplasia
Failure of a tissue or organ to develop.

Aplastic anemia
A blood disease characterized by a drastic reduction of all types of blood cells formed in the bone marrow.

Apnea
Cessation of breathing, either momentarily, or for a prolonged period, which is life-threatening.

Apocrine glands
The sweat glands found in the armpits and groin area.

Appendectomy
Surgical removal of the *appendix* to treat *appendicitis*.

Appendicitis
Inflammation of the *appendix*.

Appendix
A short, blind-ended tube that branches off the *large intestine* and has no known function.

Applanation tonometry
A method of measuring the pressure of fluids inside the eye; it is used to diagnose *glaucoma*.

Aqueous humor
The watery fluid that fills the front chamber of the eye.

Arachnoid membrane
The middle of the three membranes enclosing the brain and the *spinal cord*.

Arbovirus
A virus transmitted from one person to another or from an animal to a person by an insect.

ARC
AIDS-related complex.

Areola
The pigmented area surrounding the nipple.

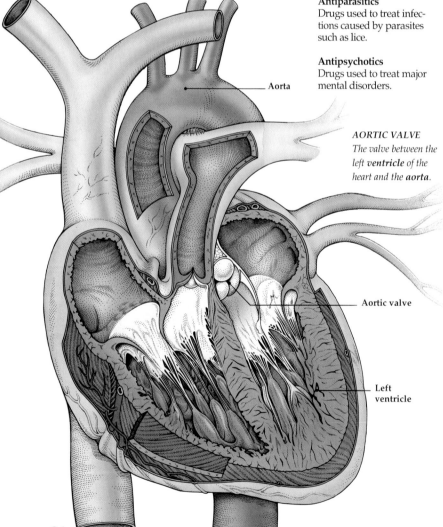

AORTIC VALVE
The valve between the left ventricle of the heart and the aorta.

Aorta

Aortic valve

Left ventricle

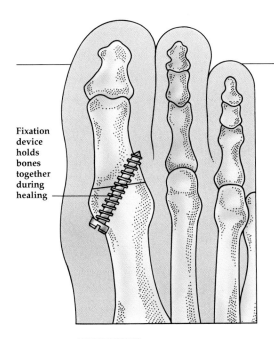

Fixation device holds bones together during healing

ARTHRODESIS
A surgical procedure in which the bones that meet
at a damaged joint are fused to provide support
or relieve pain. The weight-bearing surfaces of the
joint are removed and the bones unite as they heal.

Arrhythmia
An abnormality in the
rhythm or rate of the
heartbeat.

Arteriole
A small branch of an artery.

Arteriosclerosis
A disorder characterized
by thickening and loss of
elasticity in artery walls.

**Arteriovenous
malformation**
An abnormal network of
blood vessels between an
artery and a vein; it may be
present at birth or develop
as a result of an injury or
infection.

Arteritis
Inflammation of the wall
of an artery.

Artery
One of the large blood
vessels that carry oxygen-
filled blood away from the
heart to organs and tissues.

Arthralgia
Pain in a joint.

Arthritis
Inflammation of a joint,
characterized by pain,
swelling, and stiffness.

Arthrocentesis
Removal of a sample of fluid
from a joint for laboratory
analysis.

Arthrodesis
See illustration above left.

Arthrography
An X-ray technique used to
examine the inside of a joint
after injecting a *contrast
medium* into it.

Arthroscopy
See illustrations above right.

Artifact
An irrelevant, unwanted
feature that has appeared
in an image or other type
of test result.

Artificial insemination
The introduction of semen
into the *cervix* by artificial
means rather than by sexual
intercourse.

Artificial respiration
Artificial ventilation.

Artificial ventilation
See illustration at right.

Asbestosis
A chronic lung disorder
caused by inhalation of
asbestos fibers.

Ascariasis
Infestation of the intestines
with a type of large
roundworm.

Ascites
Excessive fluid in the
abdominal cavity that can
cause swelling.

Ascorbic acid
Vitamin C.

Asepsis
The absence of disease-
causing *microorganisms.*

Aseptic meningitis
A mild form of *meningitis*
that is caused by one of
many viruses.

Aspergillosis
A lung infection caused by a
fungus that is often found in
old buildings and decayed
vegetation.

Aspermia
Failure to produce or
ejaculate semen.

Asphyxia
Suffocation.

Aspiration
Removal of a fluid from
the body by suction, or the
accidental inhalation of a
solid or liquid.

Aspiration pneumonia
A form of *pneumonia* caused
by breathing something
other than air into the lungs.

Asthma
A respiratory disorder
characterized by spasms and
inflammation of the airways,
often accompanied by
wheezing and coughing.

Astigmatism
A distortion or blurring
of vision caused by
an irregularly
shaped *cornea.*

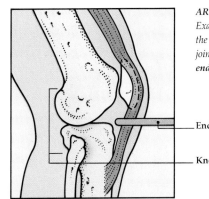

ARTHROSCOPY
*Examination of
the interior of a
joint using an
endoscope.*

Endoscope

Knee joint

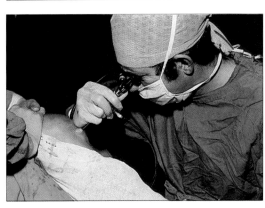

ARTIFICIAL VENTILATION
*The manual or mechanical introduction of
air into the lungs of a person who has
stopped breathing.*

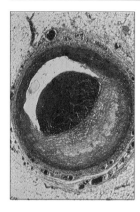

ATHEROSCLEROSIS
*A disease in which the inner layer of the arterial wall becomes inflamed and thickened with **atheromatous plaques**, causing narrowing of the artery and impairing blood flow. In the photograph above, the pink area is an atheromatous plaque; the bright red area indicates bleeding into the plaque.*

Astringent
A substance, usually applied locally, that causes tissue to dry and shrink by reducing its ability to absorb water.

Asymptomatic
Without symptoms.

Ataxia
Inability to coordinate the muscles, affecting balance and gait, limb or eye movements, and/or speech.

Atelectasis
Collapse of part or all of the lung caused by obstruction of an airway.

Atheroma
Fatty deposits on the inner lining of an artery that can lead to *atherosclerosis*.

Atheromatous plaque
A hardened patch of *atheroma* that is characteristic of *atherosclerosis*.

Atherosclerosis
See illustration above left.

Athletes' foot
See illustration above right.

ATP
Adenosine triphosphate.

Atresia
The absence at birth of a normal body opening, canal, or duct.

Atrial fibrillation
An abnormal heartbeat in which the upper chambers of the heart beat irregularly and very rapidly.

Atrial flutter
An abnormal heartbeat in which the upper chambers of the heart beat very rapidly but regularly.

Atrial septal defect
A hole in the wall between the two upper chambers of the heart.

Atrioventricular node
A small area of the heart muscle, between the upper and lower chambers, that helps coordinate the electrical signals controlling the heartbeat.

Atrium
Either of the two upper chambers of the heart; the plural form is atria.

Atrophy
Shrinking or wasting of an organ or tissue.

ATHLETES' FOOT
A fungal infection of the skin between the toes, causing itching and soreness.

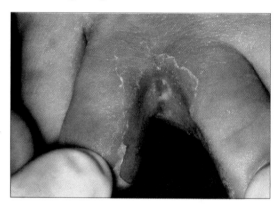

Attention-deficit disorder
A disorder characterized by learning and behavior disabilities primarily affecting children and adolescents.

Audiogram
A record of a person's hearing ability.

Audiology
The study of hearing, especially impaired hearing.

Audiometry
See illustration below left.

Auditory
Related to hearing.

Auditory cortex
The part of the brain that receives and interprets signals from the ears.

Auditory nerve
Part of the *cranial nerve* that connects the ear and brain; it conducts signals concerned with hearing.

Aura
A warning sensation that precedes a *migraine* attack or an epileptic *seizure*.

Aural
Relating to the ear.

Auscultation
The technique of listening to sounds inside the body to assess the functioning and condition of an organ.

Autism
A mental disorder of unknown cause that is characterized by extreme withdrawal and an inability to relate to people.

Autoantibody
An *antibody* that reacts against normal body tissues.

Autograft
Tissue transplanted from one site to another in the same person.

Autoimmune disease
A disease caused by the reaction of a person's *immune system* against his or her own tissues.

Autologous transfusion
A procedure in which blood is removed from a person, temporarily stored, and then reinfused back into that person during surgery.

Autologous transplant
A transplant procedure using a person's own bone marrow or *stem cells*.

Automatism
A state in which behavior is not consciously controlled; it occurs in some types of *epilepsy* and during sleepwalking.

Autonomic nervous system
The part of the nervous system that controls involuntary activities of body functioning, such as the heartbeat.

Autopsy
An examination of a body after death.

Autosomal dominant
Describes a *gene* on an *autosome* that produces an effect whenever it is present; also describes a trait or disorder caused by a gene of this type.

AUDIOMETRY
Measurement of hearing using specific tests.

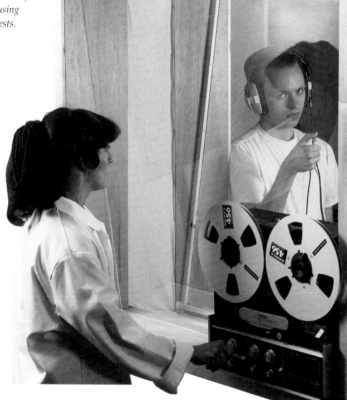

Autosomal recessive
Describes a *gene* on an *autosome* that produces an effect only when two copies of it are present; also describes a trait or disorder caused by a gene of this type.

Autosome
Any *chromosome* other than the two *sex chromosomes*.

Avascular
Describes a tissue that lacks blood vessels and, therefore, has no blood supply.

Avulsion
The tearing away of a body structure from its point of attachment.

Axilla
The armpit.

Axillary artery
An *artery* that passes through the armpit and supplies blood to the arm.

Axon
A long, fiberlike extension of a nerve cell that conducts impulses away from the cell.

Bacillus
A type of rod-shaped *bacterium*.

Bacteremia
The presence of *bacteria* in the bloodstream.

Bactericidal
Describes a substance that kills *bacteria*.

Bacteriostatic
Describes a substance that inhibits the growth or multiplication of *bacteria*.

Bacterium
See illustration at top right.

Bacteriuria
The presence of *bacteria* in urine, which often indicates a *urinary tract* infection.

Ball-and-socket joint
A type of joint, such as the hip joint, in which the end of one of the bones forming the joint is ball-shaped and fits into a cuplike space in the other bone.

Balloon angioplasty
See illustration below.

Balloon catheter
A *catheter* with a balloon near its tip used to open a narrowed artery or intestine or to drain an obstructed organ such as the bladder.

Balloon valvuloplasty
The technique of using a *balloon catheter* to widen a narrowed *heart valve*.

Barbiturates
A group of sedatives that work by depressing activity in the brain; because these drugs are habit-forming, they are strictly regulated.

Barium enema
A *barium X-ray examination* in which barium is inserted into the *colon* and *rectum* in order to investigate disorders of these organs.

Barium X-ray examination
Any of a group of imaging procedures that are used to diagnose and monitor diseases of the *gastrointestinal tract*; barium sulfate is used as a *contrast medium*.

Barr body
A single inactive X *chromosome* found in the cells of normal females.

Barrett's syndrome
A disorder in which cells of the lower part of the *esophagus* change as a result of chronic irritation from backflow of stomach acids.

Barrier method of contraception
A method of preventing pregnancy by blocking the passage of sperm to the uterus using a device such as a *diaphragm* or a *condom*.

Bartholin's glands
A pair of pea-sized glands that secrete a fluid that lubricates the vagina during sexual arousal.

Basal body temperature
The temperature of the body at absolute rest.

Basal cell carcinoma
A type of skin cancer that usually occurs on the face, neck, or arms; it is caused by prolonged, excessive exposure to the sun.

Basal ganglia
Paired clusters of nerve cells deep inside the brain that are involved in the control of movement.

Basal metabolic rate
The minimum rate at which a person expends energy to maintain vital body functions such as breathing.

Base pair
A pair of linked *nucleotide bases* that forms a single "rung" in the ladderlike structure of *DNA*.

Base triplet
A group of three *nucleotide bases* found in *DNA* and *RNA* that is the code for a specific *amino acid* in *protein* production.

Basophil
A type of *white blood cell* that is thought to play a role in some *allergic reactions*; it stains blue when prepared for microscopic study.

B cell
A type of *lymphocyte* that manufactures *antibodies* to fight infection.

BCG vaccine
A *vaccine* that provides immunity against *tuberculosis*; it is also used as a treatment for bladder cancer.

Becker's muscular dystrophy
A genetic disorder similar to *Duchenne type muscular dystrophy* but starting later in childhood and progressing more slowly.

Bell's palsy
A type of *facial palsy*.

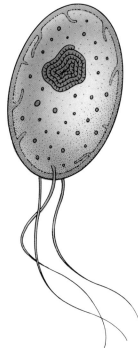

BACTERIUM
*A single-celled **microorganism** that multiplies by simple division. Many different types of bacteria exist, some of which cause disease.*

Artery

Atheromatous plaques are compressed, causing them to split

Inflated balloon

BALLOON ANGIOPLASTY
*A technique to reopen arteries narrowed by **atheromatous plaques** by inserting and inflating a **balloon catheter** inside the blood vessels.*

Bends
Decompression sickness.

Benign tumor
A type of tumor that, unlike a cancerous tumor, does not spread to other parts of the body; it may, however, grow to a large size and become life-threatening.

Benzene
A widely used industrial chemical that is poisonous and may cause cancer after prolonged exposure.

Benzodiazepines
A group of drugs that are used to relieve anxiety or to induce sleep.

Beriberi
A disorder caused by a deficiency of *thiamine* (vitamin B₁) in the diet.

Berry aneurysm
A small saclike swelling in one of the arteries in the brain that may rupture, causing a *subarachnoid hemorrhage*.

Beryllium
A metallic element used in high technology industries that, if inhaled over many years as dust or fumes, can lead to lung damage.

Beta blockers
A group of drugs used mainly to treat heart disorders and high blood pressure; they work by reducing the force and rate of the heart's contractions.

Beta carotene
A type of pigment found in orange-colored fruits and vegetables that is converted into *vitamin A* in the body; it may protect against cancer.

Beta lactamase
An *enzyme* produced by some bacteria that blocks the action of penicillin and some other *antibiotics*.

Biceps muscle
A muscle in the upper arm or back of the thigh that controls some movements of an arm or leg.

Bifocal
Describes a vision-correcting lens that has two parts with different focusing powers.

Bifurcation
The site at which a single structure, such as the *trachea*, splits into two branches.

Bilateral
Affecting or appearing on both sides of the body.

Bile
A yellow-green liquid secreted by the liver; it removes waste products and helps break down fats during digestion.

Bile duct
Any of the ducts by which bile is carried from the liver to the *gallbladder* and then to the *small intestine*.

Biliary atresia
A *birth defect* in which the *bile ducts* fail to develop or are underdeveloped; a liver transplant in infancy may be lifesaving.

Biliary cirrhosis
A form of *cirrhosis of the liver* that results when inflammation blocks the flow of bile through the liver; treatment is rarely effective but a liver transplant may be lifesaving.

Biliary colic
A severe pain in the upper right area of the abdomen usually caused by the *gallbladder's* attempts to expel *gallstones* or the passage of a stone through a *bile duct*.

Biliary tract
The organs and ducts in which bile is formed, concentrated, and carried from the liver to the *small intestine*.

Bilirubin
The orange-yellow pigment of *bile*, which causes jaundice when it accumulates in the blood or skin; its measurement in the blood is used to diagnose liver disease and *hemolytic anemia*.

Bimanual compression
A technique used to make the uterus contract after childbirth to control bleeding; the doctor compresses the uterus with one hand on the woman's abdomen and the fingers of the other hand in her vagina.

Binging and purging
Bouts of overeating followed by self-induced vomiting or purging with laxatives; it is characteristic of the eating disorder *bulimia*.

Bioequivalent
Describes two drugs having essentially the same effect on the body.

Biofeedback
A technique in which a person uses information about an involuntary body function, such as blood pressure, to try to gain control over that function.

Biopsy
See illustration at left.

Biotin
A *vitamin* – found in foods such as egg yolks, peanuts, and cauliflower – that aids the action of various *enzymes* in cells.

Bipolar disorder
Manic-depressive disorder.

Bird handlers' disease
A type of *hypersensitivity pneumonitis* caused by an *allergic reaction* to a *protein* in bird droppings.

Birth canal
The passage extending from the *cervix* to the vaginal opening through which a baby passes during childbirth.

Birth control pill
A drug that is taken orally to prevent pregnancy; it contains a synthetic form of *progesterone*, often combined with a synthetic form of *estrogen*.

Birth defect
An abnormality that is present at birth; it may be genetic in origin or acquired during fetal development or during *labor* and delivery.

Birthmark
An area of discolored skin present from birth; it is usually benign but may develop into a cancer.

Birth rate
The number of babies born during a given period compared with the total population.

Bisexuality
Sexual attraction to persons of both sexes.

Blackhead
A black-tipped plug of semisolid *sebum* that blocks the opening of a *hair follicle*.

Bladder
A hollow, muscular organ in the *pelvis* that is a reservoir for urine.

Blastocyst
An early stage in the development of an *embryo*, consisting of a two-layer sphere of cells surrounding a fluid-filled cavity.

Blastomycosis
An infection caused by a fungus found in rotting wood and soil; it may take the form of *pneumonia* or a long-term illness affecting the lungs, skin, and bones.

Bleeding time
The time required for a tiny wound to stop bleeding; one measure of the blood's clotting ability.

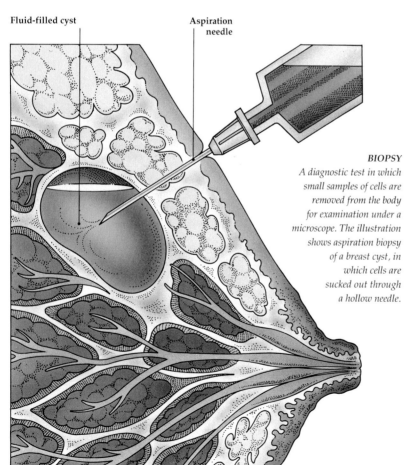

Fluid-filled cyst

Aspiration needle

BIOPSY

A diagnostic test in which small samples of cells are removed from the body for examination under a microscope. The illustration shows aspiration biopsy of a breast cyst, in which cells are sucked out through a hollow needle.

BLEPHARITIS
Inflammation of the eyelids.

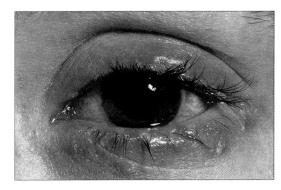

Blepharitis
See illustration above.

Blepharoplasty
Plastic surgery to remove wrinkled, drooping skin on the eyelids.

Blind spot
A small area on the *retina* of the eye that is not sensitive to light, causing a gap in vision.

Blood-brain barrier
A double layer of cells that prevents certain substances carried in the bloodstream from entering brain tissues.

Blood clot
A semisolid plug of blood that forms at a break in a blood vessel, helping to seal the damaged vessel and prevent blood loss.

Blood count
The number of *red blood cells*, *white blood cells*, and *platelets* in 1 cubic millimeter of blood; a test often used to diagnose disease.

Blood group
Blood type.

Blood poisoning
Septicemia.

Blood pressure
The pressure exerted by the flow of blood as it is pumped by the heart through the main arteries.

Blood smear
The examination under a microscope of a drop of blood that has been smeared onto a glass slide.

Blood transfusion
See illustration at right.

Blood type
The classification of a person's blood according to the presence of different marker *proteins* on the surface of *red blood cells*.

Blue baby
An infant born with a heart or lung defect that reduces the level of oxygen in the blood, giving the infant a bluish complexion.

B lymphocyte
A type of *lymphocyte* that makes *antibodies*.

Boil
See illustrations above right.

Bone
The dense, hard tissue that makes up the skeleton.

Bone density
The concentration of *protein* and mineral salts in bone; a low concentration is an indication of *osteoporosis*.

Bone graft
A surgical procedure in which a piece of bone is taken from one part of the body to repair bone damage in another part.

Bone marrow
Soft tissue found inside bone cavities that is the site of blood cell production.

Bone marrow transplant
The infusion of *bone marrow* from a healthy donor to replace a person's own defective marrow.

Bone spur
An abnormal, often painful, outgrowth of bone, most often found on the heel.

BOIL
*An inflamed, pus-filled area of skin, usually an infected **hair follicle**.*

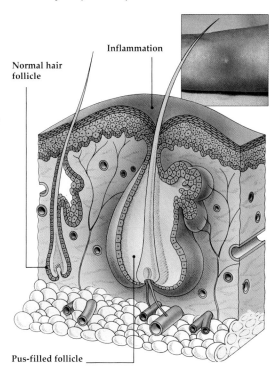

Normal hair follicle

Inflammation

Pus-filled follicle

BLOOD TRANSFUSION
The infusion of blood or blood components directly into the bloodstream to replace blood lost from surgery, injury, or disease.

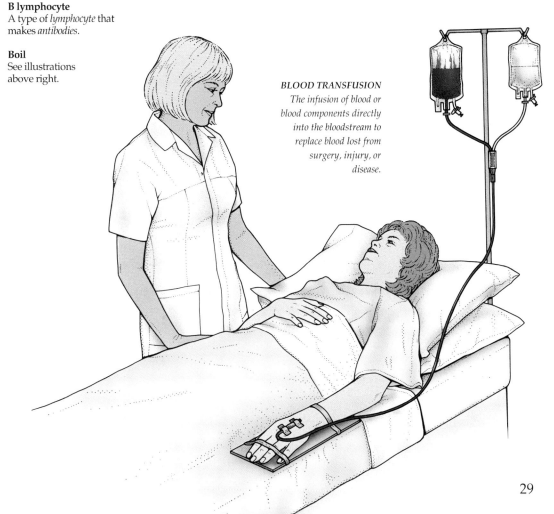

Booster
A followup dose of a *vaccine* given weeks, months, or years later to reinforce the effect of the first.

Botulism
A serious type of *food poisoning* acquired by eating improperly preserved or canned food that is contaminated with a powerful bacterial *toxin*.

Bowel
The *intestine*.

Bowleg
An outward curving of bones in the legs.

Brachial plexus
An interlacing network of nerves in the upper part of the chest that control muscles in the arms.

Bradycardia
An adult heart rate of less than 60 beats per minute; it may be normal (in some people who are physically fit) or abnormal.

Brain damage
Degeneration or death of nerve cells in the brain.

Brain death
The irreversible cessation of all brain function while the heart continues beating.

Brain stem
The lowest part of the brain, which controls basic functions such as breathing.

Braxton Hicks contraction
A brief, relatively painless tightening of the uterus during pregnancy.

Breakthrough bleeding
Vaginal bleeding or spotting between menstrual periods, which can occur when taking an *oral contraceptive*.

Breech birth
See illustration below.

Broad-spectrum antibiotic
An *antibiotic* that is effective against several different types of *bacteria*.

Broca's area
An area of the brain that controls speech.

Bronchial tree
See illustration above right.

Bronchiectasis
A disorder in which the walls of the air passages in the lungs are stretched and damaged.

Bronchiolitis
A life-threatening viral infection of the smallest airways in the lungs, mainly affecting young children.

Bronchitis
Inflammation of the airways connecting the *trachea* and lungs, resulting in coughing, the production of *sputum*, and occasionally wheezing and shortness of breath.

Bronchoconstrictor
A substance that causes the airways in the lungs to narrow, or constrict.

Bronchodilator
A drug that widens constricted air passages to improve breathing.

Bronchogenic carcinoma
A cancerous tumor in the lungs that originates in one of the air passages and is almost always caused by cigarette smoking.

Bronchopneumonia
The most common form of *pneumonia* in which inflammation spreads in small patches throughout the lungs.

Bronchoscopy
Visual examination of the main airways of the lungs using a flexible viewing instrument.

Bronchospasm
An irregular contraction of the smooth muscle of the airways in the lungs, causing the airways to narrow.

Brucellosis
A bacterial infection that is acquired from farm animals or consumption of unpasteurized dairy products.

Bruit
An abnormal sound made in the heart, arteries, or veins when blood circulation becomes turbulent or flows at an abnormal speed.

Bruxism
Unconscious grinding or clenching of the teeth.

Bubonic plague
The most common form of *plague*, characterized by painful buboes (swollen *lymph nodes*) in the armpits, groin, or neck.

Budd-Chiari syndrome
A disorder in which the veins draining blood from the liver become blocked or narrowed.

Buerger's disease
A disease of smokers in which blood vessels in the legs become inflamed and obstructed, sometimes resulting in *gangrene* and the need for amputation.

Bulimia
An illness characterized by bouts of gross overeating often followed by self-induced vomiting.

Bundle-branch block
A type of *heart block* in which the interruption to the flow of electrical impulses in the heart occurs in one or both of the heart's *ventricles*.

BRONCHIAL TREE
The branching, treelike structure of air passages in the lungs.

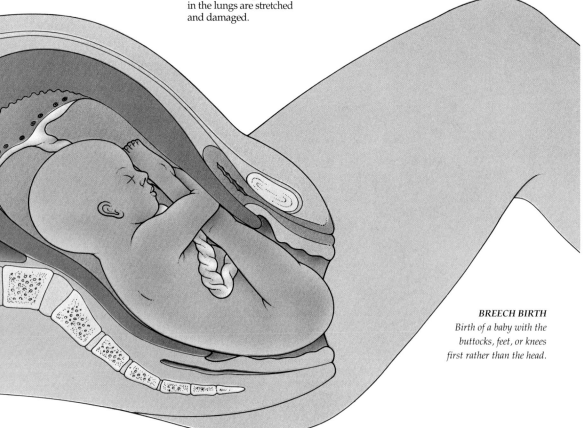

BREECH BIRTH
Birth of a baby with the buttocks, feet, or knees first rather than the head.

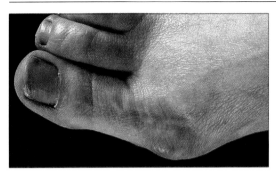

BUNION
A thickened, fluid-filled pad overlying the joint at the base of the big toe.

Bunion
See illustration above left.

Burkitt's lymphoma
A cancer of *lymphoid tissue* characterized by a tumor in the jaw or abdomen.

Burr hole
A hole made to relieve pressure inside the skull or to gain access to the brain.

Bursa
A fluid-filled pad that acts as a cushion at a pressure point in the body, often near joints.

Bursitis
Painful inflammation of a *bursa* that can result from arthritis, infection, or injury.

Butterfly bandage
A small piece of adhesive tape, with broad wing-shaped ends, that is used for holding the edges of a superficial wound together.

Bypass
A surgical procedure to divert the flow of blood or other body fluids.

Byssinosis
An occupational lung disease caused by an *allergic reaction* to dust produced during the processing of flax, cotton, or hemp.

Cachexia
General ill health marked by extreme weight loss and a wasted appearance.

Café au lait spots
Slightly darker than normal patches of skin.

Calcification
The buildup of calcium salts in body tissues, such as occurs normally in bone development or abnormally in the arteries in *atherosclerosis*.

Calcitonin
A hormone produced by the *thyroid gland* that helps control the level of calcium in the blood and enhances bone formation.

Calcium
A *mineral* essential for many body functions, including transmission of nerve impulses and muscle contractions.

Calcium channel blocker
A drug used to treat many heart and circulation disorders, including *angina pectoris* and *hypertension*.

Calculus
A hard deposit on the teeth or an abnormal formation (such as a *gallstone* or *kidney stone*) in body tissues that can cause blockage and inflammation.

Callus
New soft bone that forms across and around a fracture as it heals; or an area of thickened skin that develops at a point of regular or prolonged pressure or friction.

Caloric test
See illustration above right.

Calorie
A unit of the energy content of foods or the amount of energy expended by an organism.

Canal
A narrow, tubular passage, such as the ear canal.

Cancer
Any of a group of diseases caused by unrestrained multiplication of cells in an organ or tissue that can spread throughout the body.

Cancer grading
The examination of cancer tissue under a microscope to establish the degree of malignancy.

Cancer staging
The process of determining how advanced a cancer is.

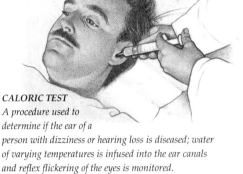

CALORIC TEST
A procedure used to determine if the ear of a person with dizziness or hearing loss is diseased; water of varying temperatures is infused into the ear canals and reflex flickering of the eyes is monitored.

Candidiasis
A common vaginal or oral yeast infection.

Canker sore
A small, painful sore that occurs in the mouth.

Cannula
A thin, flexible tube inserted into the body to withdraw or introduce fluids.

Capillary
See illustration below.

Capsulotomy
A surgical incision into a body capsule, such as into the lens of the eye to remove a cataract.

Carbohydrates
Substances – including starches and sugars – that provide the body with its main energy source.

Carbon dioxide
A colorless, odorless gas that is an important by-product of cell functions; it is exhaled from the lungs.

Carbuncle
A cluster of painful, pus-filled, inflamed sores on the skin that usually starts as an infected hair follicle.

Carcinoembryonic antigen
A *protein* that, if found to be at an elevated level in the body, may indicate recurrence of some cancers.

Carcinogen
An agent capable of causing cancer; tobacco smoke and some forms of radiation are carcinogens.

CAPILLARY
One of the tiny vessels that carry blood between the smallest arteries and the smallest veins.

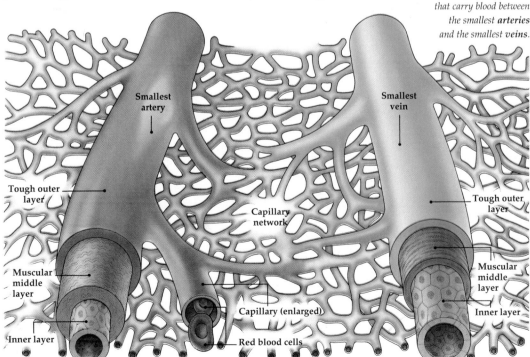

Smallest artery

Smallest vein

Capillary network

Tough outer layer

Tough outer layer

Muscular middle layer

Muscular middle layer

Inner layer

Inner layer

Capillary (enlarged)

Red blood cells

Carcinoma
A cancerous tumor that arises from cells in the surface layer or lining membrane of an organ; carcinomas include the most common cancers of the lungs, skin, breast, cervix, and prostate gland.

Carcinoma in situ
A *cancer* that has not spread beyond the layer of cells from which it originated.

Cardiac arrest
A sudden cessation of the heart's pumping action.

Cardiac catheterization
See illustration at right.

Cardiac glycoside
A drug used to treat people with heart rate and rhythm disorders, *heart failure*, or a heart muscle weakened from a heart attack.

Cardiac output
The volume of blood pumped by the heart in a specified time (usually per minute); it is a measure of the heart's efficiency.

Cardiogenic shock
A life-threatening reduction of blood flow that results from a heart attack or *pulmonary embolism*.

Cardiomegaly
Enlargement of the heart, which occurs in disorders that cause the heart to work harder than normal.

Cardiomyopathy
Any disease that affects the heart muscle.

Cardiopulmonary resuscitation
See illustration below right.

Cardiovascular fitness
The capacity of the heart to pump blood and of the blood vessels to carry blood throughout the body.

Cardiovascular system
The network of structures, consisting of the heart and blood vessels, that pumps blood and transports it throughout the body.

Carditis
Inflammation of any part of the heart or its linings.

Carotene
An orange pigment found in carrots and other colored plants that is converted in the liver to *vitamin A*.

Carotid artery
Any of the four principal arteries supplying blood to the neck and head.

Carotid endarterectomy
A surgical procedure to restore normal blood flow by removing the lining of a *carotid artery* narrowed by *atherosclerosis*.

Carpal bone
One of the eight bones that make up the wrist.

Carpal tunnel syndrome
See illustration below left.

Carrier
A person who does not have symptoms of an infection but can pass it on to others; or a healthy person who carries a defective *recessive gene* that can cause a *genetic disorder* in offspring who inherit two copies of the gene.

Cartilage
A type of *connective tissue* that forms an important structural component of many parts of the skeletal system, such as the joints.

Caruncle
A small, fleshy projection, such as the bump at the inner corner of the eye.

Cast
A rigid casing applied to part of the body to hold a broken bone or dislocated joint in place during healing.

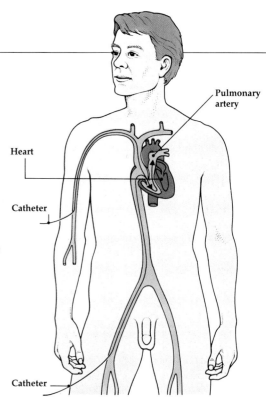

CARDIAC CATHETERIZATION
*A diagnostic procedure in which a **catheter** is threaded through a blood vessel into the heart to monitor its function and to inject a **contrast medium** for imaging. The illustration shows two routes for inserting the catheter into the heart. In some cases, the catheter is manipulated into the **pulmonary artery**.*

CARPAL TUNNEL SYNDROME
*Numbness, tingling, and pain in the wrist and hand caused by compression of the **median nerve** as it passes between the bones and a **ligament** at the front of the wrist; in most cases, it is a **repetitive strain injury**.*

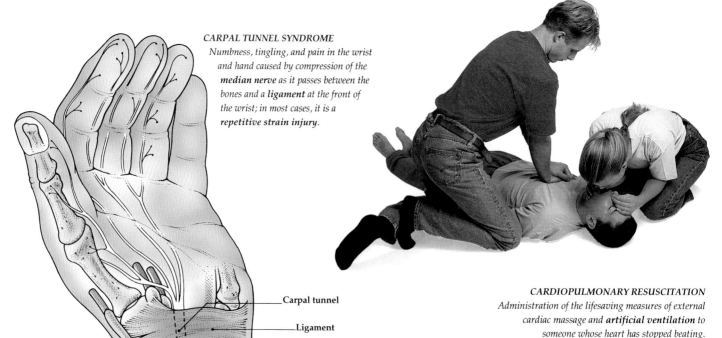

CARDIOPULMONARY RESUSCITATION
*Administration of the lifesaving measures of external cardiac massage and **artificial ventilation** to someone whose heart has stopped beating.*

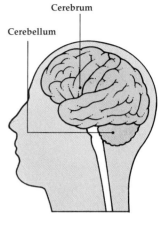

CEREBRUM
The largest and most developed part of the brain; it performs sensory and motor functions and various mental activities.

Castration
The surgical removal of one or both *testicles* or *ovaries*.

Catabolism
The processes in living cells by which complex chemicals are broken down into simpler forms to produce energy and by-products such as water and carbon dioxide.

Catalepsy
An abnormal, trancelike state in which the muscles of the face, body, and limbs remain in a rigid position.

Cataract
Loss of transparency of the *lens* of the eye.

Catecholamines
A group of chemicals produced in the body – including *dopamine* and *epinephrine* – that regulate various functions such as the response to stress.

Catheter
A hollow, flexible tube inserted into the body.

Catheterization
Insertion of a *catheter* into the body to drain or inject fluids or to perform some medical procedures such as widening narrowed blood vessels.

Cat-scratch fever
An uncommon illness that develops after a scratch or bite by a cat and is thought to be caused by a *bacterium*.

Cauliflower ear
Deformity of the ear, caused by repeated injury such as that experienced by boxers.

Cauterization
Application of a very hot instrument or caustic chemical to tissues in order to destroy them, to stop them from bleeding, or to promote their healing.

Cecum
A saclike chamber that is located at the beginning of the *large intestine*.

Celiac artery
An artery that branches from the *aorta* and supplies blood to digestive organs of the upper abdomen.

Celiac sprue
A condition in which the lining of the *small intestine* is damaged by a protein found in wheat, rye, and some other cereals.

Cell
The basic structural unit of the body.

Cellular membrane
The envelope surrounding each body cell that controls the passage of substances into and out of the cell.

Cellulitis
A bacterial infection of the skin and the tissues beneath it that, if untreated, can lead to tissue damage and blood poisoning.

Central nervous system
One of the two main parts of the nervous system, consisting of the brain and the *spinal cord*.

Cephalic vein
One of the main superficial veins of the arm.

Cephalosporins
A group of *antibiotics* derived from a fungus; they are used to treat a wide variety of infections.

Cerebellum
The region at the back of the brain concerned with the maintenance of posture and balance and the coordination of movement.

Cerebral angiography
See illustration below.

Cerebral artery thrombosis
Blockage of one of the arteries in the brain by a blood clot; a cause of *stroke*.

Cerebral cortex
The outer surface of the brain that is concerned with mental functions, such as thinking and remembering, and voluntary movement and sensation.

Cerebral embolism
Blockage of one of the arteries to the brain by an *embolus*, which is usually a blood clot that forms at a distant site and travels to the brain; a cause of *stroke*.

Cerebral hemisphere
One of the halves of the *cerebrum*.

Cerebral hemorrhage
Bleeding inside the brain caused by a ruptured blood vessel; a cause of *stroke*.

Cerebral palsy
A general term for disorders of movement and posture caused by brain damage that occurs before birth, during birth, or in early life.

Cerebrospinal fluid
The fluid flowing inside and around the brain and *spinal cord* that provides support and nutrition.

Cerebrovascular disease
Any disease affecting an artery that supplies blood to the brain.

Cerebrum
See illustration at right.

Cervical cap
A thimble-shaped, rubber contraceptive device that fits tightly over the *cervix*.

Cervical dysplasia
Changes in the cells on the surface of the *cervix* that are usually precancerous.

Cervical eversion
A condition in which mucus-producing cells, similar to those usually found inside the *cervix*, form a layer on its outside surface.

Cervical factor
Any quality in the mucus produced by the *cervix* that makes it hostile to sperm, thereby inhibiting fertility.

Cervical incompetence
Abnormal weakness of the *cervix* that can cause recurrent *miscarriages*.

Cervical mucus method
A *natural method of family planning* that is based on observing changes in the mucus secreted by the *cervix* to determine the time of *ovulation*.

Cervical osteoarthritis
A degenerative disorder of the joints between the bones in the neck, causing neck pain and stiffness.

Cervical smear
A specimen of tissue removed from the *cervix* for examination under a microscope to detect cell abnormalities; it is also called a Pap smear.

Cervical spine
The uppermost part of the spine, consisting of seven *vertebrae*.

Cervical stitch
A surgical stitch that is tied like a drawstring around a weakened *cervix* in order to prevent *miscarriage*.

Cervicitis
Inflammation of the *cervix*.

Cervix
The small, cylindrical lower part and neck of the uterus that separates the body of the uterus from the vagina.

Cesarean section
A surgical procedure to deliver a baby from the uterus through an incision in the lower abdomen.

Chancre
A painless sore, usually on the genitals, that develops during the first stage of *syphilis*.

Chancroid
An increasingly common *sexually transmitted disease* characterized by painful sores on the genitals.

Cheilitis
Inflammation, cracking, and dryness of the lips.

Chelating agent
A chemical used in the treatment of poisoning by metals such as lead, arsenic, and mercury.

Chemotherapy
Treatment of infections or cancers using drugs.

Chickenpox
A common, infectious, childhood disease, characterized by a rash of fluid-filled blisters and a slight fever.

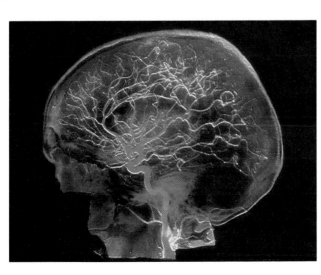

CEREBRAL ANGIOGRAPHY
*X-ray examination of the blood vessels of the brain after a **contrast medium** has been injected into them.*

Chimerism
The presence in a person of cells that are genetically different because they are derived from two different fertilized eggs; it does not cause any health problems.

Chlamydia
See illustration below.

Chloasma
Blotches of discoloration that may appear on the forehead, nose, and cheeks during pregnancy or in women taking *oral contraceptives*.

CHLAMYDIA
A type of bacterium (green and yellow specks) that causes various infections in humans, including **nongonococcal urethritis, pelvic inflammatory disease,** *and* **psittacosis.**

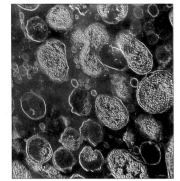

CHORIONIC VILLUS SAMPLING
A prenatal diagnostic procedure, performed in the ninth to 11th week of pregnancy, in which some fetal cells are withdrawn from the **placenta** *and studied for genetic abnormalities. The procedure is guided by* **ultrasound scanning.**

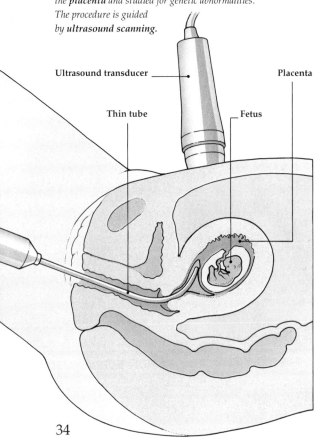

Ultrasound transducer

Placenta

Thin tube

Fetus

Cholangiocarcinoma
A cancerous growth in the *bile ducts*.

Cholangiography
An X-ray procedure for examining the *bile ducts* after they have been filled with a *contrast medium*.

Cholangitis
Inflammation of the *common bile duct*.

Cholecystectomy
Surgical removal of the *gallbladder*.

Cholecystitis
Inflammation of the *gallbladder*.

Cholera
A bacterial infection acquired from contaminated water and food; it causes severe diarrhea that can lead to rapid dehydration and death if untreated.

Cholestasis
Obstruction to the flow of *bile* inside the liver, which can cause *jaundice* and liver damage.

Cholesterol
A fatlike substance that is an important constituent of cells; it is involved in the formation of *hormones* and *bile* and in the transport of fats in the blood. A high level of cholesterol in the blood increases the risk of *atherosclerosis*.

Chondritis
Inflammation of a *cartilage*, usually caused by mechanical pressure, stress, or injury.

Chondroma
A noncancerous tumor of *cartilage* cells on the surface of or inside bones.

Chondromalacia patellae
A painful knee disorder, most common in adolescent athletes, in which the *cartilage* directly behind the kneecap is damaged.

Chondrosarcoma
A cancerous growth of *cartilage* that usually affects the long bones, the *pelvis*, and the collarbone.

Chorea
A condition characterized by involuntary, rapid, jerky movements, or fidgeting, usually affecting the face, limbs, and trunk.

Choriocarcinoma
A rare cancerous tumor that develops inside the uterus from the *placenta*.

Chorion
The outermost of the two membrane layers containing the *amniotic fluid* and the *fetus*; it gives rise to the *placenta*.

Chorionic gonadotropin
Human chorionic gonadotropin.

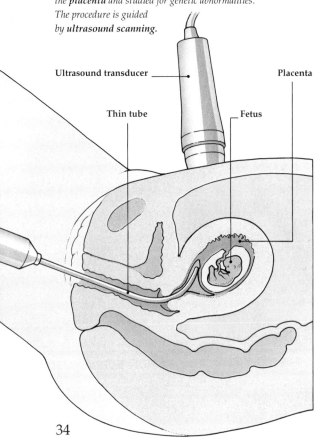

CHROMOSOMES
Threadlike structures inside the nuclei of cells that contain **genes.** *The chromosomes above are magnified 1,500 times. The enlarged chromosome is magnified 10,000 times.*

Chorionic villus sampling
See illustration below left.

Choroiditis
Inflammation of the blood vessels in the middle layer of the eye.

Christmas disease
A rare, inherited bleeding disorder; it is also called hemophilia B.

Chromatin
The material inside cells, consisting of *DNA* and *protein*, from which *chromosomes* are formed.

Chromosomes
See illustrations above.

Chromosome abnormality
An abnormality in the number or structure of *chromosomes* inside a person's cells, which can cause a serious birth defect.

Chromosome analysis
Study of the *chromosomes* inside a person's cells to learn whether he or she has a *chromosome abnormality* or to establish its nature.

Chronic
Describes a disorder that persists for a long time.

Chronic active hepatitis
A type of *hepatitis* characterized by progressive inflammation and destruction of cells in the liver; it leads to *cirrhosis of the liver*.

Chronic obstructive lung disease
A progressive disease characterized by a persistent disruption of air flow into or out of the lungs.

Cilia
Tiny, hairlike projections from the surface of some cells; they produce a wavelike motion.

Circadian rhythm
Any biological pattern based on a 24-hour cycle.

Circle of Willis
A ring of blood vessels at the base of the brain.

Circumcision
Surgical removal of the *foreskin* of the penis.

Cirrhosis of the liver
A disease, caused by widespread destruction of liver cells, in which bands of internal scarring break up the structure of the liver and harden it.

Claudication
A weakness in the leg along with cramplike pain when walking; it is usually caused by blockage or narrowing of arteries in the legs.

Claustrophobia
Intense fear of enclosed spaces or crowded areas.

Clavicle
The collarbone.

Cleft lip
A birth defect characterized by a vertical, usually off-center split in the upper lip.

Cleft palate
A birth defect characterized by a gap in the roof of the mouth, often with *cleft lip*.

Climacteric
The time span during which a woman moves from her reproductive to her nonreproductive years.

Clinical trial
A carefully monitored study on groups of people to evaluate the effectiveness and safety of a treatment.

Clitoris
A small, sensitive female genital organ, partly enclosed in the *labia*, that swells in response to sexual stimulation.

Clone
An exact copy; often applied to a group of identical *genes* or a group of genetically identical cells or organisms.

Clonus
An abnormal muscle response, in which stretching sets off a series of quick muscle contractions.

Closed fracture
A break in a bone in which the two ends of the broken bone remain under the skin.

Clostridium
A type of *bacterium* that causes infections such as *tetanus*, *botulism*, *cellulitis*, and *gas gangrene*.

Clotting factor
One of several substances in the blood that are necessary for blood to clot.

Clotting time
The time required for blood to form a clot.

Clubfoot
A foot deformity present from birth; usually the foot is bent downward and inward.

Cluster headache
A sudden, severe pain on one side of the head involving the face and neck, often occurring daily for several weeks, then ceasing for several months.

CNS
Central nervous system.

Coagulation
The conversion of blood into a jellylike solid (a blood clot).

Cobalt
A metallic element and a component of *vitamin B12*.

Cocarcinogen
A substance that by itself cannot cause cancer, but increases the activity of a cancer-causing substance.

Coccidioidomycosis
An infection resembling *tuberculosis* that is acquired by inhaling airborne fungal spores; it is also called San Joaquin Valley fever.

Coccyx
A small triangular bone consisting of four fused, smaller bones at the base of the spine.

Cochlea
See illustration below.

Cochlear implant
A device to treat deafness, consisting of electrodes implanted inside the *cochlea* to transmit sound-generated nerve impulses to the brain.

Coenzyme
An organic compound that plays an important role in activating *enzymes*.

Coitus
Sexual intercourse.

Coitus interruptus
An unreliable contraceptive method in which the man withdraws his penis before ejaculation occurs.

Cold sore
A small blister around the mouth caused by the *herpes simplex* virus.

Colectomy
The surgical removal of part or all of the *colon*.

Colic
Periodic waves of severe, spasmodic, abdominal pain.

Coliform
Relating to a group of rod-shaped *bacteria* commonly found in the intestines.

Colitis
Inflammation of the *colon*.

Collagen
The body's most common and major structural protein.

Collagen vascular diseases
A group of diseases of *connective tissues* and small blood vessels caused by malfunctioning of the *immune system*.

Collapsed lung
A condition in which a lung sags and cannot fill with air.

Collateral
A small side branch of a nerve or blood vessel.

Colon
The main part of the *large intestine*.

Colonoscopy
Examination of the inside of the *colon* using a long, flexible, viewing instrument called a colonoscope.

Color blindness
An inability to distinguish between certain colors.

Colorectal
Pertaining to the *colon* and the *rectum*.

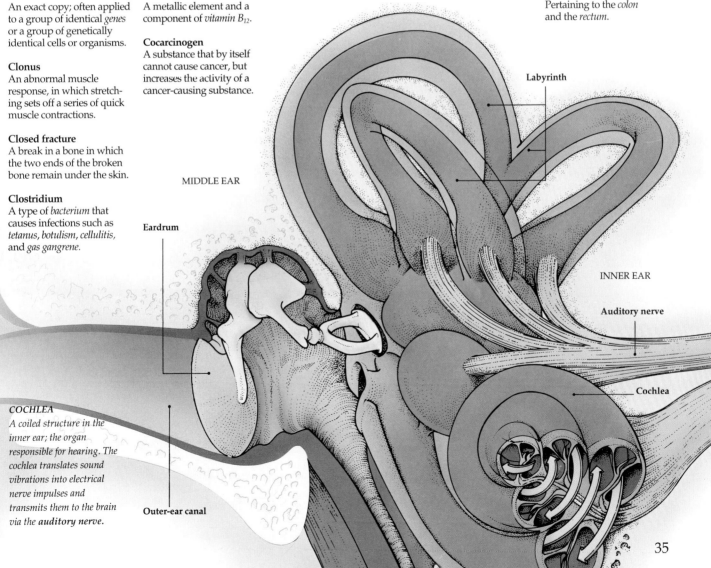

MIDDLE EAR

Eardrum

Labyrinth

INNER EAR

Auditory nerve

Cochlea

COCHLEA
A coiled structure in the inner ear; the organ responsible for hearing. The cochlea translates sound vibrations into electrical nerve impulses and transmits them to the brain via the auditory nerve.

Outer-ear canal

Colostomy
A surgical procedure in which part of the *colon* is brought through an incision in the abdominal wall and an artificial opening formed to allow the discharge of feces into a bag attached to the skin.

Colostrum
A thin, yellowish fluid produced by the breasts during late pregnancy and the first few days after childbirth; it provides infection-fighting substances to a newborn.

Colporrhaphy
A surgical procedure to stitch the vagina, either to repair a tear or to narrow it.

Colposcopy
Visual examination of the *cervix* and *vagina* using magnifying lenses.

Coma
A state of unconsciousness in which a person does not respond even to strong stimulation.

Comminuted fracture
A fracture in which the bone has **been** shattered into several pieces.

Common bile duct
The tube that carries *bile* from the *cystic duct* to the *duodenum*.

Common cold
A viral infection that causes inflammation of the *mucous membranes* lining the nose and throat, resulting in a stuffy, runny nose and sometimes a sore throat and other symptoms.

Common hepatic duct
A short tube that carries *bile* from the liver to the *cystic duct*.

Communicable disease
Any disease that can be transmitted from one person or animal to another.

Complement
A group of *proteins* in the blood that are part of the *immune system* and help the body fight infections.

Compliance
The degree to which a person follows a prescribed course of treatment; it is especially important when taking antibiotics.

Compound fracture
A break in a bone in which the broken end or ends puncture the skin.

Compression
Squeezing of a body part that occurs as the result of disease; or the application of pressure to an injured muscle or joint to reduce bleeding and swelling.

Compression bandage
A strip of gauze, elastic, or other material applied firmly around a body part to reduce bleeding and swelling after injury.

Compression fracture
A break in a short bone such as a *vertebra* in which soft bone tissue is crushed, usually as the result of a fall in a person with *osteoporosis*.

Computed tomography scanning
See illustration below.

Conception
The moment when an egg is fertilized by a sperm.

Concordance
The presence of a given trait or disorder in both members of a pair of twins.

Concussion
Brief loss of consciousness and possible confusion and other symptoms following a violent blow to the head.

Condom
See illustrations above right.

Conductive hearing loss
Difficulty hearing resulting from inadequate transmission of sound from the outer ear to the inner ear.

Cone biopsy
Surgical removal of a cone-shaped section of tissue from the *cervix* for microscopic examination.

Congenital
Present at birth.

Congenital adrenal hyperplasia
A *genetic disorder* caused by abnormal hormone production by the *adrenal glands*; it can produce male characteristics in females.

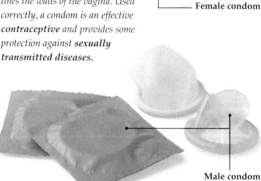

CONDOM
A thin, latex rubber device used to prevent sperm from entering the vagina. The male condom fits over the penis; the female condom fits over the **cervix** *and lines the walls of the vagina. Used correctly, a condom is an effective* **contraceptive** *and provides some protection against* **sexually transmitted diseases.**

— Female condom

Male condom

Congenital heart disease
Any structural or functional abnormality of the heart that is present from birth; the most common cause of death in newborns.

Congestive heart failure
Heart failure that results in congestion of blood in veins and excessive accumulation of fluid in body tissues.

Conjunctiva
The transparent *mucous membrane* covering the white of the eye and lining the inside of the eyelids.

Conjunctivitis
Inflammation of the *conjunctiva* resulting in redness of the eye and a thick, sticky discharge.

Connective tissue
The material that supports the structure of some parts of the body, such as bone, and binds body tissues and parts together.

Constipation
Infrequent or difficult passing of hard, dry feces.

Constriction
A narrowing in an opening or passage in the body.

Constriction ring
A band of contracted uterine muscle that sometimes develops during *labor* and prevents descent of the fetus into the birth canal.

Contact dermatitis
A rash resulting from the direct exposure of the skin to a particular substance to which a person is sensitive.

Contact tracing
The process of finding and informing the people with whom a person diagnosed as having a serious infectious disease has come into contact; the purpose is to stop the disease from spreading further.

Contagious
Describes a disease that can be transmitted from one person to another by direct or indirect contact.

Continuous positive airway pressure
Delivery of air at constant pressure to people who are otherwise unable to maintain adequate levels of oxygen in their blood.

Contraceptive
Any agent or device used to prevent pregnancy.

Contraceptive foam
A *spermicide* foam inserted into the vagina before each act of sexual intercourse to prevent pregnancy.

Contraceptive sponge
A *barrier method of contraception* in which a foam sponge that contains *spermicide* is inserted high into the vagina.

COMPUTED TOMOGRAPHY SCANNING
A diagnostic imaging technique in which X-rays (passed through the body from several angles) are detected and analyzed by a computer to produce cross-sectional images of body structures.

— Scanner

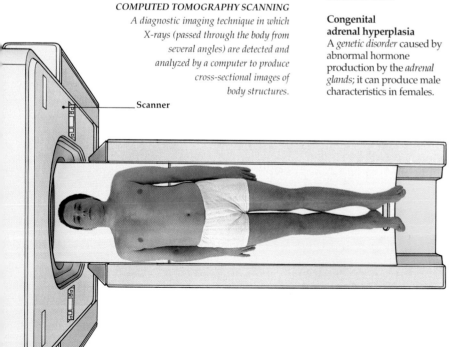

Contraction
See illustration below.

Contracture
An abnormality, usually in a joint, caused by shrinkage of scar tissue in the skin or *connective tissue*, or by irreversible shortening of muscles and tendons.

Contraindication
Any factor in a person's condition that makes it unwise for him or her to undergo a particular treatment such as drug therapy or surgery.

Contrast medium
A substance through which X-rays cannot pass.

Contrast X-ray imaging
A technique in which a *contrast medium* is introduced into hollow organs or body cavities to make them visible on X-ray film.

Controlled trial
A method of assessing the value of a drug or other therapy by monitoring its effects compared with those of another drug or therapy.

Contusion
A bruise.

Convulsion
Seizure.

Cooley's anemia
A serious form of the inherited blood disorder *thalassemia*.

Coordination
The ability of interrelated organs or body parts to function together harmoniously.

Copper
A metallic element that forms part of several *enzymes* and is an essential *mineral* in the diet.

Cord prolapse
The dropping down of the *umbilical cord* into the *cervix* or vagina during *labor*.

Corn
A small area of thickened skin on the toe, often at a joint, caused by pressure from a tight-fitting shoe.

Cornea
The transparent, thin-walled dome at the front of the eyeball that acts as a protective covering and helps focus light rays onto the *retina*.

Corneal graft
Transplantation of healthy tissue from the *cornea* of a donor eye to repair a diseased cornea.

Coronary
A term meaning "crown" that usually refers to the arteries that encircle and supply the heart; a heart attack is often called a coronary.

Coronary angiography
An X-ray technique for examining the *coronary arteries* after *cardiac catheterization* and injection of a *contrast medium*.

Coronary artery
The arteries that branch from the *aorta* and supply the heart muscle with oxygenated blood.

Coronary artery bypass
A surgical procedure to allow blood to circumvent narrowed or blocked *coronary arteries* by grafting on additional blood vessels.

Coronary heart disease
Malfunction of or damage to the heart muscle that is caused by narrowing or blockage in one or more of the *coronary arteries*.

Coronary sinus
The opening through which the blood that drains from the heart muscle enters the right *atrium*.

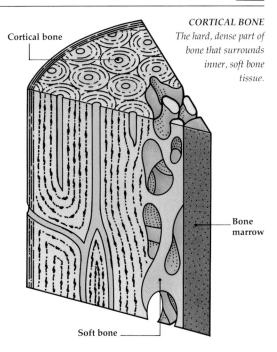

CORTICAL BONE
The hard, dense part of bone that surrounds inner, soft bone tissue.

Coronary thrombosis
Blockage of a *coronary artery* by a blood clot (*thrombus*), often causing a heart attack and, sometimes, death.

Coronaviruses
A group of viruses that can cause many respiratory illnesses, including the common cold.

Cor pulmonale
Enlargement and failure of the right side of the heart caused by a chronic lung disease that has increased blood pressure in the *pulmonary artery*.

Corpus callosum
A wide band of more than 200 million nerve fibers that connects the right and left hemispheres of the brain.

Corpuscle
Any cell in the body, particularly *red blood cells* and *white blood cells*.

Corpus luteum
A structure that grows inside an empty egg *follicle* after *ovulation* and secretes the hormone *progesterone* to prepare the uterus lining to receive a fertilized egg.

Cortex
The outer layer of an organ or other body structure.

Cortical bone
See illustration above.

Corticospinal tract
A bundle of nerve fibers that links the *cerebral cortex* of the brain with the *spinal cord* and is involved in control of the movement of muscles below the head.

Corticosteroid hormones
Several hormones – produced by the outer layer of the *adrenal glands* – that control blood pressure, the body's use of nutrients, the excretion of salts and water in the urine, the *immune system*, and the body's response to stress.

Corticosteroids
A class of synthetic drugs, similar to the natural *corticosteroid hormones* secreted by the *adrenal glands*, that have many uses including the treatment of inflammatory disorders.

Cosmetic surgery
An operation performed primarily to improve appearance rather than to improve function or to cure a disease or disorder.

Costal cartilage
Flexible *cartilage* that connects the ribs to the breastbone.

Coulter counter
An electronic device that can rapidly identify and count the red and white cells in a sample of blood.

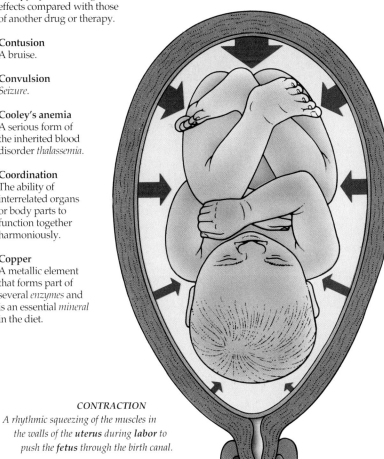

CONTRACTION
*A rhythmic squeezing of the muscles in the walls of the **uterus** during **labor** to push the **fetus** through the birth canal.*

Cowper's glands
Two small glands at the base of the inside of the penis that secrete fluid into the *urethra* during sexual stimulation.

Cowpox
A mild viral infection, causing skin blistering, that can be transmitted to humans from infected cows.

Coxsackieviruses
A group of viruses that cause a variety of illnesses, including *aseptic meningitis*, *hand-foot-and-mouth disease*, and *pleurodynia*.

CPR
Cardiopulmonary resuscitation.

Crab louse
Pubic louse.

Crackle
An abnormal crunching sound that can be heard through a stethoscope during inhalation.

Cradle cap
A condition common in babies in which thick, yellow scales occur in patches over the scalp.

Cramp
Painful, usually momentary, spasm in a muscle that often occurs during or right after exercise.

Cranial nerves
See illustration below.

Craniotomy
Opening of part of the skull to enable a surgeon to operate on the brain or to drain fluid.

Cranium
The part of the skull enclosing the brain.

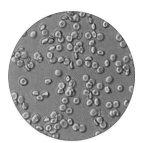
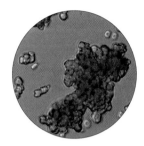

Compatible blood   Incompatible blood

CROSSMATCHING
A procedure used to determine compatibility between the blood of a person requiring a blood transfusion and that of a potential blood donor. Samples of blood from the two people are mixed together; blood that is incompatible looks clotted when viewed under a microscope.

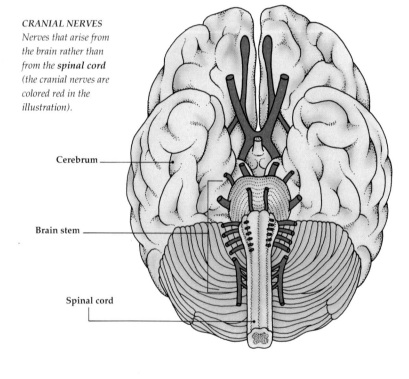

CRANIAL NERVES
Nerves that arise from the brain rather than from the **spinal cord** *(the cranial nerves are colored red in the illustration).*

Cerebrum

Brain stem

Spinal cord

Creatinine
A waste product filtered by the kidneys and excreted in the urine.

Creatinine clearance test
A test that is used to evaluate kidney function by measuring the amount of *creatinine* in the blood and in a sample of urine collected over a period of 24 hours.

Cretinism
A disorder characterized by mental retardation, stunted growth, and coarse facial features, caused by inadequate production of *thyroid hormones* at birth.

Creutzfeldt-Jakob disease
A rare, fatal condition characterized by progressive mental deterioration and muscle wasting, thought to be a *slow virus disease*.

Cricothyrotomy
See illustration at left.

Crisis intervention
The provision of immediate advice or help to a person with an acute personal or psychiatric problem.

Critical
A term used to mean seriously ill, or to describe a state of illness from which it is uncertain whether a person will recover.

Crohn's disease
A *chronic* inflammatory disease of unknown cause that can affect any part of the *gastrointestinal tract*.

Crossing over
Exchange of genetic material between pairs of *chromosomes* derived from a person's two parents during egg and sperm formation.

Crossmatching
See illustrations above.

Croup
Inflammation and narrowing of the *airways* in young children, causing a hoarse, barking cough.

Cruciate ligaments
The two *ligaments* in the knee joint that cross over each other to connect the thighbone and the shinbone and stabilize the joint.

Crush injury
An injury that crushes muscles or bones.

Cryoanesthesia
Freezing of a part of the body to deaden pain during minor surgery.

Cryocautery
Application of a substance that freezes tissue as a means of destroying it.

Cryopreservation
Preservation of living cells by freezing.

Cryosurgery
Use of low temperatures to destroy tissue by freezing.

Cryptococcosis
A rare fungal infection that can cause skin growths, *meningitis*, and *pneumonia*.

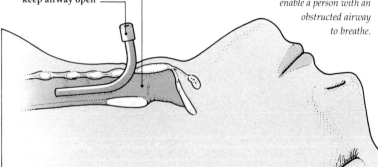

Tube inserted to keep airway open

Trachea

CRICOTHYROTOMY
Emergency surgery to create an opening in the **trachea** *to enable a person with an obstructed airway to breathe.*

Cryptosporidiosis
An *opportunistic infection* that causes severe symptoms, including chronic diarrhea, in people with *AIDS*.

CT scanning
Computed tomography scanning.

Culdocentesis
Insertion of a small needle through the vagina into the pelvic cavity to obtain a sample of blood, pus, or other fluid for examination.

Culture
A cultivation of bacteria or other *microorganisms*, cells, or tissues in the laboratory, used in diagnosing disease.

Culture medium
A substance containing nutrients that encourage the growth of *microorganisms* or cells for laboratory study.

Curet
A sharp, spoon-shaped surgical instrument used for scraping away material or tissue from an organ, body cavity, or body surface.

Curettage
Using a *curet* to scrape away abnormal tissue or take tissue for analysis from the lining of a body cavity or from the skin.

Cushing's syndrome
A disorder caused by an abnormally high level of *corticosteroid hormones* in the bloodstream; characterized by wasting of muscles, thin skin, and weakened bones.

CVS
Chorionic villus sampling.

Cyanosis
See illustration above right.

Cyst
An abnormal lump or swelling, filled with fluid or semisolid material, that may occur in any organ or tissue.

Cystadenoma
A noncancerous tumor of glandular tissue that contains *cysts*.

Cystectomy
Surgical removal of the bladder, which is often replaced with a segment of intestine; it is performed in cases of bladder cancer.

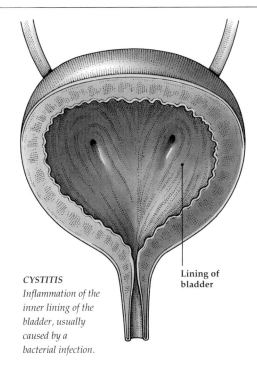

CYSTITIS
Inflammation of the inner lining of the bladder, usually caused by a bacterial infection.

Lining of bladder

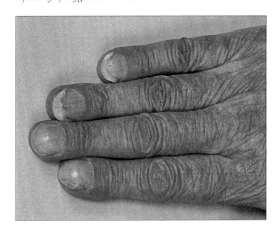

CYANOSIS
Bluish coloration of the skin and **mucous membranes** *caused by a deficiency of oxygen in the blood.*

Cystic duct
A small tube through which *bile* passes to and from the *gallbladder*.

Cysticercosis
An infection that occurs when pork *tapeworm* larvae invade body tissues after a person accidentally swallows the eggs of an adult pork tapeworm.

Cystic fibrosis
A *genetic disorder* characterized by persistent lung infections and an inability to absorb fats and other nutrients from food.

Cystic tumor
An abnormal growth that contains *cysts*.

Cystinuria
A *genetic disorder* in which excessive excretion in the urine of the *amino acid* cystine leads to the formation of kidney and bladder stones.

Cystitis
See illustration above left.

Cystocele
A swelling at the front and top of the vagina formed where the bladder pushes against weakened tissues in the vaginal wall.

Cystography
X-ray examination of the bladder after it has been filled with a *contrast medium*.

Cystometry
A procedure that measures bladder capacity and pressure changes as the bladder fills and empties.

Cystoscopy
Use of a viewing tube (a cystoscope) passed up the *urethra* to inspect the bladder and *ureters* or to perform therapeutic procedures.

Cystostomy
The surgical creation of a hole in the bladder for drainage.

Cytomegalovirus
A type of *herpesvirus* that can cause serious illness in people with weakened immune systems, such as those who have *AIDS*.

Cytoplasm
The part of a cell outside the nucleus that is the site of most of the cell's chemical activities.

Cytotoxic drugs
Drugs that kill or damage cells or prevent them from growing and dividing; they are used to treat cancer.

D and C
Dilatation and curettage.

Débridement
Surgical removal of foreign material and/or dead, damaged, or infected tissue from a wound or burn to expose healthy tissue; it is performed to speed healing.

Decalcification
The dissolving of minerals from bone or teeth caused by dietary deficiencies.

Decompression sickness
A painful, sometimes fatal illness caused by the formation of gas bubbles in body tissues, such as can occur when a diver ascends too rapidly to the surface.

Decongestant
A drug used to relieve nasal congestion.

Deep-vein thrombosis
Clotting of blood inside deep-lying veins, usually in the legs or pelvis.

Defecation
The elimination of feces from the body via the *anus*.

Defibrillation
Administration of a brief electric shock to the heart that can reverse some types of abnormalities in the heartbeat.

Defibrillator
A machine used to restore normal heart rhythm by delivering an electric shock to the heart by means of two metal plates applied to the chest.

Degenerative arthritis
Osteoarthritis.

Dehydration
A dangerous decrease in water content in a person's body or tissues.

Delirium
A state of acute mental confusion and restlessness that is often brought on by physical illness.

Delirium tremens
A state of confusion accompanied by trembling and hallucinations, occurring in chronic alcoholics when they stop drinking.

Deltoid muscle
A large, triangular muscle of the shoulder that forms the rounded flesh of the outer, upper part of the arm.

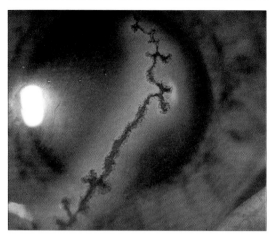

Dementia
A progressive deterioration of mental ability.

Demyelination
Breakdown of the fatty sheaths that surround and insulate nerve cells.

Dendrite
A short, threadlike extension of a nerve cell that receives chemical signals from other nerve cells.

Dendritic ulcer
See illustration above.

Dengue
An infectious disease that is caused by a *virus* carried by mosquitoes; the symptoms include fever, headache, and severe pain in the joints and muscles.

Densitometry
The measurement of the density of a substance.

Deoxyribonucleic acid
See illustration at right.

Depilatory
A chemical hair remover in the form of a cream or paste.

Depot injection
An injection of a drug that has been specifically formulated to provide for a slow, steady absorption of its active chemicals into the bloodstream.

Depression
Feelings of sadness, hopelessness, pessimism, and a general loss of interest in life, combined with a severely reduced sense of emotional well-being.

Dermabrasion
The removal of the surface layer of the skin by high-speed sanding to improve the appearance of scars or to remove tattoos.

Dermatitis
Inflammation of the skin from an allergy, an infection, stress, or (often) from no known cause.

Dermatitis artefacta
Any self-induced skin damage, such as a scratch.

Dermatitis herpetiformis
A *chronic* skin disease in which clusters of tiny, red, intensely itchy blisters occur in a symmetrical pattern on various parts of the body.

Dermatographia
Abnormal sensitivity of the skin to irritation, to the extent that firm stroking produces itchy, raised, slightly darkened areas.

Dermatomycosis
A fungal infection of the skin that usually affects moist, clothed areas of the body such as the groin.

Dermatomyositis
A rare, sometimes fatal, *autoimmune disease* in which the muscles and skin are inflamed, causing weakness of muscles and a skin rash.

Dermis
The thick inner layer of skin that contains most of its living elements.

Dermoid cyst
A noncancerous tumor inside the body with a cell structure similar to that of skin.

Desensitization
Making a person less sensitive to an *allergen* by giving a series of injections containing progressively larger doses of the allergen.

Detached retina
Separation of the *retina* from the outer layers of the eye, usually requiring surgery.

Detoxification
Treatment to diminish or eliminate the effects of a poisonous substance; or treatment aimed at freeing a person of alcohol or drug dependence.

Detrusor instability
Involuntary loss of urine (*incontinence*) caused by lack of control of the *bladder* muscle (the detrusor muscle).

Developmental delay
Failure of a child to acquire new skills or to behave in a manner appropriate for his or her age; most children catch up on their own.

Developmental disorder
A disorder that results from abnormal fetal development.

Dextrocardia
A condition in which the heart is located in the right side of the chest rather than the left, resulting from disease or a birth defect.

Dextrose
A sugar (*glucose*) that is used in intravenous *infusions* to provide nutrition.

Diabetes insipidus
A condition characterized by excessive production of urine caused by a deficiency of *antidiuretic hormone* or by insensitivity of the *kidneys* to this hormone.

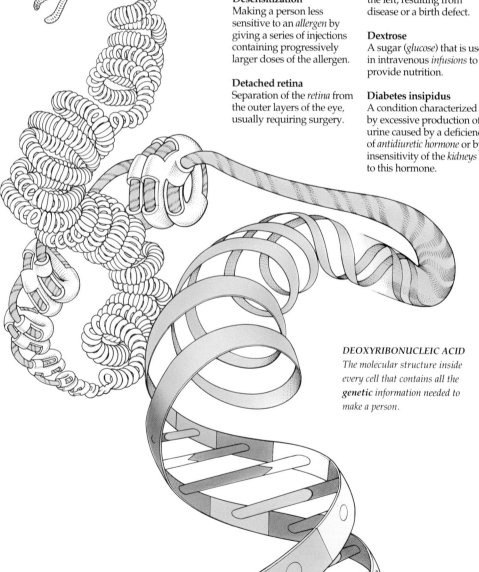

DEOXYRIBONUCLEIC ACID
*The molecular structure inside every cell that contains all the **genetic** information needed to make a person.*

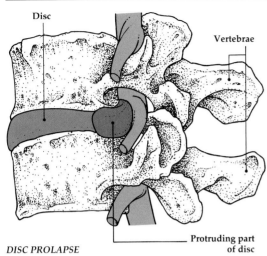

DISC PROLAPSE
*A common, painful disorder of the spine resulting when an **intervertebral disc** ruptures and part of its pulpy core protrudes.*

Diabetes mellitus
A disorder resulting from the body's inability to use the sugar *glucose*, its main energy source; its two forms are *insulin-dependent diabetes* and *non-insulin-dependent diabetes.*

Diabetic gastroparesis
A condition resulting from uncontrolled *diabetes mellitus* in which the stomach fails to empty normally because of degeneration of nerves that control stomach function.

Diabetic retinopathy
A disorder that causes blood vessels in the *retina* to bleed and, if untreated, can lead to blindness; it is a complication of *diabetes mellitus.*

Dialysis
A technique for removing substances from the blood using a membrane through which different substances pass at different rates; the procedure is used when the kidneys are not functioning normally and in some cases of poisoning or drug overdose.

Diaper rash
Inflammation of the skin in the diaper area, caused by irritation from feces, moisture, or heat; it can be prevented by keeping the area clean and dry.

Diaphragm
The dome-shaped muscle that separates the chest from the abdomen and moves up and down to aid breathing.

Diaphragm, contraceptive
A thin rubber dome with a springy rim that is inserted into the vagina to cover the opening to the uterus and block the passage of sperm, preventing pregnancy.

Diaphragmatic hernia
Protrusion of an abdominal organ through the *diaphragm* into the chest.

Diarrhea
Abnormal increase in the fluidity, frequency, and volume of bowel movements.

Diastole
The resting period of the heart muscle between heartbeats.

Diastolic pressure
The blood pressure measured during the resting period of the heart muscle between heartbeats.

Diathermy
Use of high-frequency currents to produce heat in parts of the body as a treatment for pain (such as that of arthritis) or to destroy diseased tissue.

Diastrophic
Describes a condition in which bones are curved, such as in one form of dwarfism.

Differential diagnosis
A group of diseases with similar symptoms and signs that a doctor will consider when making a diagnosis.

Differentiation
The process by which the almost identical cells of the early *embryo* gradually diversify to form specialized tissues and organs that have different functions.

Digestion
The conversion of food into a form the body can absorb and use for energy, growth, and repair.

Digestive tract
A muscular tube that carries food through the digestive process from the mouth to the anus; it includes the throat, *esophagus*, stomach, and intestines.

Digital subtraction angiography
A technique that uses a series of computer images to study blood vessels, eliminating unnecessary information and enhancing visualization.

Dilatation
Natural or artificial widening of an opening or tubelike structure in the body; also called dilation.

Dilatation and curettage
A surgical procedure (popularly referred to as D and C) in which the *cervix* is widened and the membrane lining the uterus is scraped away; it is used to diagnose and treat disorders of the uterus such as heavy, persistent, vaginal bleeding.

Diphtheria
An acute bacterial infection that causes a sore throat and fever and can lead to more serious or fatal complications if untreated.

Disc
Intervertebral disc.

Disc prolapse
See illustration at left.

Disinfection
The application of germ-killing substances to objects to prevent the spread of infection.

Dislocation
Displacement of the bones that meet at a joint so they no longer touch; it usually results from injury.

Distal
Describes a part of the body that is situated farther away from a central point of reference than another part of the body; for example, the fingers are distal to the arm with the trunk as the point of reference.

Distention
Enlargement or swelling.

Diuresis
Increased production and excretion of urine.

Diuretic
A drug that helps remove excess water from the body by increasing the amount lost in the urine.

Diurnal
Occurring on a daily basis.

Diverticulitis
Inflammation of *diverticula*, causing fever, pain, and tenderness.

Diverticulosis
The presence of *diverticula* in the gastrointestinal wall.

Diverticulum
A small sac created by a protrusion of the intestine's inner lining through its muscular layers; the plural form is diverticula.

DNA
Deoxyribonucleic acid.

DNA analysis
Genetic analysis.

DNA fingerprint
See illustration below.

DNA marker
A piece of *DNA* located at a particular site on a *chromosome* that varies detectably from person to person; DNA markers are used as landmarks to find disease-causing *genes.*

DNA replication
The process by which *DNA* copies itself in cells.

DNA sequencing
The process of determining the code of a defective *gene* and comparing it with the code of a normal gene to identify a specific defect.

DNA FINGERPRINT
*A pattern of bands on transparent film, produced by laboratory processing of a person's **DNA**, which is unique to that person; the technique is useful in **paternity testing** and in identifying crime suspects.*

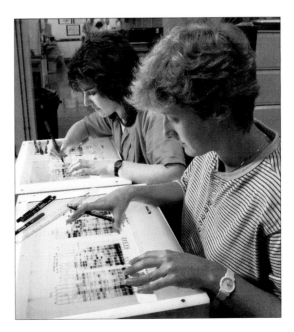

Dominant gene
A *gene* that produces an effect whenever it is present.

Dominant inheritance
A pattern of inheritance in which a child is likely to inherit a particular trait or disorder even though only one parent has it.

Dopamine
A chemical messenger in the brain that is involved in the control of movement.

Dopamine-boosting drug
A drug that is converted to *dopamine* in the brain, used to help raise an abnormally low dopamine level.

Dopamine-releasing drug
A drug that boosts *dopamine* activity by mobilizing it but does not actually increase dopamine levels.

Doppler ultrasound scanning
See illustration above right.

Dorsal
Relating to the back.

Double-blind trial
See illustration at right.

Double helix
The structure of *DNA*, which resembles a twisted ladder.

Down's syndrome
See illustration below right.

DPT vaccination
A series of injections beginning in infancy that provide immunity against *diphtheria*, *pertussis* (whooping cough), and *tetanus*.

Drug screening test
A test used to determine the type and amount of drugs taken in an overdose or to measure and monitor the levels of medications taken by a patient.

Drug tolerance
Progressively decreased sensitivity to a drug that a person has taken repeatedly, requiring higher doses to produce the desired effect.

Drug withdrawal
Unpleasant physical and mental symptoms experienced when a person stops taking a drug on which he or she has become physically dependent.

Dry eye
Inadequate lubrication of the *cornea* as a result of deficient tear production.

Duchenne type muscular dystrophy
A *genetic disorder* that occurs almost exclusively in boys and is characterized by progressive muscle weakness.

Duodenal ulcer
A raw area in the wall of the *duodenum*; the most common type of *peptic ulcer*.

Duodenitis
Inflammation of the *duodenum*.

Duodenum
The first part of the *small intestine* into which the stomach empties.

Dura mater
The outermost layer of the three protective membranes surrounding the brain.

Dust mite
A tiny, spiderlike animal that thrives in house dust and is a common cause of *allergic reactions*.

Dyschondroplasia
A birth defect characterized by the proliferation of cartilage cells inside bones, which causes limb deformities.

Dysentery
An infection of the intestines acquired from contaminated food or water that causes *diarrhea* (with blood, pus, and mucus in the feces) and abdominal pain.

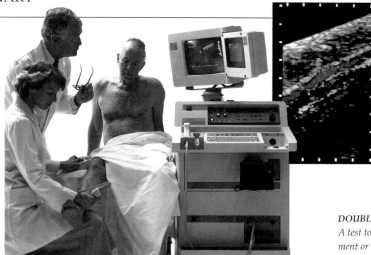

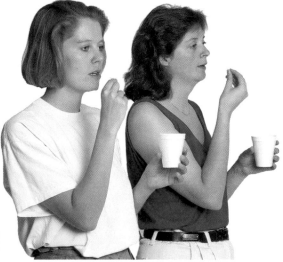

DOPPLER ULTRASOUND SCANNING
*A type of **ultrasound scanning** used to obtain information about the rate of blood flow through arteries and the heart.*

DOUBLE-BLIND TRIAL
A test to evaluate the effectiveness of a new treatment or to compare two treatments; neither the people in the study nor researchers know which treatment a given person is receiving.

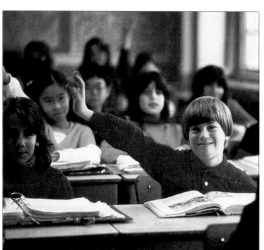

DOWN'S SYNDROME
*A **chromosome abnormality** in which a person's cells contain an extra **chromosome**, resulting in mental retardation and a characteristic appearance.*

Dysfunctional
Unable to function normally.

Dysgenesis
Abnormal development, usually during fetal growth.

Dyskinesia
Abnormal muscular movements caused by drugs or a brain disorder.

Dyslexia
A learning disability characterized by difficulty with written symbols.

Dysmenorrhea
Pain or discomfort experienced just before or during a menstrual period.

Dyspareunia
Pain experienced by a woman during sexual intercourse.

Dyspepsia
Indigestion.

Dysphagia
Difficulty swallowing.

Dysplasia
Abnormality in the growth of body structures or cells, such as the abnormal, potentially precancerous cells in the *cervix* that can be detected by a *Pap smear*.

Dyspnea
Difficult or labored breathing.

Dysrhythmia
Arrhythmia.

Dystonia
Abnormal muscle rigidity, causing painful muscle spasms or strange movement patterns.

Dystrophy
Any disorder in which cells lack nutrition and fail to develop normally or are damaged.

e

Eardrum
A thin, oval membrane (separating the *middle ear* from the outer ear) that transmits sound waves.

Echocardiography
Ultrasound scanning of the heart and its structures.

Eclampsia
A dangerous condition (for both the woman and the *fetus*) of late pregnancy, characterized by *seizures* in the woman.

ECT
Electroconvulsive therapy.

Ectopic
Occurring in an abnormal site and/or out of sequence.

Ectopic heartbeat
A heartbeat that is out of sequence and arises from an abnormal site.

Ectopic pregnancy
See illustration at right.

Ectropion
A turning outward of the eyelid, usually the lower lid.

Eczema
Skin inflammation.

Edema
An abnormal accumulation of fluid in body tissues.

EEG
Electroencephalography.

Efferent nerve
A nerve that conveys impulses away from the brain or *spinal cord* to muscles or glands.

Ejaculation
Expulsion of semen from the penis at *orgasm*.

Elective
Describes a procedure that is not an emergency, such as correction of hemorrhoids or cosmetic surgery.

Electric shock treatment
Electroconvulsive therapy.

Electrocardiography
Recording and study of the electrical activity of the heart muscle.

Electrocoagulation
The use of an electric current to seal blood vessels to prevent bleeding.

Electroconvulsive therapy
A method of treating some mental disorders, such as depression, by passing electric currents through the brain to stimulate *seizures*.

Electroencephalography
See illustration below right.

Electrolysis
Permanent removal of unwanted hair achieved by destroying hair roots with an electric current.

Electromyography
Recording and study of the electrical activity in muscle.

Electronic fetal monitoring
Measurement of the *heart rate* of the *fetus* and the woman's uterine contractions during *labor* using various electronic or pressure-sensitive devices.

Electrophoresis
A diagnostic technique to identify *proteins* or other chemicals in body fluids.

Electrosurgery
Surgery performed using electrical instruments.

ELISA
Enzyme-linked immunosorbent assay.

Embolectomy
Surgical removal of an *embolus* from a blood vessel.

Embolism
Interruption of blood flow in a blood vessel caused by obstruction by an *embolus*.

Embolus
A plug of material carried in the bloodstream (such as a *blood clot* or air bubble) that may obstruct a blood vessel.

Embryo
The developing, fertilized egg from shortly after *conception* until the end of the second month.

Emergency medical technician
A person who is trained in emergency care and is responsible for transporting and treating victims of *acute* injury or illness.

Emetic
A drug that induces vomiting.

Emphysema
A disease – almost always caused by cigarette smoking – in which the tiny air sacs in the lungs become damaged, causing shortness of breath and sometimes leading to *respiratory failure* and/or *heart failure*.

Enamel
The protective, bony, outer layer of a tooth.

Encephalitis
Inflammation of the brain, usually caused by infection with a *virus*.

Encephalomyelitis
Inflammation of the brain and *spinal cord* that can occur as a complication of some viral infections or after a *rabies* vaccination.

Encephalopathy
Any disorder of the brain that involves widespread destruction or degeneration of brain tissues.

Endarterectomy
The surgical removal of the thickened lining of a narrowed *artery* to restore normal blood flow.

Endemic
Describes a disease or disorder that is constantly present in a particular population or region.

Endocarditis
Inflammation of the lining of the heart wall or a *heart valve*, usually caused by a bacterial infection.

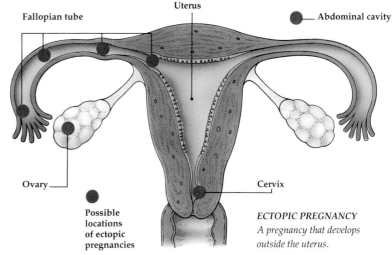

Fallopian tube · Uterus · Abdominal cavity

Ovary · Cervix

Possible locations of ectopic pregnancies

ECTOPIC PREGNANCY
A pregnancy that develops outside the uterus.

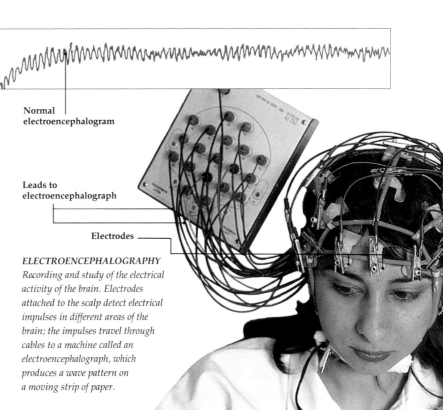

Normal electroencephalogram

Leads to electroencephalograph

Electrodes

ELECTROENCEPHALOGRAPHY
Recording and study of the electrical activity of the brain. Electrodes attached to the scalp detect electrical impulses in different areas of the brain; the impulses travel through cables to a machine called an electroencephalograph, which produces a wave pattern on a moving strip of paper.

Endocardium
The inner lining of the heart valves and the heart wall.

Endocrine gland
A gland that secretes *hormones* directly into the bloodstream.

Endocrine system
See illustration at right.

Endogenous
Developing or arising from inside the body.

Endometrial polyp
A growth arising from the lining of the *uterus;* it is usually noncancerous.

Endometriosis
A condition in which fragments of the lining of the *uterus* are found in other parts of the pelvic cavity; it sometimes causes *infertility*.

Endometritis
Inflammation of the lining of the *uterus*.

Endometrium
The membrane that lines the inside of the *uterus*; it increases in thickness during each *menstrual cycle* and is shed during *menstruation*.

Endophthalmitis
Severe inflammation of the inside of the eye, usually resulting from infection.

Endorphin
A substance produced naturally in the brain that can help control response to pain and stress and can improve mood.

Endoscope
A lighted viewing instrument used to look inside a body cavity or organ or to perform diagnostic or therapeutic procedures.

Endoscopic retrograde cholangiopancreatography
A method of producing X-ray images of the ducts that lead into the *duodenum* from the *liver, gallbladder,* and *pancreas,* after injecting a *contrast medium* into the ducts using an *endoscope*.

Endothelium
A single layer of flattened cells that lines the chambers of the heart, the blood vessels, and the vessels of the *lymphatic system*.

Endotoxin
A poison released by some *bacteria* after they die.

Endotracheal tube
A narrow, plastic tube that is threaded through the mouth or nose into the windpipe (*trachea*) in order to maintain breathing in an unconscious or anesthetized person.

Engagement
See illustrations below.

Enkephalin
A type of *endorphin*.

Enteric
Relating to the *small intestine*.

Enteric-coated tablet
An oral medication coated with a substance that prevents it from being released and absorbed until it reaches the *small intestine*.

Enteritis
Inflammation of the *small intestine*.

Enterobiasis
Infestation of the intestines by pinworms.

Enterostomy
The surgical formation of an opening in the wall of the abdomen to allow part of the *small intestine* to discharge feces into a bag attached to the skin.

Enterotoxin
A bacterial *toxin* that inflames the lining of the *intestine,* causing *diarrhea* and vomiting.

Entropion
A turning inward of the eyelid, so that the lashes rub against the eye.

Enucleation
The surgical removal of a complete eyeball, organ, or tumor from its enveloping capsule, sac, or covering.

Enuresis
The involuntary passage of urine, especially at night during sleep.

Enzyme
A *protein,* produced by living cells, that promotes or accelerates a particular chemical reaction.

Enzyme blocker
A drug that inhibits the action of an *enzyme*.

Enzyme-linked immunosorbent assay
A laboratory blood test to detect the presence of particular *antibodies* or *antigens* in the blood; the test is commonly used to diagnose *AIDS* infections.

Eosinophil
A type of *white blood cell* that is easily stained by a red dye called eosin; the number of these cells increases in *allergic reactions*.

Epicondylitis
Painful inflammation of one of the bony, prominent areas that lie on either side of the elbow, caused by overuse of the forearm muscles.

Epidemic
The sudden occurrence of a large number of cases of a disease in a particular community.

Epidermis
The thin, outermost layer of the skin.

Epididymis
A long, coiled tube at the back of each *testicle* in which *sperm* mature.

Epididymo-orchitis
Inflammation of the *epididymis* and the *testicle,* which can cause infertility.

ENDOCRINE SYSTEM
A group of ductless glands and tissues that secrete **hormones** *directly into the bloodstream to regulate the function of specific tissues or organs or of the entire body. The illustration shows the primary endocrine glands.*

Pituitary gland
Thyroid gland
Parathyroid glands
Adrenal glands
Pancreas
Ovaries (female)
Testicles (male)

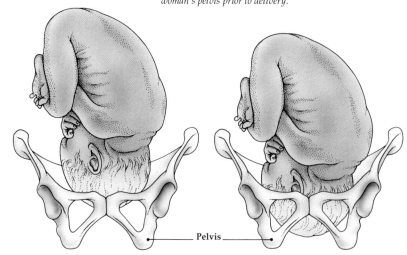

ENGAGEMENT
Entrance of the **fetus's** *head into the woman's pelvis prior to delivery.*

Pelvis

NOT ENGAGED

ENGAGED

Epidural
Outside the *dura mater*.

Epidural anesthesia
See illustrations below right.

Epidural hemorrhage
Bleeding between the *dura mater* and the inner surface of the skull.

Epigastric hernia
A protrusion through a weakness in the muscles of the central, upper part of the abdomen.

Epiglottis
A flap of *cartilage* behind the tongue that overhangs the entrance to the *larynx* and helps to prevent food or liquid from being inhaled.

Epiglottitis
Inflammation of the *epiglottis* as a result of infection.

Epilepsy
A tendency to recurrent *seizures* or temporary alteration in one or more brain functions, caused by abnormal electrical activity in the brain.

Epinephrine
A *hormone* produced by the *adrenal glands*, also called adrenaline; it increases heart rate and blood flow, improves breathing, and helps the body cope with the demands of exercise.

Epiphysis
Either of the two growing ends of one of the long bones of the arms or legs.

Episcleritis
Inflammation of the outer layers of the white of the eye and the overlying tissues.

Episiotomy
An incision made into the tissue between the vagina and the anus to facilitate childbirth.

Epispadias
A birth defect in which a boy's *urethra* opens on the upper surface of the penis rather than at its tip.

Epithelium
The coating of cells, occurring in one or more layers, that covers the entire body and lines many of the hollow structures, such as the respiratory tract.

Epstein-Barr virus
See illustration at right.

ERCP
Endoscopic retrograde cholangiopancreatography.

Erectile tissue
Spongy tissue that becomes stiff and raised when filled with blood in response to stimulation.

Ergot drug
Any of various drugs derived from ergot, a *fungus* that grows on rye and other grains; ergot drugs include a valuable treatment for *migraine* and a drug used to make the *uterus* contract after childbirth.

Erosive gastritis
An inflammatory condition characterized by multiple raw areas (that usually bleed) in the stomach lining.

Eruption
A breaking out, as in the emergence of a new tooth or the sudden appearance of a skin rash.

Erysipelas
A bacterial skin infection caused by *streptococci*, characterized by fever and inflammation of facial skin.

Erythema
Redness of the skin, which can have many causes.

Erythema multiforme
An inflammatory condition – associated with allergies, infections, and pregnancy – in which rashes of various sizes and shapes appear on the skin or *mucous membranes*.

Erythema nodosum
An inflammatory skin condition characterized by tender, red swellings under the skin, usually on the legs.

Erythrocyte
A *red blood cell*.

Erythrocyte sedimentation rate
The rate at which *red blood cells* collect at the bottom of a sample of unclotted blood; an elevated rate may be an indication of the presence of inflammation somewhere in the body but does not identify specific diseases.

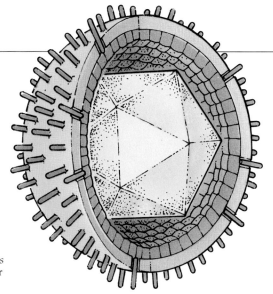

EPSTEIN-BARR VIRUS
*A **virus** that causes **mononucleosis** and is associated with **Burkitt's** lymphoma.*

Erythroplakia
Patches of red discoloration in the *mucous membranes* in the mouth, throat, or *larynx* that can develop into cancer; tobacco chewing and pipe smoking increase the risk.

Erythropoietin
A *hormone* that stimulates *red blood cell* production in the *bone marrow*.

Esophageal diverticulum
A pouch in the lining of the *esophagus* that protrudes from its outer wall.

Esophageal spasm
Uncoordinated contractions of the muscles of the *esophagus* that interfere with the effective propulsion of food into the stomach.

Esophageal stricture
Narrowing of the *esophagus*, which can sometimes cause difficulty swallowing.

Esophageal varices
Swollen veins in the lower *esophagus* and sometimes in the stomach that result from *portal hypertension*.

Esophagitis
Inflammation of the *esophagus*, caused by infection, irritation, or backflow of stomach acid.

Esophagogastro-duodenoscopy
Examination of the *esophagus*, stomach, and *duodenum* using an *endoscope*.

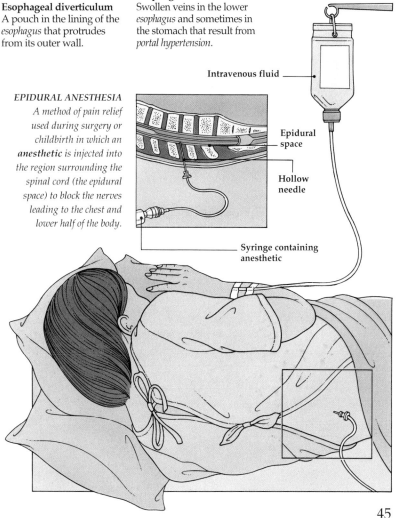

EPIDURAL ANESTHESIA
*A method of pain relief used during surgery or childbirth in which an **anesthetic** is injected into the region surrounding the spinal cord (the epidural space) to block the nerves leading to the chest and lower half of the body.*

Intravenous fluid

Epidural space

Hollow needle

Syringe containing anesthetic

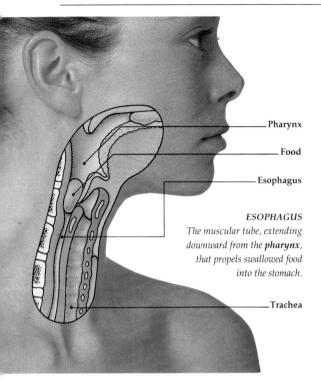

Pharynx

Food

Esophagus

ESOPHAGUS
The muscular tube, extending
*downward from the **pharynx**,*
that propels swallowed food
into the stomach.

Trachea

Esophagus
See illustration above.

Esotropia
A type of cross-eye in which
only one of the eyes is
directed inward.

Essential hypertension
Hypertension for which no
specific cause can be found.

Estradiol
The most powerful type of
naturally occurring *estrogen*.

Estrogen
Any of a group of *hormones*
secreted by the *ovaries* that
are essential for normal
female sexual development
and for the healthy
functioning of the female
reproductive system.

**Estrogen
replacement therapy**
Treatment with *estrogen* to
relieve symptoms accom-
panying *menopause*, such
as vaginal dryness, and to
protect against *osteoporosis*
and heart disease.

Eugenics
The study of ways to
improve the hereditary
characteristics of future
generations through
selective breeding.

Euphoria
A feeling or state of elation
that may be a normal
response to a situation, but
may also be drug-induced or
characteristic of some mental
disorders.

Eustachian tube
The tube that connects the
middle ear cavity to the back
of the nose; it acts as a
drainage passage and helps
maintain hearing.

Euthanasia
The deliberate act of causing
(either actively or passively)
the painless death of a
person who is suffering
from an incurable disease.

Eversion
A turning outward.

Evoked potential
A tracing of a brain wave or
nerve impulse produced in
evoked response studies.

Evoked response
A test in which the electrical
activity of the brain or *spinal
cord* in response to a specific
external stimulus is mea-
sured and recorded as a
tracing; the test is used to
diagnose some diseases and
to monitor brain activity in
patients during surgery.

Ewing's tumor
A cancerous bone tumor
affecting children.

Exanthema
Any disorder (including
many common childhood
infections such as *chickenpox*
and *measles*) that involves a
rash; it is also used as a term
for the rash itself.

Exchange transfusion
The infusion of donated
blood in exchange for most
of an infant's circulating
blood to improve its oxygen-
carrying capacity and
remove *bilirubin* in cases
of *Rh incompatibility*.

Excision
Surgically cutting off or
removing diseased tissue.

Excoriation
A tear or wound in a body
surface caused by deep
scratching.

Excretion
The discharge of waste
products from individual
cells, tissues, or organs.

Exercise stress test
See illustration at right.

Exercise thallium test
A type of imaging method
that assesses functioning of
the heart muscle during and
after an *exercise stress test*.

Exfoliation
Shedding of cells from a
surface, such as the skin.

Exfoliative dermatitis
Inflammation and excessive
shedding or peeling of the
skin, which can sometimes
be life-threatening.

Exocrine gland
A gland that secretes
substances through a duct.

Exogenous
Developing or arising
from outside the body.

Exostosis
A noncancerous growth
on the surface of a bone.

Exotoxin
A poison that is released
by some *bacteria*.

Exotropia
A type of cross-eye in which
one eye is directed outward
in relation to the other eye.

Expectorant
A medication that promotes
the coughing up of *mucus*
and other secretions.

Exstrophy
The turning inside out of an
organ, which occurs most
frequently as a birth defect
involving the *bladder*.

Extension
A joint movement in which
two adjoining bones are
straightened relative to each
other; the opposite move-
ment is flexion.

Extensor muscle
Any muscle that produces
extension of a joint when it
contracts.

External ligament
A strong, fibrous *ligament*,
connecting one bone to
another, that lies outside
the main structure of a joint.

External radiation
Radiation generated by
machines from outside the
body, used to treat cancer.

External version
A procedure in which a *fetus*
is turned inside the *uterus* to
the correct position for birth
by external manipulation
through the abdominal wall.

Extracellular
Outside a cell or cells.

**Extracorporeal shock
wave lithotripsy**
A technique in which
externally applied shock
waves are used to disintegrate *kidney stones*.

Extradural anesthesia
Loss of sensation in part
of the body achieved by the
injection of an *anesthetic* into
the space in the spinal canal
outside the *dura mater*.

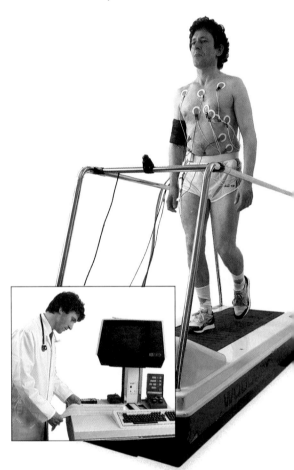

EXERCISE STRESS TEST
The use of equipment to monitor the heart during
vigorous exercise, usually while a person walks on
an exercise treadmill or rides an exercise bicycle.

Fabry's disease
A *genetic disorder* characterized by widespread damage to blood vessels.

Facial palsy
See illustration below right.

Factor VIII
A blood *protein* essential for normal blood clotting; it is deficient in the blood of people with *hemophilia*.

Failure to thrive
Lack of expected growth in an infant, which may indicate a serious disorder.

Fallopian tube
Either of a pair of funnel-shaped tubes, extending from the *uterus* to an *ovary*, through which eggs and sperm travel; the site of *fertilization*.

Familial
Occurring more often in a family than would be expected by chance; a familial disorder may be caused by *heredity* and/or environmental influences.

Familial hypercholesterolemia
A *genetic disorder* that prevents the body from adequately regulating the level of fats and *cholesterol* in the blood, leading to heart disease at an early age.

Familial polyposis
A *genetic disorder* causing multiple growths in the *colon*; affected people frequently develop colon cancer in their late 20s.

Fanconi's syndrome
A *genetic disorder* characterized by *aplastic anemia* and abnormalities of the skin, bones, and other tissues.

Farmers' lung
A type of *hypersensitivity pneumonitis* affecting farmers that results from exposure to some molds or *fungi* that grow on straw or hay.

Fasciitis
Inflammation of a layer of the sheets of *fibrous tissue* that enclose and connect the muscles, causing pain.

Fasciotomy
A surgical procedure to relieve pressure on muscles by making an incision into the band of *fibrous tissue* that surrounds them.

Fat necrosis
Death of fatty tissue in the body that results from injury or infection, leaving tough scar tissue.

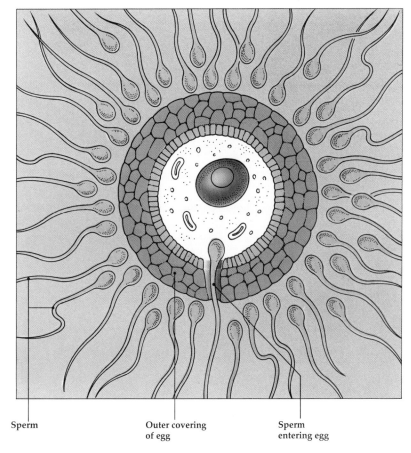

Fatty acid
One of many organic compounds that are constituents of fats; those not made in the body must be provided in the diet.

Fatty liver
An accumulation of fat inside *liver* cells, usually resulting from *hepatitis* caused by long-term high alcohol consumption.

Febrile
Feverish or related to fever.

Fecal impaction
An accumulation of hardened feces in the *rectum*.

Fecal incontinence
Inability to retain feces in the *rectum*, caused by failure of voluntary muscle control.

Fecal occult blood test
A screening test for possible signs of cancer of the *colon* or *rectum* using chemically sensitive paper to detect the presence of blood in a sample of feces.

FACIAL PALSY
*A **paralysis** of the facial muscles that is usually one-sided and temporary, caused by inflammation of a facial **nerve**.*

Fecal–oral
Describes the route of transmission of infectious organisms from feces to mouth, usually via the unwashed hands of an infected person.

Femoral artery
The main *artery* that carries blood into the leg; it extends from the groin to the knee.

Femoral hernia
Protrusion of a loop of *intestine* into the canal in the groin through which the main blood vessels to the leg pass.

Femur
A bone that extends from the *pelvis* to the knee; also called the thighbone.

Ferritin
A *protein* that plays a role in iron storage in the body.

Fertile period
The time in the *menstrual cycle* during which *fertilization* is possible; *ovulation* occurs during this time.

Fertility
The ability to reproduce.

Fertility drug
A hormonal or *hormone*-related drug used to treat male or female *infertility*.

Fertilization
See illustration below.

Fetal alcohol syndrome
A combination of seriously damaging effects on the *fetus* resulting from high alcohol consumption by the pregnant woman.

Fetal blood sampling
Testing of a *fetus's* blood to establish whether a blood transfusion is necessary in cases of *Rh incompatibility* or to determine if the fetus has a particular abnormality.

Fetal circulation
The route of blood circulation in the *fetus*, which bypasses the fetus's lungs.

Fetal distress
Physical stress experienced by a *fetus* from not receiving enough oxygen, characterized by an abnormal *heart rate* or rhythm and the passage of *meconium* from the fetus's bowels.

FERTILIZATION
The union of an egg and a sperm to produce the first cell of a new person (a fertilized egg).

Sperm   Outer covering of egg   Sperm entering egg

FIBROADENOMA

*A noncancerous tumor of glandular and **fibrous tissue**; the illustration shows a fibroadenoma in the breast.*

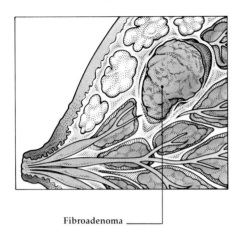

Fibroadenoma

Muscular tissue

Fibroids

Outer surface

Inner surface

Wall of uterus

Fibroid

Stalk

Fibroid

FIBROID

*A noncancerous tumor of muscular and **fibrous tissue** growing in the wall of the uterus. The illustration shows sites where fibroids can occur – under the inner or outer surfaces of the uterus, within its muscular tissue, or on a stalk.*

Cervix

Vagina

Fetal monitoring
Use of an instrument to record and/or listen to the *heart rate* of a *fetus* during pregnancy and *labor* in order to check for signs of *fetal distress*.

Fetal tissue transplant
An experimental treatment in which cells obtained from an aborted *fetus* are implanted into the brain of a person with a degenerative brain disorder such as *Parkinson's disease*.

Fetoscopy
A procedure for directly observing a *fetus* inside the uterus using a viewing instrument called a fetoscope.

Fetus
See illustration below.

Fiber
The components of plants that cannot be broken down by *enzymes* in the digestive tract; fiber helps maintain healthy bowel function.

Fiberoptics
Transmission of an image along thin, flexible fibers that convey light by internal reflection; often used to illuminate *endoscope*s.

Fibrillation
Recurrent, inefficient contraction of muscle, especially the heart muscle.

Fibrin
A stringy, insoluble *protein* that gives *blood clots* their semisolid form, enabling them to plug and seal damaged blood vessels.

Fibrinogen
A soluble *protein* that is converted into *fibrin* to form a *blood clot*; a high level in the blood is a risk factor for heart attacks.

Fibrinolytic
A drug that helps to dissolve *blood clots* by increasing the blood level of plasmin, a substance that dissolves the protein *fibrin*.

Fibroadenoma
See illustration above left.

Fibroblast
A flat, elongated cell that generates the structural protein *collagen*.

Fibrocartilage
A tough, shock-absorbing form of *cartilage*, composed of many thick bundles of *collagen* fibers, found in structures subject to stress.

Fibrocystic breast disease
The most common cause of *cysts* in the breast.

Fibroid
See illustration above.

Fibroma
A noncancerous tumor made of *connective tissue*.

Fibrosarcoma
A rare cancer containing *connective tissue*; it usually develops around a muscle or tendon, but can also affect bone.

Fibrosis
Overgrowth of *fibrous tissue*, such as scar formation after injury or as a characteristic of some disorders.

Fibrositis
Pain and stiffness in the back or in muscles around joints; it is thought to involve *fibrous tissue*.

Fibrous tissue
A form of *connective tissue* consisting of twisted, elastic fibers; it forms scar tissue and is a component of skin, *ligaments*, and *tendons*.

Fibula
The long, thin bone on the outer side of the lower leg.

Fifth disease
A childhood viral infection characterized by a widespread rash that often begins on the cheeks.

Filariasis
A group of tropical diseases transmitted by biting insects and characterized by infestation with various types of parasitic worms or their larvae.

Fissure
Any cleft or groove on a body surface.

Fistula
An abnormal channel between two internal organs or from one organ to the surface of the body.

Fitness
The state of having physical strength, flexibility, and endurance.

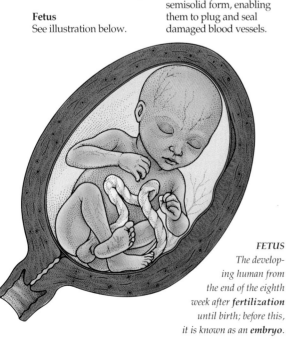

*FETUS
The developing human from the end of the eighth week after **fertilization** until birth; before this, it is known as an **embryo**.*

Fixed joint
A joint, such as those between the skull bones, that allows no movement.

Flagellum
A long, whiplike projection that extends from some single-celled *microorganisms* to help them move.

Flatulence
The presence of an excessive amount of gas or air in the intestines, and its expulsion through the *anus*.

Flexion
A movement, such as bending the knee, that decreases the angle between two adjoining bones. The opposite movement is *extension*.

Floaters
One or more spots that appear to drift in front of the eye, usually while a person is reading; they are caused by debris in the *vitreous humor* of the eye.

Floppy infant syndrome
A general term for a condition in which a baby's muscles lack normal tone.

Floppy valve syndrome
Mitral valve prolapse.

Flow cytometry
A test that reveals the arrangement and amount of *DNA* inside cells; it is used to diagnose *lymphomas* and other cancers.

Flu
Influenza.

Fluke
Any of various types of flattened worms that infest humans and animals.

Fluorescein angiography
A procedure used to highlight blood circulation in the eye by injecting a harmless dye (fluorescein) into a vein and photographing the *retina* while the dye is passing through the bloodstream.

Fluoride
A *mineral* that helps to prevent tooth decay; it has been added to the US water supply since the 1940s.

Fluoroscopy
A method for continuous viewing of internal body structures or organ function by passing X-rays through the body and onto an X-ray sensitive fluorescent screen.

Fluorosis
Poisoning with repeated large doses of *fluoride*, characterized by mottling and pitting of tooth enamel and, in extreme cases, degeneration of bones.

Folic acid
A *vitamin*, essential for cell growth and repair and for blood cell production; now considered an important nutrient during pregnancy to prevent *neural tube defects*.

Follicle
A small, pouchlike depression or cavity in a body structure.

Follicle-stimulating hormone
A *gonadotropic hormone*, secreted by the *pituitary gland*, that stimulates the maturation of eggs in the ovaries and the production of sperm in the testicles.

Folliculitis
A term that usually refers to inflammation of *hair follicles* resulting from infection with *streptococci* bacteria.

Fontanelles
Two membrane-covered gaps in a baby's skull, which close up by the age of 18 months.

Food poisoning
Any illness of sudden onset with stomach pain, diarrhea, and vomiting, caused by eating contaminated food.

Foramen
A natural opening or passage in a membranous structure or bone.

Forceps
Any of a wide variety of surgical instruments resembling a pair of tongs; they are used to grasp, secure, and manipulate.

Forceps delivery
The use of obstetric *forceps* to ease passage of a baby's head through the birth canal.

Forebrain
The term for the largest part of the brain, consisting of the *cerebrum*, the *thalamus*, and the *hypothalamus*.

Foreign body
Any object found in an organ or body cavity that should not be there.

Foreskin
A loose fold of skin that covers the head of the penis; it is removed in *circumcision*.

Fracture
See illustrations below left.

Fragile X syndrome
A *genetic disorder* caused by a defect in the *X chromosome*; the most common cause of mental retardation.

Fraternal twins
Twins that develop from two separately fertilized eggs and, therefore, are not identical; they may be of the same sex or opposite sexes.

Free radical
Oxygen free radical.

Friedreich's ataxia
A *genetic disorder* that causes loss of coordinated movement and balance; it first appears in childhood or adolescence.

Frontal bone
The bone at the front of the skull that forms the forehead and the roots of the eye sockets.

Frontal lobe
The largest part of the *cerebrum*; it influences personality and the higher mental activities such as thinking.

Frostbite
See illustration below right.

Frozen section method
A technique for preparing a *biopsy* specimen when it is necessary to establish quickly whether tissue is cancerous, such as during surgery for breast cancer when a doctor needs to know how much tissue to remove.

Fructose
A simple sugar found in honey, various fruits, sugar beet, and sugar cane.

Fulminant
Describes a severe illness that develops suddenly and progresses rapidly.

Functional disorder
A disorder in which performance is impaired, but for which there is no evidence of a physical cause.

Fungal infection
Infection in any part of the body caused by a *fungus*.

Fungicidal drugs
Drugs that are capable of killing *fungi*.

Fungus
Any of a group of organisms that are dependent on other life-forms for nourishment and that reproduce by simple division or spore formation.

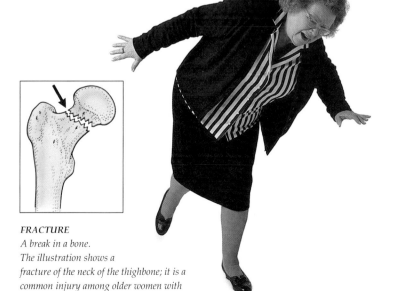

FRACTURE
A break in a bone.
The illustration shows a fracture of the neck of the thighbone; it is a common injury among older women with **osteoporosis***, usually as the result of a fall.*

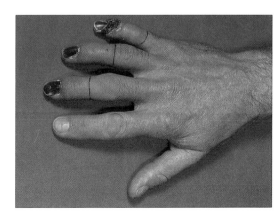

FROSTBITE
Damage caused by freezing of body tissues from exposure to extremely cold temperatures.

G6PD deficiency
Glucose-6-phosphate dehydrogenase deficiency.

Galactocele
A *cyst*like, milk-filled swelling in an obstructed milk duct in the breast.

Galactorrhea
Production of breast milk not associated with childbirth or nursing.

Galactose
A sugar derived from the milk sugar lactose.

Galactosemia
A *genetic disorder* caused by the lack of an *enzyme* in the liver that breaks down *galactose*; it can be treated with a milk-free diet.

Gallbladder
A small, pear-shaped sac under the liver that stores *bile* secreted by the liver.

Gallstone
See illustration at right.

Gallstone ileus
Blockage of the intestine caused by a *gallstone* that has passed through an abnormal channel leading from the *gallbladder*.

Gamete
A male or female reproductive cell (sperm or egg).

Gamete intrafallopian transfer
A procedure for treating *infertility* in which mature eggs are removed from a woman's *ovaries*, combined with sperm, and injected into one of the woman's *fallopian tubes*.

Gamma-aminobutyric acid
A *neurotransmitter* that controls the flow of nerve impulses in the brain by blocking the release of other neurotransmitters, such as *dopamine*.

Gamma globulin
A substance prepared from pooled blood that contains *antibodies* against many common infections; it is used mainly to immunize against *hepatitis A*.

Gamma-glutamyltransferase
An *enzyme* widely distributed in body tissues and released into the blood when tissue (especially liver tissue) is damaged.

Ganglion
A fluid-filled swelling associated with a tendon sheath or the outer lining of a joint, usually occurring on the wrist.

Gangrene
Death of tissue caused by loss of its blood supply.

Gas gangrene
Death of tissue caused by infection with a gas-forming bacterium (called *Clostridium*) found in soil.

Gastrectomy
Surgical removal of all or part of the stomach.

Gastric acid
The digestive acid secreted by glands in the stomach.

Gastric erosion
A break in the innermost layer of the membrane lining the stomach.

Gastric juice
A mixture of digestive secretions from the stomach lining that breaks down *protein* in food and destroys infectious *organisms*.

Gastric lavage
Washing out of the stomach (stomach pumping); it is used as a treatment for some types of poisoning.

Gastric ulcer
An *ulcer* located in the stomach; it may be benign or it may contain cancer cells.

Gastrin
A hormone that increases the muscular activity of the stomach and stimulates production of *gastric acid*.

Gastrinoma
A *gastrin*-secreting tumor, which is usually found in the *pancreas* and often associated with *peptic ulcers*; it causes excess acidity in the stomach and *duodenum*.

Gastritis
Inflammation of the *mucous membrane* that lines the stomach; its causes include viruses, bacteria or their *toxins*, alcohol, and nonsteroidal anti-inflammatory drugs such as aspirin.

Gastroenteritis
Inflammation of the stomach and intestines as a result of infection, causing fever, abdominal pain, diarrhea, and vomiting.

Gastroesophageal junction
The point at which the *esophagus* joins the stomach.

Gastrointestinal series
A series of *barium X-ray examinations* in which X-rays are taken at various intervals after a patient has swallowed a suspension of barium sulfate (which is visible on X-rays).

Gastrointestinal tract
The part of the digestive system consisting of the mouth, *esophagus*, stomach, and intestine.

Gastrojejunostomy
A surgically created connection between the stomach and the small intestine that bypasses the *duodenum* to prevent *gastric acid* from irritating a *duodenal ulcer*.

Gastroscopy
Examination of the lining of the *esophagus*, stomach, and *duodenum* using an *endoscope* inserted through the mouth.

Gastrostomy
A surgically created opening through the abdominal wall into the stomach to provide a permanent or temporary passage for a feeding tube or for drainage.

GALLSTONE
*A hardened mass of **cholesterol**, **bile** pigments, or calcium salts that can form in the **gallbladder** or in a **bile duct**.*

Gaucher's disease
A *genetic disorder* caused by an *enzyme* deficiency that leads to enlargement of the liver and *spleen*, bone damage, and *anemia*.

Gavage
Feeding of liquids through a tube threaded through the nose into the stomach.

Gay bowel syndrome
A group of disorders (such as diarrhea) affecting the *anus*, *rectum*, *colon*, and small intestine that occurs most frequently, but not exclusively, in male homosexuals.

Gene
The basic, functional unit of *heredity*; each gene contains the instructions to make a specific *protein*.

Generic drug
A drug marketed under its official, chemical name rather than under a patented brand name.

Gene therapy
An experimental technique to treat *genetic disorders* by identifying disease-causing *genes* and replacing them with healthy ones.

Gene tracking
The study of *DNA markers* to establish the transmission pattern of a specific disease-causing *gene* in a family.

Genetic analysis
Laboratory study of *DNA* to diagnose *genetic disorders*.

Genetic code
The set of instructions that directs the development and functioning of a person; the universal key by which genetic information is recorded and translated in all life-forms.

Genetic counseling
Providing information and advice to prospective parents about their risk of having a child with a *birth defect* or *genetic disorder*.

Genetic disorder
Any disorder resulting from a defect in a single *gene*, a *chromosome abnormality*, or a combination of environmental and genetic factors.

Genetic engineering
Manipulation of genes to make useful drugs (such as insulin) or *vaccines* that protect against some viruses (including hepatitis B).

Genetic fingerprint
DNA fingerprint.

Genetic mapping
A technique for locating the site of particular *genes* on *chromosomes*.

Genetic probes
Labeled fragments of *DNA* that can be used to detect the presence of matching fragments in a sample of a person's DNA; they are used to diagnose *genetic disorders*.

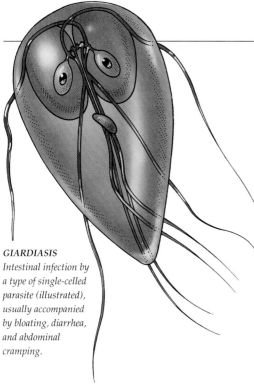

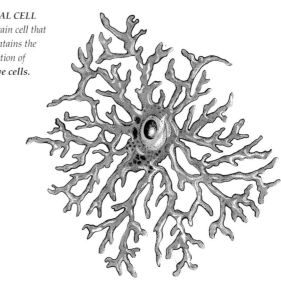

GIARDIASIS
Intestinal infection by a type of single-celled parasite (illustrated), usually accompanied by bloating, diarrhea, and abdominal cramping.

GLIAL CELL
*A brain cell that maintains the function of **nerve cells**.*

Genital herpes
An infection with the virus that causes *herpes simplex*, which is acquired through sexual contact; it is characterized by fluid-filled blisters on the *genitals*.

Genital tract
The group of organs that make up the male or female *reproductive system*.

Genital wart
A *wart* growing in or around the vagina and anus or on the penis, caused by a virus spread by sexual contact, a cause of cervical cancer.

Genitals
The male and female sex, or reproductive, organs, both internal and external.

Genitourinary
Referring to the *genitals* and the *urinary tract*.

Genome
The complete set of *genes* that makes up the master set of instructions for the growth, development, and functioning of an *organism*.

Genotype
The entire genetic makeup of a person.

Geographic tongue
A harmless disorder in which patches of the surface cells coating the tongue break down, producing a maplike pattern.

German measles
Rubella.

Germ cell
A sperm or egg cell or a cell that divides to form a sperm or egg.

Gestation
The period of time from *fertilization* to birth.

Giant cell tumor
A tumor arising in some bone cells that may be cancerous or benign.

Giardiasis
See illustration above left.

GIFT
Gamete intrafallopian transfer.

Gigantism
Excessive body growth caused by overproduction of *human growth hormone* in childhood or adolescence.

Gilbert's syndrome
A common inherited disorder that sometimes causes mild *jaundice*.

Gingivae
The gums.

Gingivectomy
An operation to remove a diseased or infected portion of the gums.

Gingivitis
Inflammation of the gums, usually caused by poor dental hygiene.

GI series
Gastrointestinal series.

Gland
An organ or a collection of cells that manufactures and releases chemical substances, such as *enzymes* and *hormones*, for use by the body; the two main types are the *endocrine glands* and the *exocrine glands*.

Glans penis
The conelike head of the penis.

Glaucoma
A condition in which the pressure of the fluid inside the eye becomes abnormally high, causing internal damage and affecting vision if untreated.

Glial cell
See illustration above right.

Gliding joint
See illustration below.

Metatarsal-
phalangeal joint

GLIDING JOINT
*A joint, such as the metatarsal-phalangeal joints in the foot, in which bone surfaces lie almost flat against each other, bound together by **ligaments** in a way that allows only a gliding motion.*

Glioblastoma multiforme
The most common, fastest-growing, and deadliest type of brain tumor.

Glioma
A tumor of the *glial cells* that can vary widely in its degree of malignancy and rate of growth.

Globulins
A group of *proteins* that play important roles in the formation of *antibodies*; they are involved in allergies, in fighting infections, and in *autoimmune diseases*.

Globus hystericus
The uncomfortable sensation of having a "lump in the throat" that cannot be swallowed; it often accompanies emotional conflict or acute anxiety.

Glomerulonephritis
Inflammation of the filtering units of the kidneys, which can seriously hamper kidney function.

Glomerulosclerosis
Scarring that develops as a result of damage to the filtering units of the kidneys, sometimes occurring with severe *glomerulonephritis*.

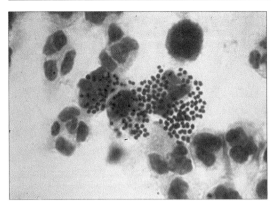

GONORRHEA
*A common **sexually transmitted disease**, caused by* Neisseria gonorrhoeae *bacteria (small red dots shown above).*

Glossectomy
Surgical removal of part or all of the tongue as a treatment for cancer of the tongue.

Glucagon
A hormone secreted by the *pancreas* that stimulates the release of *glucose* into the bloodstream; its action opposes that of *insulin*.

Glucocorticoids
A group of hormones, produced by the *adrenal glands*, that suppress inflammation and raise the level of *glucose* in the blood.

Glucose
A simple sugar found in honey, fruit, and the healthy blood of animals; it is the chief source of energy for living organisms.

Glucose-6-phosphate dehydrogenase deficiency
A *genetic disorder* in which lack of a particular *enzyme* affects the chemistry of *red blood cells*, making them prone to damage during infectious illness or after a person ingests certain foods or drugs.

Glucose tolerance test
A test of the body's response to a dose of *glucose* after a period of fasting, used to diagnose *diabetes mellitus*.

Glutamate
A *neurotransmitter* in the brain, thought to play a part in memory.

Gluten
A *protein* found in wheat and other grains.

Gluteus maximus muscle
The large, powerful muscle in each of the buttocks that gives them their rounded shape and moves the thigh sideways and backward.

Glycerol
A constituent of many fats; it is released from food during digestion and absorbed on its own or in combination with *fatty acids*.

Glycogen
A complex sugar formed from *glucose*; it is the main *carbohydrate* stored in the body, primarily in the liver and in muscle cells.

Glycosuria
The abnormal presence of *glucose* in the urine, which usually results from *diabetes mellitus*.

Goiter
Enlargement of the *thyroid gland* from any cause, visible as a swelling on the neck.

Gonad
An organ – such as the *testicle* and the *ovary* – that produces sperm or eggs.

Gonadotropic hormones
A group of hormones that stimulate cell activity in the *ovaries* and *testicles* and are essential for both male and female fertility.

Gonadotropin-releasing hormones
Hormones that stimulate the release of *gonadotropic hormones*.

Gonorrhea
See illustration above left.

Gout
See upper illustration below.

Graft
Healthy tissue taken from one part of the body, or from a donor, and surgically implanted in another part of the body to repair or replace damaged tissue.

Graft-versus-host disease
A complication of a *bone marrow transplant* that results when *antibodies* formed in the donor's transplanted marrow attack the recipient's own cells.

Gram negative
Describes specific types of bacteria – as identified by the *Gram's stain* – that cause infections in the *genitourinary* and *gastrointestinal tracts*.

Gram positive
Describes specific types of bacteria – as identified by the *Gram's stain* – that cause infections on the skin and in the respiratory tract .

Gram's stain
See lower illustration below.

Grand mal
A type of *seizure* characterized by loss of consciousness (lasting up to 15 minutes) and involuntary movement.

Granulation tissue
A mass of tissue that develops in a wound during the healing process.

Granuloma
A mass of *granulation tissue* associated with inflammation, injury, or infection.

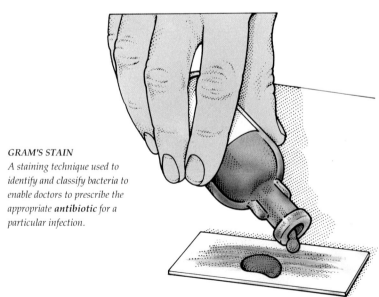

GOUT
*A disorder of **metabolism** characterized by high levels of **uric acid** in the blood, which can cause attacks of **arthritis** (joint pain and inflammation), usually in a single joint.*

Graves' disease
An *autoimmune disease* characterized by an overactive and enlarged *thyroid gland*, excessive production of thyroid hormones, weight loss, and bulging eyes.

Gray matter
The gray portion of the brain and *spinal cord* that is composed of the bodies of nerve cells.

Greenstick fracture
An incomplete fracture in which a bone is bent but splintered only on the upper curve of the bend.

Group therapy
A form of therapy in which people meet to discuss common emotional or psychological problems under the guidance of a trained counselor.

Growing pains
Vague aches and pains of unknown cause that affect the muscles and joints of children or adolescents.

Guillain-Barré syndrome
An abnormal condition in which nerves in the *peripheral nervous system* become inflamed, impairing movement and sensation.

Guthrie test
A blood test performed on all newborns to detect *phenylketonuria*.

GRAM'S STAIN
*A staining technique used to identify and classify bacteria to enable doctors to prescribe the appropriate **antibiotic** for a particular infection.*

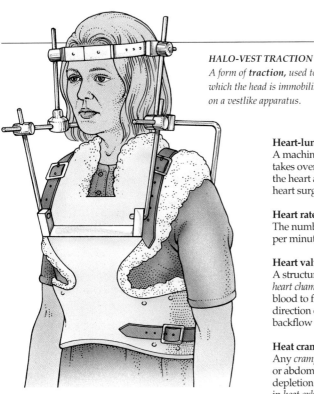

HALO-VEST TRACTION
*A form of **traction**, used to treat fractures of the neck, in which the head is immobilized by a halo of metal mounted on a vestlike apparatus.*

h

Hair follicle
A tiny pit in the skin from which a hair grows.

Halitosis
Bad breath.

Hallucination
A sensory perception that occurs without an external stimulus; it may involve any of the senses.

Halo-vest traction
See illustration above.

Hammer toe
A deformity in which the toe (usually the second toe) is permanently flexed.

Hamstring muscle
Any of three muscles, extending down the back of the thigh, that bend the knee.

Hand-foot-and-mouth disease
A viral infection of preschoolers that is characterized by blistering of the palms of the hands, the soles of the feet, and the inside of the mouth.

Hardening of the arteries
Arteriosclerosis.

Hashimoto's disease
An *autoimmune disease* in which the body's immune system develops *antibodies* that attack the *thyroid gland*, preventing it from producing its hormones.

Hay fever
Allergic rhinitis.

HDL
High-density lipoprotein.

Heart attack
Myocardial infarction.

Heart block
An interruption in the passage of electric impulses through the heart's conduction system that regulates the heartbeat.

Heartburn
A painful, burning sensation in the chest, just below the breastbone, usually occurring after overeating, eating spicy food, or drinking alcohol.

Heart chamber
Any of the four contracting regions inside the heart that regulate blood flow.

Heart failure
The inability of the heart to maintain its work load of pumping blood to the lungs and the rest of the body.

Heart-lung machine
A machine that temporarily takes over the functioning of the heart and lungs during heart surgery.

Heart rate
The number of heartbeats per minute.

Heart valve
A structure at the exit of a *heart chamber* that allows blood to flow in one direction only, preventing backflow of blood.

Heat cramp
Any *cramp* in the arm, leg, or abdomen caused by depletion of water and salt in *heat exhaustion.*

Heat exhaustion
A condition characterized by dizziness, nausea, exhaustion, and *dehydration* from overexposure to heat; untreated, it can develop into *heat stroke.*

Heat stroke
A condition in which body temperature reaches a dangerously high level; it results from overexposure to extreme heat that disrupts the body's heat-regulating mechanisms.

Heel spur
An abnormal, often painful, bony outgrowth on the back surface of the heel bone.

Heimlich maneuver
See illustration at right.

Helper T cells
White blood cells (also called CD4 cells) that regulate other cells of the *immune system*; they are the main cells attacked by the *AIDS* virus.

Hemangioblastoma
A rare, slow-growing, noncancerous brain tumor made up of blood vessel cells.

Hemangioma
A red-purple *birthmark* caused by an abnormal distribution of blood vessels in the skin; it can be either flat or raised.

Hemarthrosis
Bleeding into a joint, usually resulting from injury, that causes the joint to swell.

Hematemesis
Vomiting blood.

Hematocrit
The percentage of the total blood volume that *red blood cells* occupy, determined by laboratory testing; an abnormally high or low volume may be a sign of disease or injury.

Hematoma
A collection of blood inside the body, caused by bleeding from an injured blood vessel.

Hematuria
The presence of *red blood cells* in the urine, which can result from an infection or from cysts, tumors, or stones that develop in the *urinary tract.*

Hemiballismus
Irregular and uncontrollable flinging movements of the arm and leg on one side of the body, caused by disease in part of the brain.

Hemicolectomy
Surgical removal of a part of the *colon*, usually to treat cancer of the colon, *ulcerative colitis, diverticulitis,* or an obstructed blood vessel.

Hemiparesis
Partial *paralysis* affecting one side of the body.

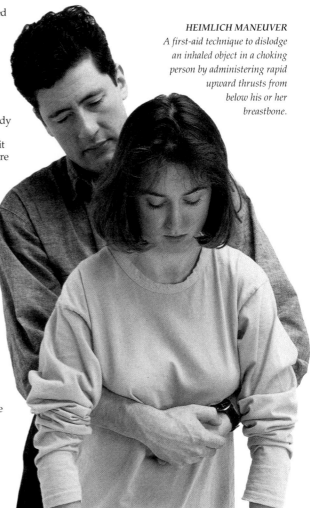

HEIMLICH MANEUVER
A first-aid technique to dislodge an inhaled object in a choking person by administering rapid upward thrusts from below his or her breastbone.

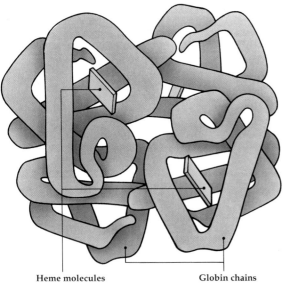

Heme molecules   Globin chains

HEMOGLOBIN

*The pigment in **red blood cells** that carries **oxygen**. Hemoglobin consists of four chains of globin (linked **protein** molecules), each surrounding a molecule of heme (a chemical structure with an atom of iron at its center).*

HEMOPHILIA

*A **genetic disorder** characterized by deficiency of a **protein (factor VIII)** necessary for blood clotting, leading to abnormal bleeding; it almost always affects males. The swelling in the right knee of a person with hemophilia in the photograph below is caused by bleeding into the joint.*

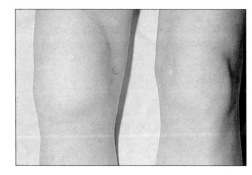

Hemolytic anemia
A form of *anemia* in which the rate of *red blood cell* production is normal or high, but the cells are destroyed abnormally fast.

Hemolytic disease of the newborn
Excessive *red blood cell* destruction in a *fetus* or newborn infant, resulting from *Rh incompatibility* between mother and child.

Hemophilia
See illustration at left.

Hemorrhage
Bleeding.

Hemorrhoidectomy
Surgical removal of a *hemorrhoid*.

Hemorrhoid
See illustration below left.

Hemosiderosis
A general increase in the body's supply of iron, usually as a result of multiple blood transfusions.

Hemospermia
The presence of a small amount of blood in *semen*.

Hemostasis
The stoppage of bleeding after injury, either surgically or by the body's own blood-clotting process.

Hemostatic drugs
Drugs that stop bleeding; they are used to treat bleeding disorders such as *hemophilia*.

Hemothorax
A collection of blood in the space between the chest wall and the lung, which is usually caused by injury.

Hepatectomy
Surgical removal of the liver, which is performed as part of a liver transplant.

Hepatic
Relating to the liver.

Hepatic artery
The artery that carries blood from the heart to the liver.

Hepatitis
Inflammation of the liver, which may be caused by a viral infection, by some drugs (including alcohol), or by poisons.

Hemiplegia
Complete *paralysis* affecting one side of the body.

Hemochromatosis
A *genetic disorder* resulting in an accumulation of iron in the liver and other organs that, if untreated, can lead to *cirrhosis of the liver*.

Hemodialysis
A form of *dialysis*, used to treat kidney failure, in which blood is passed through a machine and purified before being returned to the body.

Hemoglobin
See illustration above left.

Hemoglobinopathy
A term for a variety of inherited blood disorders – including *sickle cell anemia* and the *thalassemias* – characterized by errors in *hemoglobin* production.

Hemoglobinuria
The abnormal presence of *hemoglobin* in the urine.

Hemolysis
The breakdown of *red blood cells*; it occurs as a normal process at the end of their life span, but occasionally occurs prematurely, leading to *anemia* and *jaundice*.

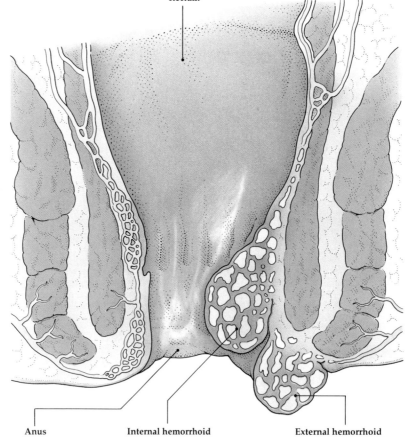

Rectum

Anus   Internal hemorrhoid   External hemorrhoid

HEMORRHOID

A bulging vein in the lining of the anus (external hemorrhoid) or lower part of the rectum (internal hemorrhoid) caused by increased pressure, such as that from straining to defecate or from pregnancy.

Hepatitis A
Hepatitis caused by the hepatitis A virus, which is spread directly from an infected person's feces or indirectly from contaminated food or water.

Hepatitis B
See illustration at right.

Hepatitis C
A type of *hepatitis* caused by the hepatitis C virus; it is transmitted sexually, by needle-sharing among drug abusers, and by other types of blood-to-blood contact.

Hepatitis D
A type of *hepatitis* that causes symptoms only if a person already has *hepatitis B*.

Hepatocyte
The most common type of liver cell.

Hepatoma
The most common type of cancerous tumor of the liver, usually occurring in people who have *hepatitis* or *cirrhosis of the liver*.

Hepatomegaly
Enlargement of the liver.

Hereditary spherocytosis
A *genetic disorder* in which *red blood cells* are fragile and spherical rather than doughnut-shaped; it causes periodic episodes of *hemolytic anemia*.

Heredity
The transmission of *traits* and disorders from parents to children through *genes*.

Heritability
A measure of the degree to which a *trait* or disorder is determined by *genes*.

Hermaphroditism
A condition present at birth in which a person has both *testicles* and *ovaries* and the external *genitals* are not clearly male or female.

Hernia
Protrusion of a portion of an organ or tissue through a weak area in the muscle wall that normally contains it.

Herniated disc
A *disc prolapse*.

Herniorrhaphy
Surgical repair of a *hernia*.

Herpes encephalitis
Inflammation of the brain caused by the spread of a *herpes simplex* infection; it is potentially life-threatening.

Herpes genitalis
Genital herpes.

Herpes simplex
Infection with the herpes simplex virus, which causes blisterlike sores on the face, lips, mouth, or genitals, and occasionally affects the eyes, fingers, or brain.

Herpes zoster
Shingles.

Herpesviruses
A group of viruses that includes the *herpes simplex* virus, *varicella-zoster virus*, *Epstein-Barr virus*, and *cytomegalovirus*.

Herpetic whitlow
See illustration below right.

Heterosexuality
Sexual attraction to members of the opposite sex.

Heterozygous
Possessing two different forms of a *gene* that controls a specific inherited *trait*, in contrast to being *homozygous*.

Hiatal hernia
A condition in which part of the stomach protrudes upward into the chest through an opening in the *diaphragm*.

Hiccup
A sudden, involuntary contraction of the *diaphragm* followed by rapid closure of the vocal cords, producing a characteristic sound.

High-density lipoprotein
A type of *protein* molecule carried in the blood that removes *cholesterol* from tissues and appears to protect against *coronary heart disease;* popularly referred to as the "good" cholesterol.

Hinge joint
A joint, such as the knee or elbow, in which the two bone surfaces fit tightly, allowing backward and forward movement only.

Hippocampus
A structure in the brain that is thought to be involved in memory.

Hirschsprung's disease
A disorder present at birth in which the nerve cells that control rhythmic contractions fail to develop in a part of the intestine; the segment becomes narrowed, blocking the movement of feces.

Hirsutism
Excessive body hair, especially in women.

Histamine
A chemical present in some body cells that is released during an *allergic reaction* and produces the symptoms of inflammation.

H₁ (histamine) blocker
An *antihistamine* that is widely used in the treatment of *allergic reactions*.

H₂ (histamine) blocker
An *antihistamine* that prevents *histamine* from triggering *gastric acid* production; the drug is used to treat *peptic ulcers*.

Histocompatibility antigens
A group of genetically determined *proteins* on many cells that are the major compatibility problem in unsuccessful organ transplants; they also play a role in susceptibility to *autoimmune diseases*.

Histoplasmosis
An infection acquired by inhaling the spores of a *fungus* found in areas contaminated with bird or bat droppings.

HIV
Human immunodeficiency virus.

Hives
An itchy, raised rash of white lumps on the skin, surrounded by areas of inflammation, that results from an *allergic reaction*.

HLA
Human leukocyte antigen.

Hodgkin's disease
A cancer of *lymphoid tissue*, causing enlarged *lymph nodes*, weight loss, and *anemia*.

HEPATITIS B
A type of hepatitis caused by the hepatitis B virus (illustrated below); it is transmitted sexually, or by needle-sharing among drug abusers or other types of blood-to-blood contact.

HERPETIC WHITLOW
Blistering of the skin on the fingers caused by infection with the herpes simplex virus.

Holter monitor
A portable device that makes a continuous recording of heart activity; it is often used to detect an irregular heartbeat.

Homeostasis
The constant internal environment, necessary for health, that is maintained by active processes in the body despite external changes.

Homocystinuria
A *genetic disorder* that leads to the abnormal presence of a substance called homocystine in the blood and urine; it usually causes skeletal deformities.

Homosexuality
Sexual attraction to members of the same sex.

Homozygous
Possessing two identical forms of a *gene* that controls a specific inherited *trait*, in contrast to being *heterozygous*.

Hookworm
A blood-sucking worm with hooklike teeth that infests the intestines, causing *anemia* in severe cases.

Hormonal implant
An *implant* placed under the skin that slowly releases a dose of a synthetic *hormone*.

Hormone
A chemical, such as *insulin*, that is produced by the body and released directly into the bloodstream to perform a specific range of functions.

Hormone antagonist
A drug that blocks the action of a particular *hormone*.

Hormone replacement therapy
The use of manufactured or natural hormones to treat diseases or disorders.

Hospice
A hospital or part of a hospital devoted to caring for people who are dying.

Hot flash
Reddening of the face, neck, and upper trunk, accompanied by a sensation of heat and often followed by sweating; it is usually associated with decreased *estrogen* production after *menopause*.

HTLV
Human T-cell lymphotrophic virus.

Human chorionic gonadotropin
A hormone that is produced by the *placenta* in early pregnancy; its measurement is the basis of most pregnancy tests.

Human growth hormone
A chemical produced by the *pituitary gland* that stimulates normal body growth and development.

Human immunodeficiency virus
See illustration below right.

Human leukocyte antigens
One of the main types of *histocompatibility antigens* that are studied to determine tissue compatibility between donors and recipients for transplants; many are associated with specific diseases or conditions.

Human T-cell lymphotrophic virus
A virus closely resembling the *human immunodeficiency virus* and one that infects the same immune cells (*T lymphocytes*); it is associated with adult *T-cell leukemia* and T-cell *lymphomas*.

Humerus
The bone of the upper part of the arm.

Hunter's syndrome
A *genetic disorder* that causes dwarfism and mental retardation.

Huntington's chorea
A fatal *genetic disorder* that causes degeneration of nerve cells in the brain, resulting in involuntary jerking movements (*chorea*) and *dementia*; the symptoms of the disease usually do not appear until the person is 30 or older.

Hurler's syndrome
A *genetic disorder* that causes severe mental retardation.

Hyaline cartilage
Smooth, semi-transparent *cartilage* that is the most common type in the body.

Hydatid disease
An infestation caused by the larva stage of a *tapeworm*, usually found in dogs; in people, the larvae form *cysts* in the lungs, liver, brain, and other organs.

Hydatidiform mole
A rare, usually noncancerous tumor, resembling a bunch of grapes, that develops early in pregnancy from tissue of the *placenta* in which an *embryo* has failed to develop.

Hydramnios
Excess *amniotic fluid* in the uterus during pregnancy.

Hydrocele
See illustration at right.

Hydrocephalus
Excessive accumulation of *cerebrospinal fluid* inside the skull of an infant, usually causing increased pressure and abnormal enlargement of the head; it can result from a birth defect, infection, injury, or a brain tumor.

Hydrochloric acid
A strong acid that is a major component of *gastric juice*.

Hydrocortisone
A *corticosteroid* that is used to treat inflammatory and allergic disorders.

Hydrophobia
A rarely used term for *rabies*, meaning "fear of water," that refers to the drinking difficulty that is one of the symptoms of rabies.

Hydrotherapy
The use of water (in exercise pools, whirlpool baths, and showers) to treat muscle and joint problems.

Hygiene
The science and practice of promoting and preserving health; the term is often equated with cleanliness.

Hymen
A thin, membranous ring surrounding the opening to the vagina; it is usually torn by tampon use or during first sexual intercourse.

Hyperacidity
Excessive production of *gastric acid* by the stomach; it occurs with *duodenal ulcers* and sometimes with *gastric ulcers* and indigestion.

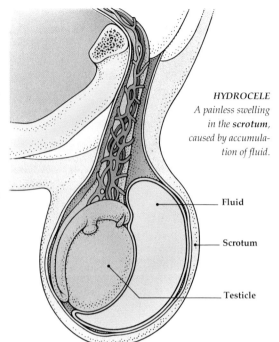

HYDROCELE
A painless swelling in the scrotum, caused by accumulation of fluid.

Fluid

Scrotum

Testicle

Hyperactivity
A high level of restlessness and low level of concentration; in children it is a characteristic of *attention-deficit disorder*.

Hyperalimentation
Providing nutrients in excess of the amount required by the body to people who are unable to take food by mouth or who are undernourished because of illness.

Hyperbaric oxygen treatment
Increasing the oxygen supply in the tissues by exposing a person to oxygen at a higher-than-normal atmospheric pressure.

Hyperbilirubinemia
An excessive concentration of *bilirubin* in the blood, which may lead to *jaundice*.

Hypercalcemia
An abnormally high level of calcium in the blood which, untreated, can be fatal; it is caused by disorders such as bone cancer, *hyperparathyroidism*, and *osteoporosis*.

Hypercholesterolemia
Abnormally high levels of *cholesterol* in the blood that may result from eating a high-fat diet or from an inherited disorder such as *familial hypercholesterolemia*.

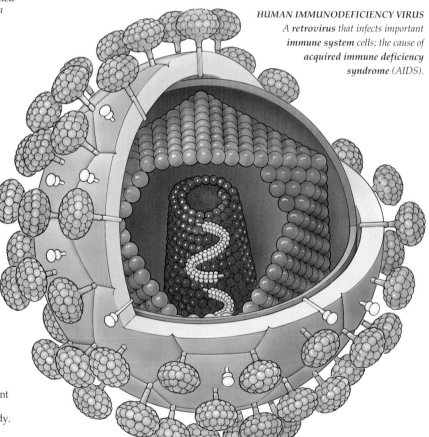

HUMAN IMMUNODEFICIENCY VIRUS
A retrovirus that infects important immune system cells; the cause of acquired immune deficiency syndrome (AIDS).

ICHTHYOSIS
A condition, which may be inherited, that is characterized by thick, dry, scaly skin.

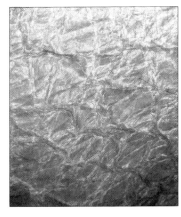

Hyperextension injury
An injury caused by the straightening of a joint beyond its normal limits.

Hyperglycemia
An abnormally high level of the sugar *glucose* in the blood; it is a feature of untreated or inadequately controlled *diabetes mellitus*.

Hyperlipidemia
A term for abnormally high levels of *lipids*, including *cholesterol*, in the blood.

Hyperparathyroidism
Overactivity of the *parathyroid glands*, usually caused by a noncancerous tumor of one or more of the glands, resulting in increased calcium in the blood and a decrease of calcium in bones; it can lead to *osteoporosis* and *kidney stones*.

Hyperplasia
An abnormal increase in the size of an organ caused by an increase in the number of its constituent cells.

Hypersensitivity
An overreaction of the *immune system* to a *protein* it recognizes as foreign.

Hypersensitivity pneumonitis
Inflammation of the lungs caused by an *allergic reaction* from inhaling dust containing various animal or plant materials.

Hypertension
A condition characterized by persistently raised blood pressure, even when a person is resting.

Hyperthermia
Extremely high body temperature.

Hyperthyroidism
Overactivity of the *thyroid gland*, leading to overproduction of *thyroid hormones*, which speeds up body processes and causes a variety of symptoms including nervousness, weight loss, fatigue, and diarrhea.

Hypertrophic cardiomyopathy
A *genetic disorder* that causes overgrowth of muscle fibers in the heart; it often causes sudden death.

Hypertrophy
An increase in the size of an organ that is caused by an increase in the size of its constituent cells rather than in their number.

Hyperuricemia
An abnormally high level of *uric acid* in the blood, which can lead to *gout*, arthritis, or *kidney stones*.

Hyperventilation
Abnormally deep, rapid, or prolonged breathing.

Hypnosis
A trancelike state of altered consciousness in which a person becomes extremely responsive to suggestion.

Hypnotic
A drug that induces sleep.

Hypochondriasis
A person's persistent and irrational fear that he or she is ill, despite medical reassurance to the contrary.

Hypodermic needle
A hollow needle attached to a syringe that is used to inject medication under the skin, into a muscle, or directly into blood vessels.

Hypoglycemia
An abnormally low level of *glucose* in the blood that usually results when a person with *diabetes mellitus* takes too much *insulin*, but also, rarely, when a pancreatic tumor secretes too much insulin or a person drinks large amounts of alcohol.

Hypoglycemic drugs
Drugs that lower *glucose* levels in the blood; they are used to treat *non-insulin-dependent diabetes* that cannot be controlled by diet.

Hypogonadism
Underactivity of the *gonads*, resulting in low production of *sex hormones*, or in a failure to produce sperm or eggs.

Hypoparathyroidism
Insufficient production of *parathyroid hormone*, resulting in abnormally low levels of calcium in the body.

Hypophysectomy
Surgical removal of the *pituitary gland* to eradicate a tumor or to slow the growth of some breast, ovary, or prostate cancers.

Hypoplasia
Failure of an organ or tissue to develop fully or to reach its normal adult size.

Hypospadias
A birth defect in which the *urethra* opens on the underside of the penis rather than at the tip.

Hypotension
Abnormally low blood pressure that reduces blood flow to the brain, causing dizziness and fainting.

Hypothalamus
See illustration below.

Hypothermia
A dangerous drop in body temperature to below the normal level (98.6°F), which causes drowsiness and reduced breathing and heart rates and may lead to unconsciousness and death.

Hypothyroidism
Underactivity of the *thyroid gland*, and consequent underproduction of *thyroid hormones*, usually caused by an *autoimmune disease*.

Hypoventilation
A reduced breathing rate.

Hypoxemia
Lack of a sufficient supply of oxygen in the blood.

Hypoxia
An inadequate level of oxygen in a tissue.

Hysterectomy
Surgical removal of the uterus.

Hysteria
A term that is applied to a wide range of physical or mental symptoms that are attributed to mental stress in someone who does not have a *psychosis*.

Hysterosalpingography
An X-ray examination of the uterus and *fallopian tubes*, used to investigate *infertility*.

Hysteroscopy
Examination of the *cervix* and the interior of the uterus using a viewing instrument called a hysteroscope.

Iatrogenic
A term applied to any disease or disorder that has resulted from medical treatment, such as an infection acquired in a hospital; it literally means "physician-produced."

Ichthyosis
See illustration above left.

Idiopathic
Of unknown cause.

Ileostomy
An operation in which the *ileum* is brought through an incision in the abdominal wall and formed into an artificial outlet to allow discharge of feces into a bag attached to the skin.

Ileum
The final, longest, and narrowest part of the *small intestine*.

Iliac artery
Either of two large arteries into which the *aorta* divides in the lower part of the abdomen; the iliac arteries supply blood to the pelvic region and the legs.

Ilium
One of the two bones on either side of the body that form the hips.

Imaging
The use of magnetic fields, sound waves, or radiation, often combined with computers, to produce images of structures inside the body.

Immune deficiency
Reduced effectiveness of the *immune system*, which most frequently occurs in people who are malnourished, infected with the *AIDS* virus, or undergoing *chemotherapy* for the treatment of cancer.

HYPOTHALAMUS
A small structure at the base of the brain that activates and controls the **autonomic nervous system**, *the hormonal system, and many body functions including water and food intake, body temperature, and sleep.*

Hypothalamus ———

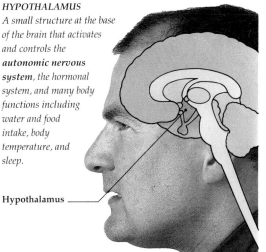

Immune system
A collection of body structures, cells, and substances that works to protect the body from harmful disease-causing *organisms* and from the development of cancer.

Immunity
A state of resistance to a disease through the defensive activities of the *immune system*.

Immunity, active
Resistance to infection acquired as the result of previous infection with a disease-causing *organism* or after a vaccination.

Immunity, passive
The injection of *antibodies* into a person to provide temporary protection against a disease-causing *organism*.

Immunization
See illustration above right.

Immunoassay
A group of laboratory techniques used to detect *antibodies*, *antigens*, or other substances in a person's blood or tissue to diagnose infectious diseases.

Immunodeficiency disorder
Any disorder in which the *immune system* fails to fight infection or the development of tumors.

Immunoglobulin
Any of five different *antibodies* found in *serum* and tissue fluids.

Immunology
The study of the functioning of the *immune system*.

Immunostimulant
A drug that is used to increase the efficiency of the *immune system*.

Immunosuppressant
A drug that reduces the activity of the *immune system*.

Immunotherapy
Preventive therapy to build up a person's *immunity* to something to which he or she is allergic (such as bee venom); it is also used as a form of cancer treatment.

Impacted fracture
A break in a bone in which the fragmented ends of the bone have been forced into one another; this type of fracture is difficult to set.

Impacted tooth
A tooth that has failed to emerge fully or at all from the gum, usually caused by overcrowding of teeth.

Impedance audiometry
A test for determining if hearing loss is caused by damage to the *middle ear*.

Imperforate anus
A disorder, present at birth, in which the opening at the *anus* is malformed; the defect must be corrected surgically.

Impetigo
A highly contagious skin infection, most common in children, that is caused by bacteria; it usually occurs around the nose and mouth.

Implant
Any object or material (either natural or artificial) that is inserted into the body surgically.

Impotence
Inability to achieve or maintain an erection.

Inborn error of metabolism
A *genetic disorder* in which a deficiency of or a defect in a specific *enzyme* blocks a particular chemical process in the body, causing illness.

Incest
Sexual intercourse between close relatives.

Incisor tooth
One of the eight teeth at the front of the mouth that are used for cutting through (incising) food.

Incompetent cervix
See illustration at left.

Incomplete miscarriage
A *miscarriage* in which not all of the fetal and placental tissue has been expelled from the uterus.

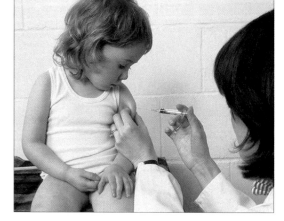

IMMUNIZATION
*The process of inducing **immunity** as a preventive measure against specific infectious diseases; it is performed by injecting **antibodies** into the body or priming the **immune system** to make its own antibodies.*

Incontinence
Inability to control the passing of urine or feces.

Incubation period
The time during which an infectious disease develops, from the point when the disease-causing *organism* enters the body until the appearance of symptoms.

Incubator
A transparent plastic container in which oxygen, temperature, and humidity levels are controlled to provide premature or sick infants with ideal conditions for survival.

Indigestion
A term describing a variety of symptoms (such as burning discomfort in the upper part of the abdomen) brought on by eating.

Induction of labor
The use of artificial means (such as drugs) to initiate the process of childbirth.

Infarction
Death of tissue caused by a deficient blood supply.

Infection
The invasion of the body by disease organisms that reproduce and multiply, causing illness by entering and destroying cells or secreting a *toxin*; these activities produce an *immune response* in the body.

Infective arthritis
Disease in joints resulting from the invasion of bacteria, including those that cause *gonorrhea*, *typhoid*, and *salmonella* infections.

Inferior
Located below a point of reference; for example, the legs are inferior to the trunk.

Infertility
The inability of a couple of reproductive age to produce offspring, despite having regular unprotected sexual intercourse; the success of treatment for infertility varies with its cause.

Infestation
The presence of animal parasites, such as lice or mites on the skin or hair, or worms inside the body.

Inflammation
Redness, swelling, heat, and pain in a tissue that results from the body's protective response to injury or infection.

Inflammatory bowel disease
Either of two chronic inflammatory disorders (*Crohn's disease* and *ulcerative colitis*) that affect the intestine; the cause of these disorders is unknown.

Inflammatory joint disease
Any type of *arthritis* in which joints are inflamed.

Uterus

Membranes bulging through cervix

Cervix

INCOMPETENT CERVIX
*An abnormal condition of pregnancy in which the **cervix** opens prematurely; as a result, the membranes surrounding the fetus may bulge down through the cervix, which can result in a **miscarriage.***

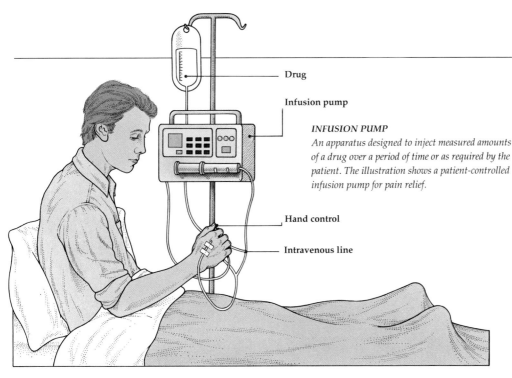

Drug

Infusion pump

INFUSION PUMP
An apparatus designed to inject measured amounts of a drug over a period of time or as required by the patient. The illustration shows a patient-controlled infusion pump for pain relief.

Hand control

Intravenous line

Influenza
A sometimes severe viral infection that causes a cough, fever, headache, muscle aches, and weakness.

Informed consent
Consent to a surgical or diagnostic procedure after receiving a thorough explanation of the procedure and the risks involved.

Infrapatellar bursitis
Inflammation of the fluid-filled pad (*bursa*) just below the kneecap.

Infusion
The introduction of a fluid, drug, nutrient, or other substance directly into a blood vessel or body cavity.

Infusion pump
See illustration above.

Ingestion
The act of taking any substance into the body through the mouth.

Ingrown toenail
A common, painful condition resulting when one or both edges of the nail of the big toe press into the adjacent skin; it can lead to infection and inflammation.

Inguinal hernia
Protrusion of part of the intestine into the muscles of the groin; it is usually repaired surgically.

Inhalation
The act of breathing in air.

Inhaler
See illustration below right.

Inheritance
The transmission of traits or disorders from parents to children through the influence of *genes*.

Injection
Introduction of a drug or *vaccine* from a syringe into the body through a needle; it may be administered into a vein, muscle, or joint or under the skin.

Insemination
The introduction of *semen* into a woman's vagina, *cervix*, or uterus.

In situ
A term meaning "in place"; it usually refers to cancers that have not spread from their site of origin.

Insoluble fiber
Any form of dietary *fiber* that passes through the digestive tract unchanged.

Insomnia
Difficulty getting to sleep or remaining asleep.

Insulin
A *hormone* produced by the *pancreas* that is vital to the body's use of the sugar *glucose* as an energy source.

Insulin-dependent diabetes
A form of *diabetes mellitus* requiring regular injections of *insulin*; it usually begins in childhood.

Insulinoma
A tumor of the *pancreas* that secretes excessive amounts of *insulin* into the blood-stream, causing a dangerous drop in the amount of *glucose* in the blood, which can lead to collapse and *coma*.

Intensive care
Close monitoring of a seriously ill patient in the hospital, allowing for immediate treatment to be given if his or her condition deteriorates.

Interferon
A group of *proteins*, produced naturally by body cells, that provide a defense against viral infections and some cancers.

Interleukin-1
A substance, released by *white blood cells* during an infection, that resets the brain's thermostat to a higher level, causing a fever.

Interleukin-2
A substance, made naturally by certain types of *white blood cells*, that is used in the treatment of kidney cancer and is being investigated for its possible use in treating other types of cancer.

Internal fixation
A method of holding together the parts of a broken bone using various metal rods, wires, plates, or screws, which are inserted surgically when the fracture is being set.

Internal mammary artery bypass
A method of *coronary artery bypass* surgery in which a blood vessel in the chest (called the internal mammary artery) is used to bypass the narrowed *coronary artery*.

Interstitial
Pertaining to or located between parts of the body or in the space between tissues.

Interstitial cystitis
Chronic inflammation of the lining and muscle of the bladder, which causes pain and a frequent urge to urinate; it is difficult to treat effectively and the cause is unknown.

Interstitial lung disease
Any disease of the *connective tissues* surrounding the air sacs in the lungs that causes a dry, unproductive cough, lung scarring, and shortness of breath.

INHALER
A device used for administering a drug in powder or vapor form to treat respiratory disorders.

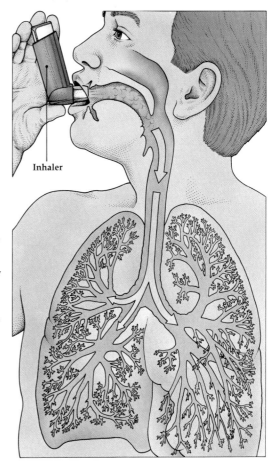

Inhaler

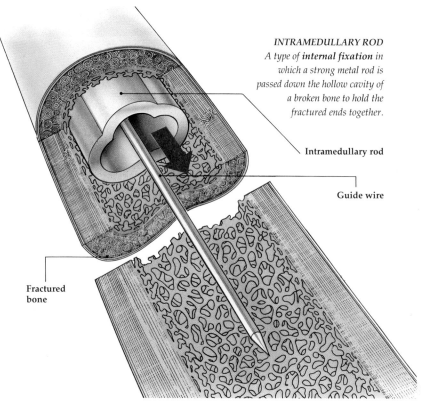

INTRAMEDULLARY ROD
*A type of **internal fixation** in which a strong metal rod is passed down the hollow cavity of a broken bone to hold the fractured ends together.*

Intramedullary rod

Guide wire

Fractured bone

Interstitial pulmonary fibrosis
Scarring and thickening of the *connective tissues* inside the lung, leading to shortness of breath.

Interstitial radiation therapy
Treatment of a cancer by inserting radioactive material into or around the cancerous growth.

Intervertebral discs
Discs containing fibrous *cartilage* with a jellylike core that act as shock absorbers between *vertebrae*.

Intestinal bypass
An operation in which a loop near the beginning of the *small intestine* is joined to a loop near its end to reduce food absorption in severely obese people; the procedure is rarely performed because of serious side effects.

Intestinal polyposis
The presence of multiple growths (*polyps*) in the intestine.

Intestine
A long tube, extending from the exit of the stomach to the *anus*, that forms the largest part of the *digestive tract*.

Intra-aortic balloon pump
A device inserted into the *aorta* to provide temporary assistance to a failing heart by inflating between contractions of the heart muscle, helping to circulate the blood.

Intracerebral hemorrhage
Bleeding from a ruptured blood vessel into the tissues of the brain.

Intractable
Unresponsive to treatment.

Intramedullary rod
See illustration above.

Intramuscular
Inside or into a muscle.

Intraocular pressure
The pressure inside the eyeball necessary to maintain its shape and allow normal functioning.

Intrauterine device
A device, usually made of molded plastic, that is inserted into the uterus to prevent pregnancy.

Intravenous
Inside a vein.

Intravenous drip
An *infusion* into a vein.

Intravenous pyelography
See illustration below right.

Intrinsic
Located in or originating from a tissue or organ.

Intubation
Passage of a tube into any organ or tubular structure in the body, such as insertion of a breathing tube into the *trachea* for *artificial ventilation*.

Intussusception
A condition in which one part of the intestine telescopes in on itself, like a shirt sleeve pulled partially inside out.

Invasive
Describes either a medical procedure in which body tissues are penetrated by an instrument or a cancer that has a tendency to spread beyond its site of origin.

Inverted uterus
A turning of the uterus inside-out; it happens in rare cases if attempts are made to remove the *placenta* after childbirth while it is still attached to the uterine wall.

In vitro
Performed in a laboratory; the term means "in glass."

In vitro fertilization
A method of treating *infertility* in which an egg is removed from a woman, fertilized in the laboratory, and reinserted into her uterus or a *fallopian tube*.

In vivo
Occurring in the body.

Involuntary
Occurring without conscious control or will (such as the beating of the heart).

Iodine
A substance essential to the formation of *thyroid hormones*; seafood is the best dietary source of iodine.

Ion
An atom or group of atoms that carries a positive or negative electric charge.

Ionizing radiation
A type of *radiation* that may cause genetic and cellular damage; it is used in *radiation therapy* to destroy cancerous tumors and in X-ray imaging.

IQ
Intelligence quotient – the measure of a person's intelligence, based on the results of special tests.

Iridectomy
Surgical removal of part or all of the *iris* of the eye.

Iris
See illustration on page 61.

Iritis
Inflammation of the *iris*, which can impair vision.

Iron
A *mineral* that is essential for many *enzymes* and for the formation of *hemoglobin*.

Iron-deficiency anemia
A form of *anemia* caused by excessive loss of iron from bleeding, by poor absorption of iron from food, or by an inadequate intake of iron in the diet.

Irrigation
Cleansing a wound or body cavity by flushing it with water or other fluids.

Irritable bladder
Intermittent, uncontrolled contractions of muscles in the bladder.

Irritable bowel syndrome
A combination of intermittent abdominal pain and irregular bowel habits (such as constipation and/or diarrhea) that frequently occurs in otherwise healthy adults; the condition is usually associated with stress.

Ischemia
Decreased blood supply to an organ or tissue.

Islets of Langerhans
Groups of cells located inside the *pancreas* that secrete the hormones *insulin* and *glucagon*.

Isolation
Separating a patient from other people to prevent him or her from infecting them or from being infected by them.

Isometric exercise
Active exercise that strengthens muscles by applying pressure against resistance, such as pressing the hands together.

IUD
Intrauterine device.

IVF
In vitro fertilization.

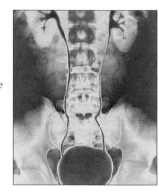

INTRAVENOUS PYELOGRAPHY
An X-ray procedure to view the kidneys and their drainage tracts after injecting a dye into the bloodstream. In the color-enhanced pyelogram at left, the urine-collecting ducts of the kidneys and the drainage tracts are outlined in red.

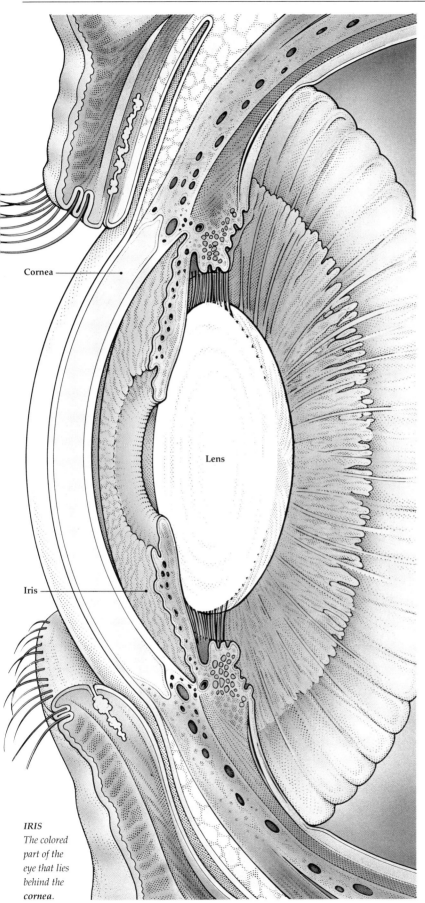

Cornea

Iris

Lens

IRIS
The colored
part of the
eye that lies
behind the
cornea.

j

Jakob-Creutzfeldt disease
Creutzfeldt-Jakob disease.

Jaundice
Yellowing of the skin and the whites of the eyes; it is caused by excessive accumulation in the blood of the pigment *bilirubin*, which spreads into and stains tissues and body fluids.

Jock itch
A fungal infection in the groin area.

Joggers' nipple
Painful inflammation of the nipples caused by rubbing against clothes during long-distance running.

Juvenile rheumatoid arthritis
A form of inflammatory *arthritis* that usually affects the larger joints of children under 16.

Kaposi's sarcoma
A type of cancer, characterized by purple-red skin tumors that begin on the feet and spread; it affects many people with *AIDS*.

Karyotype
A standardized classification of a person's *chromosomes* by number, according to size.

Kawasaki disease
A disease of infants and children that causes a fever, swollen *lymph nodes*, a rash, red eyes, peeling of the skin on the arms and legs, and complications affecting the heart and brain.

Keloid
A raised, firm, irregularly shaped scar on the skin resulting from an abnormal healing response.

Keratin
A fibrous *protein* that is the main component of the outermost layer of the skin, nails, and hair.

Keratitis
Inflammation of the *cornea*.

Keratoconjunctivitis
A severe inflammation of the *conjunctiva* and the *cornea*, usually caused by a virus; it sometimes leads to blindness.

Keratolytics
Drugs that cause peeling and softening of the outer layer of skin, used to treat skin and scalp disorders such as warts and dandruff.

Keratopathy
Any disorder of the *cornea*.

Keratoplasty
A surgical reshaping or replacement of the *cornea*.

Keratosis
A skin growth caused by overproduction of *keratin*.

Ketoacidosis
A life-threatening complication of untreated or inadequately controlled *diabetes mellitus* in which excessive amounts of substances called ketones accumulate in the body.

Kick chart
A record of fetal movements kept by a woman during later stages of pregnancy.

Kidney
Either of two organs at the back of the *abdominal cavity* that filter the blood and excrete waste products and excess water in the form of urine; they control blood volume and *acid-base balance*.

Kidney stone
A hardened accumulation (usually of mineral salts) that has formed in a kidney.

Killer T cells
White blood cells that target and destroy invading germs and cancer cells.

Kilocalorie
The amount of energy needed to raise the temperature of 1 kilogram of water by 1°C – the same as the calorie applied to food energy values.

Kimmelstiel-Wilson syndrome
A kidney disorder associated with *diabetes mellitus* that can lead to *albuminuria*, swelling in parts of the body, high blood pressure, and kidney failure.

Klinefelter's syndrome
A collection of abnormalities in a male – including breast enlargement and inability to produce sperm – that result from the presence of one or more extra *X chromosomes* in his cells.

Knee-jerk reflex
A simple test of nervous system function; when the area just below the kneecap is tapped, activation of a simple nerve pathway causes a muscle in the thigh to contract and the lower leg jerks upward.

Kyphoscoliosis
A combination of *kyphosis* and *scoliosis* (curvature of the spine to one side).

Kyphosis
Abnormal outward curvature of the spine that usually occurs in the upper part of the back.

Labia
The folds of skin at the opening of the vagina.

Labor
The process of birth, from the first uterine contraction to delivery.

Labyrinthitis
Inflammation of the three interconnecting fluid-filled chambers in the inner ear that play an important part in balance; the condition causes *vertigo* and nausea.

Laceration
A torn, jagged wound.

Lacrimal apparatus
A system of glands and ducts that produces tears and drains tears away from the inner corners of the eyes to the back of the nose.

Lactase deficiency
An inherited disorder caused by deficiency of the *enzyme* lactase, making a person unable to digest the milk sugar lactose.

Lactate dehydrogenase
An *enzyme* that is released into the blood when heart muscle cells are damaged in a heart attack; measurement of its level in the blood helps doctors assess the severity of the attack.

Lactation
See illustration above.

Lactation suppression
The suppression of milk production during pregnancy by high levels of *estrogen* in the blood.

Lactic acid
A weak acid produced by cells during *anaerobic exercise* that contributes to muscle cramps in the arms or legs.

Lactose
A form of sugar that is found in milk and milk products.

Lactose intolerance
An inability to digest *lactose*, caused by *lactase deficiency*; drinking milk or eating milk products can cause bloating, nausea, diarrhea, and abdominal cramps.

Lactose intolerance test
A test used to check for *lactose intolerance* by measuring glucose levels in a person's blood before and after the person has drunk a solution of *lactose*.

Lamaze method
A method of preparing for childbirth that includes relaxation, physical conditioning techniques, and breathing exercises.

Laminectomy
Surgical removal of one or more pieces of bone from a *vertebra*, usually to relieve pain caused by pressure on a compressed nerve.

Lanugo hair
Fine, soft, downy hair that covers a *fetus* and is shed before birth.

Laparoscope
A tube, usually with a tiny camera at its tip, inserted into the *abdominal cavity* to view or treat internal organs while the surgeon watches the image on a screen.

Laparoscopic cholecystectomy
Removal of the *gallbladder* using a *laparoscope*.

Laparoscopic surgery
Any surgical procedure performed through a tiny incision into the *abdominal cavity* using a *laparoscope*.

Laparoscopy
See illustration at left.

Laparotomy
Any operation in which the abdomen is opened up.

Large-cell carcinoma
One of the four main types of lung cancer.

Large intestine
The part of the *digestive tract* extending from the end of the *small intestine* to the *anus*.

Larva
The immature form of a worm or other parasite, or of an insect.

Larva migrans
An infestation with *larvae* that move through the skin or internal tissues.

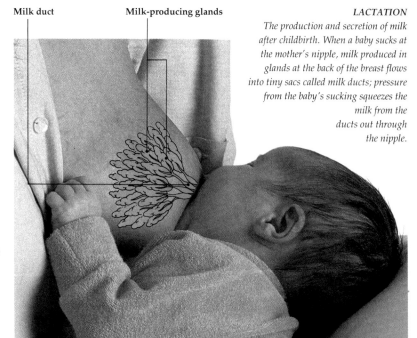

LACTATION

The production and secretion of milk after childbirth. When a baby sucks at the mother's nipple, milk produced in glands at the back of the breast flows into tiny sacs called milk ducts; pressure from the baby's sucking squeezes the milk from the ducts out through the nipple.

Milk duct   Milk-producing glands

LAPAROSCOPY
*Examination of the interior of the **abdominal cavity** using a **laparoscope**. The viewing instrument is inserted through a small incision in the abdomen and the image is usually displayed on a TV-like screen.*

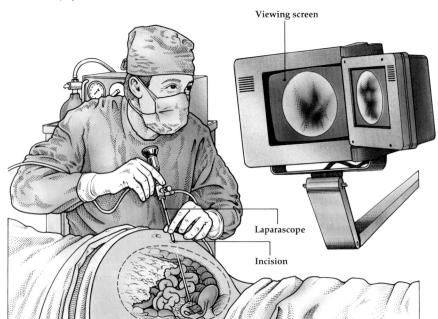

Viewing screen

Laparoscope

Incision

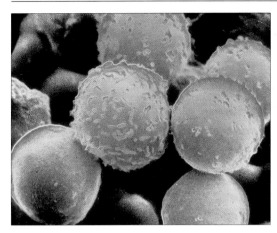

LEUKEMIA

*Any of various forms of cancer characterized by disorganized proliferation and production of **white blood cells** in the body's bone marrow. The color-enhanced photograph (magnified 2,500 times) shows the abnormal white blood cells of a person with acute lymphoblastic leukemia.*

Laryngectomy
Surgical removal of all or part of the *larynx* to treat cancer; the procedure may be performed alone or along with *radiation therapy*.

Laryngitis
Inflammation of the *larynx* that results in hoarseness.

Laryngoscopy
Examination of the *larynx* with a mirror or with a viewing tube called a laryngoscope.

Larynx
The organ at the top of the *trachea* that contains the *vocal cords* and produces voice sounds; it is popularly referred to as the voice box.

Laser treatment
The use of a concentrated beam of light to perform a number of surgical procedures, such as cutting through or destroying tissues; it reduces blood loss and the need for more *invasive* surgery.

Lassa fever
A usually fatal viral infection, confined mainly to Africa, that causes symptoms such as chills, fever, and severe diarrhea and vomiting.

Latent infection
An infection that remains inactive in the body for months or years but that may reappear.

Lateral
Situated on one side.

Lazy eye
A visual defect that can result from untreated *strabismus* in a child.

LDL
Low-density lipoprotein.

Lead poisoning
Swallowing or inhaling lead in an amount that can damage the brain, *nerves, red blood cells,* and digestive system; it is most common in children who have licked or eaten lead-containing paint.

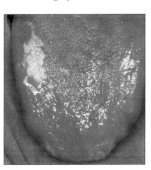

LEUKOPLAKIA
*Raised, white patches on the **mucous membranes** of the mouth, or on the penis or **vulva**, that have the potential to develop into cancer. The photograph shows leukoplakia affecting the tongue.*

Learning disability
Any of a range of physical and psychological disorders, such as hearing problems or *dyslexia*, that can interfere with learning.

Legionnaires' disease
A serious form of *pneumonia* caused by a bacterium that can sometimes contaminate water and air-conditioning systems.

Leiomyoma
A noncancerous tumor of smooth muscle, usually inside the uterus.

Leishmaniasis
Any of a variety of diseases caused by infection with single-celled parasites that are spread from person to person by sandfly bites.

Lens
The internal component of the eye that adjusts focus.

Lens implant
An artificial lens that is used to replace a *lens* affected by a *cataract*.

Leprosy
A chronic infectious disease, caused by a bacterium that primarily affects nerves in the face and limbs.

Leptospirosis
A serious infection caused by contact with a bacterium that is carried by rats and excreted in their urine.

Lesbian
A woman who is sexually attracted to other women.

Lesch-Nyhan syndrome
A *genetic disorder* characterized by mental retardation and self-mutilation.

Lesion
A localized abnormality.

Lethality
The ability of a disease to cause death.

Leukemia
See illustration above left.

Leukocyte
A white blood cell.

Leukocyte count
The number of *white blood cells* in a person's blood; it is used as an indicator of health or possible disease.

Leukodystrophy
Any of a group of inherited childhood diseases in which the protective coverings around many nerves are damaged or destroyed.

Leukoplakia
See illustration below left.

LH
Luteinizing hormone.

Lichen planus
A skin disease of unknown cause characterized by small, shiny, itchy, pink or purple, raised spots on the wrists, forearms, or lower parts of the legs.

Ligament
See illustration below.

Ligation
The process of tying off with thread or other material any structure including a blood vessel (to prevent bleeding) or a duct (to close it).

Limbic system
A part of the brain that is thought to control various emotions and instincts and to perceive odors.

Linkage
The tendency of two *genes* that are close to each other on the same *chromosome* to be passed on together from a parent to a child; this kind of association is used by scientists to discover *genetic disorders* and to track their transmission in a family.

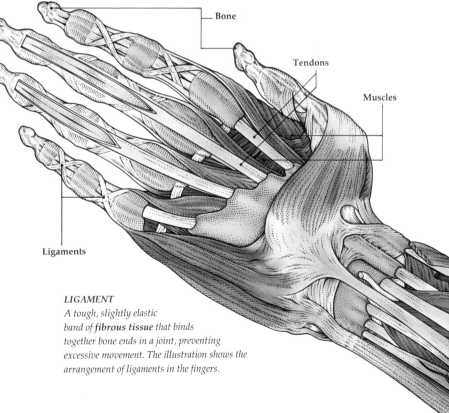

Bone

Tendons

Muscles

Ligaments

LIGAMENT
*A tough, slightly elastic band of **fibrous tissue** that binds together bone ends in a joint, preventing excessive movement. The illustration shows the arrangement of ligaments in the fingers.*

Lipase
An *enzyme* secreted by the *pancreas* that breaks down fats in food so they can be used by the body.

Lipase deficiency
Reduced *lipase* secretion by the *pancreas*, causing fats to pass undigested through the intestine and resulting in stools that are bulky, greasy, and foul-smelling.

Lipid-lowering drug
A drug used to lower the amount of specific fats in blood to reduce a person's risk of *atherosclerosis*.

Lipidosis
A general term for disorders of *metabolism* that result in excessive accumulation of some fats (*lipids*) in the body; some of the disorders, such as *Gaucher's disease* and *Tay-Sachs disease*, are inherited.

Lipids
A group of fats that play an important part in body chemistry; they are stored in the body and used for energy.

Lipoma
A noncancerous tumor of fatty tissue beneath the skin that usually requires no treatment.

Lipoproteins
Substances that are made of *lipids* and *protein*; most fats, including *cholesterol*, are carried in the blood in the form of lipoproteins.

Liposarcoma
A cancerous tumor of fatty tissue.

Liposuction
A form of *cosmetic surgery* in which localized areas of fat are removed from underneath the skin using a suction-pump device.

Listeriosis
An infection contracted by eating undercooked meat, soft cheese, or other foods that have been contaminated with a particular type of bacterium.

Lithotripsy
A new technology that uses focused and concentrated ultrasonic shock waves to disintegrate stones formed in the urinary system.

Lithotriptor
A machine used to perform *lithotripsy*.

Liver
See illustration below.

Liver failure
The life-threatening final stage of severe liver disease, for which a liver transplant may be considered.

Liver fluke
A small flatworm that causes liver enlargement and *jaundice* if it infests the liver.

Lobe
A well-defined subdivision in an organ such as the brain, liver, or lungs.

Lobectomy
Surgical removal of a *lobe*.

Local anesthesia
The direct administration of pain-killing drugs into a small part of the body to prevent pain during surgical or diagnostic procedures.

Locked joint
A joint that cannot be moved out of a particular position because of fragments of bone or cartilage trapped between the bone ends or because of joint disease such as *osteoarthritis*.

Lockjaw
A painful spasm of the jaw muscles that makes opening the mouth difficult; it occurs as a symptom of *tetanus*.

Locomotor system
The parts of the body – the bones, muscles, joints, and parts of the nervous system – that are responsible for all of the body's skeletal movement.

Loin
The part of the back on each side of the spine that is located between the lowest pair of ribs and the top of the pelvis.

Loose body
A fragment of bone or *cartilage* that has chipped off from a surface inside a joint as a result of degeneration of the joint.

Lordosis
The inward curvature of the spine in the neck and in the lower part of the back.

Lou Gehrig's disease
Amyotrophic lateral sclerosis.

Low-density lipoprotein
A type of *lipoprotein* that carries a high proportion of *cholesterol*; high levels in the blood are associated with *atherosclerosis* and *coronary heart disease*; popularly referred to as the "bad" cholesterol.

Low-impact aerobics
A type of aerobic exercise that involves little strain on the joints.

Lumbago
Pain in the lower part of the back, usually caused by *arthritis* or a strained muscle or *ligament*.

Lumbar plexus
An interlacing network of nerves located on either side of the spine in the lower back region.

Lumbar puncture
A diagnostic procedure in which a hollow needle is inserted into the lower part of the spinal canal to withdraw *cerebrospinal fluid* or to inject drugs.

Lumbar spine
The part of the spine located between the lowest pair of ribs and the top of the *pelvis*; it consists of five lumbar *vertebrae*.

Lumbosacral spasm
Prolonged or intermittent tightening of the muscles that surround the lower part of the spine; it can cause back pain and result in temporary *scoliosis*.

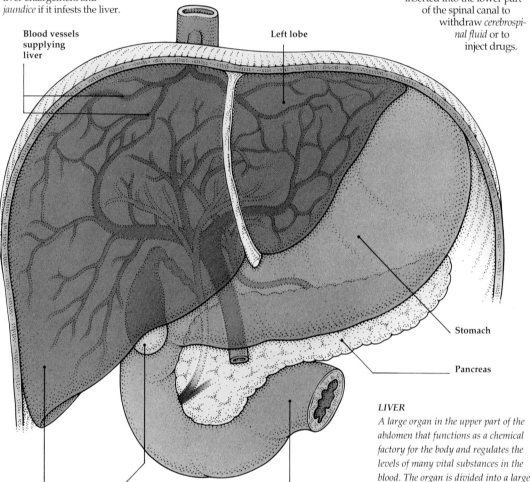

Blood vessels supplying liver

Left lobe

Stomach

Pancreas

Right lobe Gallbladder Duodenum

LIVER

*A large organ in the upper part of the abdomen that functions as a chemical factory for the body and regulates the levels of many vital substances in the blood. The organ is divided into a large right **lobe** and a smaller left lobe.*

Lumpectomy
A surgical procedure for breast cancer in which only the tumor itself and a small rim of surrounding tissue are removed.

Lung
Either of the two organs in the chest whose function is to extract oxygen from the air for use by the body and to expel *carbon dioxide*.

Lung collapse
A condition in which a lung cannot inflate, which causes *atelectasis*.

Lupus erythematosus
A chronic *autoimmune disease* that causes inflammation of *connective tissue*; it is much more common in women than men.

Luteinizing hormone
A hormone secreted by the *pituitary gland* that stimulates secretion of sex hormones by the *ovaries* and *testicles* and is involved in the maturation of eggs and sperm.

Luteinizing hormone-releasing hormone
A hormone released by the *hypothalmus* that stimulates the *pituitary gland* to release both *luteinizing hormone* and *follicle-stimulating hormone*.

Lyme disease
An infectious disease caused by a bacterium transmitted by tick bites; it causes a rash, fever, and joint and heart inflammation.

Lymph
A milky body fluid that plays an important part in the immune system and in the absorption of fats from the intestine.

Lymphadenopathy
Swollen *lymph nodes*.

Lymphangiography
A diagnostic procedure that enables a part of the *lymphatic system* to be seen on X-ray film after a *contrast medium* has been injected.

Lymphatic system
See illustration below.

Lymph node
A small gland that lies along the course of a vessel in the *lymphatic system*; it filters *lymph* and acts as a barrier to the spread of infection.

Lymphocyte
A type of *white blood cell* that plays an important part in the body's *immune system*.

Lymphocytic leukemia
A type of *leukemia* characterized by a proliferation of *white blood cells* called *lymphocytes*; it develops slowly, usually in older people.

Lymphogranuloma venereum
A *sexually transmitted disease* that is common in tropical countries; it results from infection with *chlamydia* bacteria.

Lymphoid tissue
A tissue rich in *lymphocytes* that is found in *lymph nodes* and in the *spleen*.

Lymphomas
A group of cancers of *lymphoid tissue* that can occur in any part of the body and can spread.

Lymphosarcoma
A *non-Hodgkin's lymphoma*.

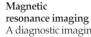

Parasites   **Skin**   **Blood vessel**

Liver

Infected red blood cells

LYMPHATIC SYSTEM
*A system of organs, vessels, nodes, and ducts that drains **lymph** from the body's tissues back into the bloodstream; it plays an important part in the body's **immune system**. The illustration shows lymph drainage channels, along which lie **lymph nodes**.*

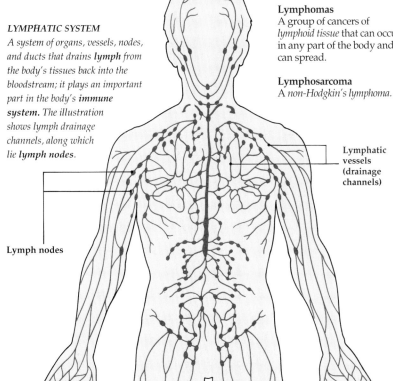

Lymph nodes

Lymphatic vessels (drainage channels)

m

Macrophage
A cell of the *immune system* that engulfs and destroys bacteria and other foreign particles.

Macula
A small, flat, usually colored spot on the skin or in the eye.

Macular degeneration
A blood vessel disorder in which the central part of the *retina* in the eye deteriorates, causing partial loss of vision; further degeneration can sometimes be stopped with *laser treatment*.

Magnesium
An essential *mineral* that plays several vital roles in the body such as transmission of nerve signals.

Magnetic resonance imaging
A diagnostic imaging technique that uses powerful magnetic fields and radio waves to produce images without the use of radiation.

Malabsorption
Impaired absorption of nutrients through the lining of the *small intestine*.

Malaria
See illustration above.

Malformation
A structural defect that occurs during organ or tissue formation in early fetal development.

MALARIA
*A group of parasitic diseases confined mainly to the tropics and spread from person to person by the bites of mosquitoes. When a mosquito carrying malaria parasites bites a person, parasites in the mosquito's saliva enter the person's bloodstream and travel to the liver, where they multiply before reentering the bloodstream and invading **red blood cells**. Symptoms of malaria appear only when infected red blood cells burst.*

Malignant
Describes a condition such as cancer that tends to become progressively worse and can be fatal.

Malignant hyperthermia
A *genetic disorder* that results in powerful muscle contractions and a dangerously high fever when an affected person is anesthetized with certain gases before surgery.

Malignant melanoma
See illustration below.

Mallory-Weiss syndrome
A condition in which violent vomiting tears the lower end of the *esophagus*, causing severe bleeding.

Mammography
An X-ray procedure for detecting breast cancer at an early stage.

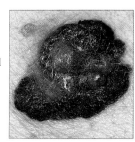

MALIGNANT MELANOMA
*The most serious type of skin cancer; it usually develops from an existing **mole** that undergoes change. A malignant melanoma, such as the one shown above, bleeds easily and is dark and of irregular color and shape.*

Mammoplasty
A surgical procedure to reduce or increase the size of the breasts (usually for cosmetic reasons) or to reconstruct a breast after surgery for cancer.

Mandible
The lower jaw.

Mania
A mental disorder characterized by episodes of extreme excitement and elation, *hyperactivity*, and agitation.

Manic-depressive disorder
A mental disorder characterized by alternating episodes of *mania* and *depression*.

MAO inhibitor
Monoamine oxidase inhibitor antidepressant.

Marasmus
A severe form of malnutrition that occurs primarily in famine conditions.

Marfan's syndrome
A *genetic disorder* affecting *connective tissue* that results in abnormalities of the skeleton, heart, and eyes.

Mast cell
A type of cell that plays a role in the *immune system* and in *allergic reactions*; it releases inflammatory substances in response to the presence of *allergens*.

Mast cell stabilizers
Drugs that prevent the release of inflammatory substances from *mast cells*; they are used to prevent *allergic reactions*.

Mastectomy
Surgical removal of all or part of the breast, usually to treat breast cancer.

Mastitis
Inflammation of breast tissue, often caused by a bacterial infection.

Maxilla
One of a pair of bones that form the upper jaw.

Measles
See illustration above.

Meconium
The thick, sticky, greenish-black feces passed by a fetus or by an infant during the first day or two after birth.

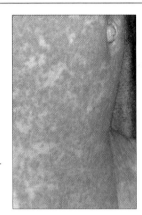

MEASLES
A viral illness, mainly affecting children, that causes a characteristic rash (shown at left) and a fever.

Medial
Located in or toward the middle of the body.

Median nerve
A nerve in the arm that controls movement of muscles in the forearm and hand and conveys sensation from a part of the hand.

Mediastinoscopy
Investigation of the central region of the chest using a flexible viewing tube inserted through an incision in the neck.

Medulla
The lower part of the *brain stem*, containing centers that control breathing, blood pressure, and other vital functions.

Medullary canal
The cavity, containing *bone marrow*, that runs down the center of a long bone; or the central canal in the spine, containing the *spinal cord*.

Medulloblastoma
A cancerous brain tumor that usually arises in the back of the brain and is most common in children.

Megacolon
A grossly swollen *colon*, usually accompanied by severe, chronic constipation; it occurs as a life-threatening complication of *ulcerative colitis* or as a *birth defect*.

Megaloblastic anemia
A type of *anemia* characterized by the presence of enlarged *red blood cells* and caused by a deficiency of *vitamin B_{12}* or *folic acid*.

Meiosis
Cell division that produces eggs or sperm, which each contain half the *genes* of the original cell.

Melanin
The pigment that gives skin, hair, and eyes their color.

Melanocyte
A cell in the skin that forms *melanin*.

Melanocyte-stimulating hormone
A hormone secreted by the *pituitary gland* that stimulates dispersion of *melanocytes* in the skin and their production of *melanin*.

Melanoma
A tumor composed of *melanocytes*; *malignant melanoma* is the most life-threatening type.

Menarche
The onset of *menstruation*.

Mendelian inheritance
The inheritance of *traits* or disorders according to the relatively simple laws of probability discovered in 1865 by Gregor Mendel.

Meniere's disease
A disorder of the inner ear characterized by *vertigo*, hearing loss, and *tinnitus*.

Meninges
See illustration below.

Meningioma
A rare, noncancerous brain tumor that develops from the *meninges*.

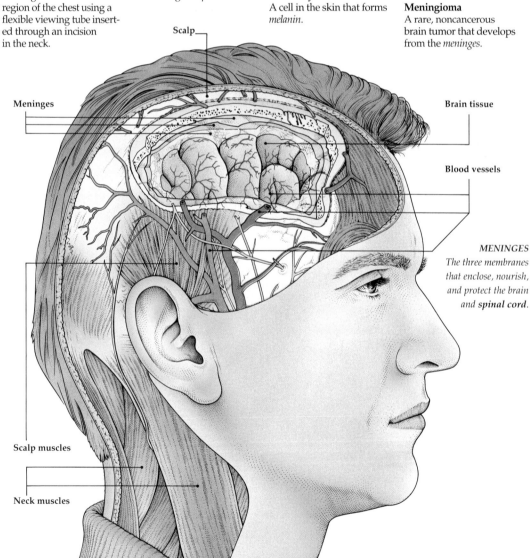

Scalp

Meninges

Brain tissue

Blood vessels

Scalp muscles

Neck muscles

MENINGES
*The three membranes that enclose, nourish, and protect the brain and **spinal cord**.*

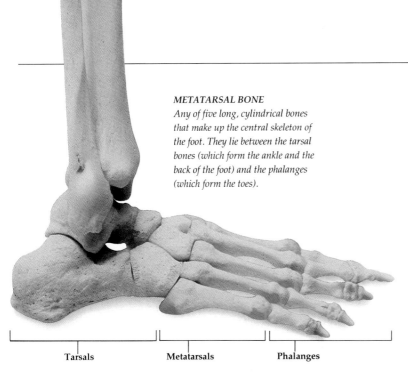

METATARSAL BONE
Any of five long, cylindrical bones that make up the central skeleton of the foot. They lie between the tarsal bones (which form the ankle and the back of the foot) and the phalanges (which form the toes).

Tarsals   Metatarsals   Phalanges

Metacarpal bone
See lower illustration below.

Metastasis
The spread of cancer from its original site to another site in the body; or a tumor that has developed in this way.

Metatarsal bone
See illustration at left.

Metatarsalgia
A pain in the metatarsal region of the foot.

Metered dose inhaler
A type of *inhaler* that delivers a preset quantity of a drug with each use.

Methyl alcohol
A highly poisonous liquid, derived from wood, that is chemically related to ethyl alcohol, the alcohol in alcoholic beverages.

Microbe
A *microorganism*, particularly one that causes disease.

Microcephaly
A birth defect characterized by an abnormally small head and some degree of mental retardation.

Microdiscectomy
A surgical treatment for *disc prolapse* in which the protruding part of the disc is removed using magnification and specialized instruments inserted through the skin of the back.

Microorganism
Any tiny, usually microscopic, life-form such as a bacterium or virus.

Microsurgery
Surgery aided by a specialized microscope that permits the surgeon to operate on tiny, delicate, or not easily accessible tissues.

Micturition syncope
A disorder in which a person (usually an older man) faints or feels faint while standing at the toilet, caused by *arrhythmia* or a drop in blood pressure.

Middle ear
A cavity on the inside of the eardrum containing three tiny bones that transmit sound vibrations as part of the hearing mechanism.

Meningitis
Inflammation of the *meninges* caused by infection, usually with bacteria but sometimes with a virus.

Meningocele
A form of *spina bifida* in which the membranes covering the spinal cord protrude under the skin.

Meniscectomy
Surgical removal of the *meniscus* from a joint, usually the knee joint.

Meniscus
A pad of *cartilage* found in some joints.

Menopause
The cessation of *menstruation*, usually at some time between ages 45 and 60, when the *ovaries* reduce their production of *estrogen* and stop producing eggs.

Menorrhagia
Excessive loss of blood during *menstruation*.

Menstrual cycle
The recurring sequence of changes, brought about by hormonal fluctuations and interactions, that occur approximately monthly in a woman's body.

Menstruation
The periodic cyclical shedding of the lining of the *uterus*, accompanied by bleeding, that occurs in a woman who is not pregnant.

Mesenteric infarction
See illustration at right.

Mesenteric lymphadenitis
Inflammation of *lymph nodes* in the membrane attaching organs to the abdominal wall (the mesentery), causing acute abdominal pain; it mostly affects children.

Mesothelioma
A rare, cancerous tumor of the membrane covering the lungs and lining the chest cavity; it is associated with exposure to asbestos.

Mesothelium
A type of surface cell layer that lines the *peritoneum* and the *pleura* and makes up the *pericardium*.

Messenger RNA
An *RNA* molecule that conveys *DNA* instructions out of a cell's nucleus to be translated into chains of *amino acids* to make *proteins*.

Metabolic rate
The amount of energy used by the body in a given amount of time.

Metabolism
The sum of all the chemical processes that take place in the body.

Metabolite
Any substance that is part of a chemical process in the body.

MESENTERIC INFARCTION
A life-threatening condition in which part of the intestine dies when its blood supply is blocked, for example by a blood clot.

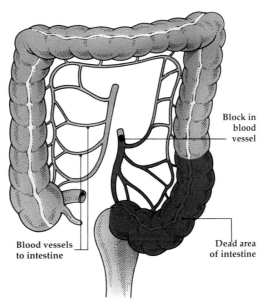

Block in blood vessel

Blood vessels to intestine

Dead area of intestine

METACARPAL BONE
Any of five long, cylindrical bones in the middle of the hand. They run from the carpals at the wrist to the phalanges, which form the fingers and the thumb.

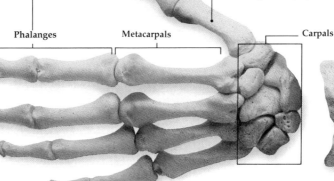

Metacarpal bone

Phalanges   Metacarpals   Carpals

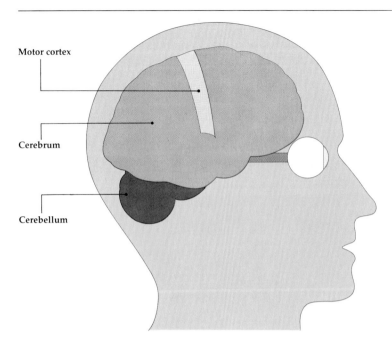

Motor cortex

Cerebrum

Cerebellum

MOTOR CORTEX

An area of the brain that sends instructions to muscles, permitting voluntary movement such as writing or forming the sounds of speech. It is located in both halves, or hemispheres, of the cerebrum in the position shown at left. Motor nerve cells that originate in one hemisphere stimulate muscles on the opposite side of the body.

Middle ear effusion
An accumulation of fluid in the *middle ear*, which can impair hearing.

Midwifery
The profession concerned with the care and assistance of women in pregnancy and childbirth.

Migraine
A severe headache, often occurring on only one side, accompanied by disturbances of vision and/or nausea and vomiting.

Milk-alkali syndrome
A rare, but potentially serious, disturbance of body chemistry caused by long-term excessive intake of *antacids* and milk.

Mineral
A chemical element (for example, iron, calcium, or phosphorus) that must be present in the diet for the maintenance of health.

Minipill
A type of *oral contraceptive* whose sole active ingredient is a drug related to the hormone *progesterone*.

Minnesota Multiphasic Personality Inventory
A psychological test used to construct a profile of an individual's personality and to detect various mental disorders, including *schizophrenia* and *depression*.

Miotics
Drugs that cause the *pupil* of the eye to constrict; they are used to treat *glaucoma*.

Miscarriage
The spontaneous termination of a pregnancy before the *fetus* has developed enough to survive outside the uterus.

Mite
A tiny, eight-legged animal, some species of which are parasites on humans.

Mitosis
A simple form of cell division that is the usual way the body grows and repairs itself; the genetic material inside a dividing cell is duplicated into two identical daughter cells.

Mitral insufficiency
Leaking of the *mitral valve*, which reduces the heart's pumping efficiency; the valve can be replaced surgically.

Mitral stenosis
Narrowing of the *mitral valve*, which puts a strain on the left side of the heart and may eventually cause symptoms such as shortness of breath.

Mitral valve
The valve that allows blood to flow only one way between the two chambers on the left side of the heart.

Mitral valve prolapse
A common, usually minor deformity of the *mitral valve* that can cause the valve to leak to some degree.

Modified radical mastectomy
A surgical procedure for breast cancer in which the breast and adjacent muscle, together with *lymph nodes* under the arm, are removed.

Molar tooth
Any of the 12 large, strong teeth at the back of the jaws.

Mole
See illustration below right.

Molecule
The smallest unit that can retain the characteristic properties of a substance.

Molluscum contagiosum
See illustration above right.

Monarthritis
Inflammation of one joint.

Mongolian spot
A flat, smooth, brown to blue-black spot, of varying size, present on the lower part of the back and the buttocks at birth; it usually disappears before age 5.

Monoamine oxidase inhibitor antidepressant
An *antidepressant* that works by blocking the action of an *enzyme* that breaks down *neurotransmitters* in the brain.

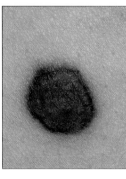

MOLLUSCUM CONTAGIOSUM

A harmless viral infection of the skin characterized by numerous tiny, pearly-white lumps on the skin (shown above).

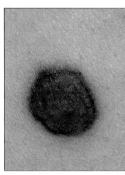

MOLE

A colored mark or blemish on the skin, usually brown, which may be flat or raised and of varying size.

Monoclonal antibodies
Antibodies that are mass-produced in the laboratory to target specific *antigens*; they are used to diagnose and treat some cancers, including *malignant melanoma*.

Mononucleosis
An acute viral infection characterized by a high fever, sore throat, swollen *lymph nodes* (particularly in the neck), and a large number of abnormal *white blood cells*.

Monounsaturated fat
A type of fat, found in high quantities in olive oil and peanut oil, that is thought to provide some protection against heart disease.

Morbidity
Illness or disease.

Morning sickness
Episodes of nausea and vomiting common in early pregnancy.

Mortality
The death rate, indicating the number of deaths per unit of population per year from a specific disease, or for a specific age group, country, or other classification.

Mosaicism
The presence of two or more genetically different groups of cells in one person, all derived from the same fertilized egg.

Motor cortex
See illustration at top of page.

Motor nerve
A nerve that carries signals that cause a muscle contraction.

Motor neuron disease
A group of diseases of unknown cause in which nerves in the brain and *spinal cord* that control muscle activity degenerate, causing muscle weakness and wasting.

Mouth-to-mouth resuscitation
A method of *artificial ventilation* in which the rescuer breathes air into the victim's lungs while sealing his or her lips over the victim's mouth.

MRI
Magnetic resonance imaging.

MS
Multiple sclerosis.

Mucocele
A swollen sac or cavity filled with *mucus* secreted from cells in its inner lining.

Mucolytic
A drug that works by making *mucus* in the lungs less sticky and easier to cough up.

Mucosa
A *mucous membrane.*

Mucous membrane
The thin, soft, pink, skinlike layer that lines many cavities and tubes in the body, such as the inside of the mouth, the stomach, and the urinary and genital passages.

Mucus
A thick, slimy fluid secreted by a *mucous membrane* to lubricate and protect that part of the body.

Multifactorial inheritance
The inheritance pattern of characteristics or disorders determined by the interaction of many *genes* with environmental factors.

Multi-infarct dementia
A type of *dementia* caused by destruction of brain tissue following multiple *strokes*.

Multiple endocrine neoplasia
A *genetic disorder* in which tumors form in hormone-secreting glands.

Multiple-gated acquisition scan
An imaging technique in which blood flow into and out of the heart is recorded to help doctors evaluate the efficiency of the heartbeat.

Multiple myeloma
A cancer characterized by the uncontrolled prolifera-tion of a type of *white blood cell* in the *bone marrow.*

Multiple pregnancy
See illustration below.

Multiple sclerosis
A disorder in which progressive degeneration of the protective coverings of nerve cells impairs the functioning of the nervous system; symptoms range from numbness and tingl-ing to paralysis.

Mumps
See illustration below right.

Murmur
The sound of turbulent blood flow through the heart, as heard through a stethoscope.

Muscle fiber
See illustration at right.

Muscle relaxants
Drugs used in *anesthesia* and *artificial ventilation*; they are also used to treat low back pain and disorders that cause muscle spasm.

Muscle tone
The natural, balanced tension in muscles.

Muscle wasting
Loss of bulk in a muscle, caused by disease or starvation.

Muscular dystrophy
A group of *genetic disorders* characterized by progressive de-generation of *muscle fibers* and loss of muscle strength.

Mutagen
A chemical or environmental agent that can cause a *mutation.*

Mutation
A change in a *gene.*

Myalgia
Muscle pain.

Myasthenia gravis
An *autoimmune disease* in which muscles – particularly in the face, throat, and limbs – become weak and tire easily.

Mycobacterium
A type of slow-growing bacterium; different mycobacteria cause *tuberculosis* and *leprosy.*

Mycoplasma
A group of *microorganisms* that are similar to, but smaller than, bacteria; one species is a cause of respiratory diseases.

Mycoplasmal pneumonia
A form of *pneumonia,* popularly referred to as walking pneumonia, that is caused by *mycoplasma.*

Mycosis
Any disease that is caused by a *fungus.*

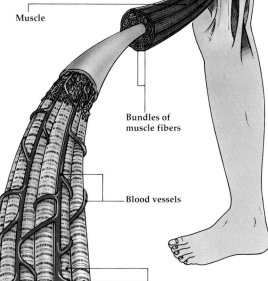

MUSCLE FIBER
One of the specialized cells in muscles that contract to create movement of the skeleton or the body's internal organs. The illustration shows skeletal muscle fibers.

Muscle

Bundles of muscle fibers

Blood vessels

Muscle fibers

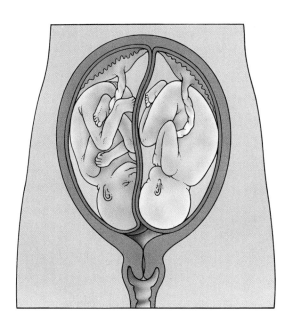

MULTIPLE PREGNANCY
*A pregnancy in which there is more than one **fetus** in the uterus.*

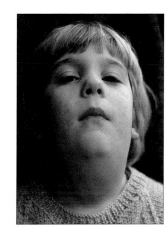

MUMPS
*A viral infection characterized by inflammation and swelling of the **salivary glands** on one or both sides of the face, which produces a thick-necked appearance; it primarily affects children.*

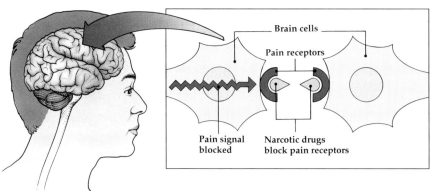

Brain cells

Pain receptors

Pain signal blocked

Narcotic drugs block pain receptors

*NARCOTIC
ANALGESICS
Painkilling drugs used
in the treatment of
moderate and severe
pain; regular use often
leads to addiction.
Narcotic analgesics
diminish perception of
pain by combining
with pain receptors on
brain cells and block-
ing the transmission
of pain signals.*

Mycosis fungoides
A rare cancer of unknown origin characterized by multiple, scaly plaques or flat growths on the skin that may persist for years.

Mydriatic
A drug that, when instilled into the eye, causes widening of the *pupil*.

Myelin sheath
A fatty covering that provides protection and electrical insulation around the conducting fibers of nerve cells.

Myelitis
Inflammation of the *spinal cord*.

Myelocele
A severe form of *spina bifida* in which part of the *spinal cord* protrudes under the skin on the back.

Myelography
An X-ray examination of the *spinal cord*, nerves, and other tissues and structures inside and around the spinal canal after injection of a *contrast medium*.

Myeloid leukemia
A type of *leukemia* that results from uncontrolled proliferation of *white blood cells* called granulocytes; its outlook has been improved with the use of *chemotherapy* and *bone marrow transplants*.

Myeloma
A cancer composed of cells that are normally found in *bone marrow*; it is often used as an abbreviation for *multiple myeloma*.

Myelosclerosis
An increase of *fibrous tissue* inside the *bone marrow*, which impairs the production of blood components.

Myocardial infarction
Death of part of the heart muscle, resulting from loss of its blood supply, which usually causes chest pain and sometimes shock or a fatal *arrhythmia*; it is also called a heart attack.

Myocarditis
Inflammation of the heart muscle.

Myocardium
The heart muscle.

Myofibril
A delicate, cylindrical thread that is the basic contractile element of a *muscle fiber*; bundles of myofibrils make up one muscle fiber.

Myomectomy
Surgical removal of a noncancerous muscle tumor, such as a *fibroid*.

Myopathy
Any disease of muscle.

Myopia
Nearsightedness.

Myositis
A painful inflammation of muscle, which may be caused by infection, injury, or a disorder of the body's *immune system*.

Myringotomy
The surgical opening of a hole in the eardrum to allow drainage of the *middle ear*, usually performed on children to treat persistent *middle ear effusion*.

Myxoma
A noncancerous, jellylike tumor, usually occurring under the skin, that may grow very large.

n

Narcolepsy
A condition of unknown cause, characterized by sudden collapses into sleep.

Narcosis
A state of stupor caused by a drug or chemical.

Narcotic
A substance that produces insensibility and stupor.

Narcotic analgesics
See illustration above.

Narcotic antidiarrheals
Mild *narcotic* drugs used to treat diarrhea by slowing the passage of liquid stool and allowing more time for water to be absorbed into the body; this effect reduces the frequency, volume, and consistency of bowel movements.

Nasal septum
The central, dividing partition inside the nose, made of *cartilage* and covered by *mucous membranes*.

Nasogastric tube
A narrow, plastic tube that is passed through the nose, down the *esophagus*, and into the stomach to introduce fluids into or remove secretions from the stomach.

Nasopharyngeal swab
A specimen of mucus taken from the back of the throat using a sterile, cotton-tipped stick called a swab.

Nasopharynx
The passage connecting the cavity behind the nose to the top of the throat.

Natural childbirth
Techniques to enable a woman to give birth with a minimum of medical intervention; also called prepared childbirth.

Natural methods of family planning
Methods used to determine when a woman is ovulating to allow a couple to time intercourse either to avoid conception or to maximize their chances of conception.

Nausea
The sensation of needing to vomit.

Nebulizer
See illustration below.

Necrosis
Death of tissue cells.

Needle aspiration
Removal of fluid for examination by suctioning it through a hollow needle attached to a syringe.

Needle biopsy
Removal of a piece of tissue for examination by cutting it out with a wide-diameter hollow needle.

Neonatal ophthalmia
Inflammation of the eye in a newborn resulting from an infection acquired during the birth process.

Neonate
An infant from birth to 1 month of age.

Neoplasm
A *tumor*.

Nephrectomy
Surgical removal of one or both kidneys.

Nephritis
Inflammation of one or both kidneys that may result from an infection, an abnormal immune response, or some disorders such as *gout*.

Nephroblastoma
A fast-growing cancerous tumor of the kidneys that occurs in children; it is usually referred to as Wilms' tumor.

Nephrolithotomy
The surgical removal of a kidney stone.

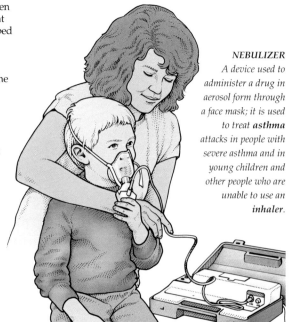

*NEBULIZER
A device used to
administer a drug in
aerosol form through
a face mask; it is used
to treat **asthma**
attacks in people with
severe asthma and in
young children and
other people who are
unable to use an
inhaler.*

Nephrons
The microscopic units in the kidneys that filter waste products from the blood and regulate the excretion of salts and water in the urine.

Nephrosclerosis
A process in which normal kidney structures are replaced with scar tissue.

Nephrostomy
Introduction of a small tube into the kidney to drain urine to the abdominal surface, bypassing the *ureter*; the procedure is sometimes performed to allow the ureter to heal after surgery.

Nephrotic syndrome
A collection of symptoms and signs that results from kidney damage.

Nerve
A bundle of fibers that transmit electrochemical messages back and forth between the brain and the *spinal cord* and other parts of the body.

Nerve block
The injection of a pain-killing drug into or around a nerve to produce loss of sensation in a part of the body supplied by that nerve.

Nerve cell
See illustration at right.

Nerve compression
Pressure on a nerve from outside the body or from surrounding structures, causing nerve damage and muscle weakness.

Nerve growth factor
A substance that influences differentiation, growth, and maintenance of nerve cells.

Neuralgia
Pain caused by irritation of, or damage to, a nerve.

Neural tube
The tube running along the back of an early *embryo* that develops into the *spinal cord* and brain.

Neural tube defects
A group of *birth defects* – including *spina bifida* – that result from failure of the *spinal cord* or brain to develop normally in an *embryo*.

Neuritis
A condition characterized by inflammation of a nerve.

Neuroblastoma
A cancerous tumor that usually originates in the *adrenal glands*; it is most common in children under the age of 4.

Neurofibromatosis
A *genetic disorder* characterized by numerous soft, fibrous swellings that grow from nerves in the skin.

Neuroleptic
Antipsychotic.

Neuroma
A noncancerous tumor of nerve tissue.

Neuromuscular junction
See illustration at right.

Neuron
Nerve cell.

Neuropathy
Disease, inflammation, or damage to any of the peripheral nerves that carry messages between the brain and *spinal cord* and the rest of the body.

Neurosis
A term used to describe a range of relatively mild emotional disorders, such as *phobias* and *panic disorder*.

Neurotoxins
Chemicals that damage nerve tissue.

Neurotransmitters
Chemicals that carry messages from brain or nerve cells to other cells.

Neurotrophic factors
Proteins that stimulate growth of nerve cells during normal fetal development and after injury; they are essential for maintaining nerve cells.

Neutrophil
The most common type of *white blood cell.*

Nevus
A *birthmark.*

Newborn respiratory distress syndrome
A disorder of premature babies characterized by difficulty breathing; it results from lack of surfactant, a chemical that prevents the lungs from collapsing.

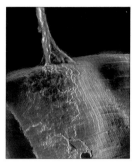

NEUROMUSCULAR JUNCTION
*The point at which the impulse carried in a **motor nerve** fiber is transmitted to a **muscle fiber**, making it contract. The color-enhanced photograph above (magnified 300 times) shows the junction between a motor nerve fiber (pink) and a skeletal muscle fiber (yellow).*

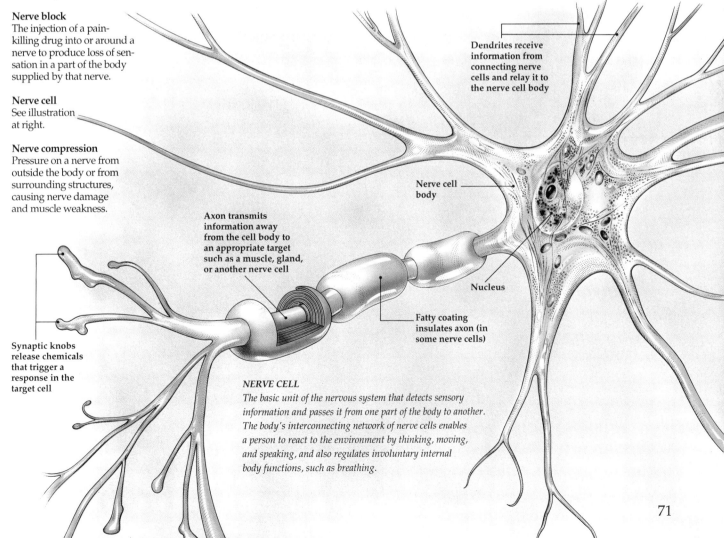

Dendrites receive information from connecting nerve cells and relay it to the nerve cell body

Nerve cell body

Nucleus

Axon transmits information away from the cell body to an appropriate target such as a muscle, gland, or another nerve cell

Fatty coating insulates axon (in some nerve cells)

Synaptic knobs release chemicals that trigger a response in the target cell

NERVE CELL
The basic unit of the nervous system that detects sensory information and passes it from one part of the body to another. The body's interconnecting network of nerve cells enables a person to react to the environment by thinking, moving, and speaking, and also regulates involuntary internal body functions, such as breathing.

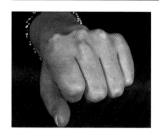

NODULE

A small, rounded mass of tissue that may protrude from the skin or form deep under the skin.

Niacin
A *vitamin*, widely distributed in foods, that plays a role in many chemical processes in the body.

Night terrors
A temporary disorder, occurring mainly in children, characterized by abrupt arousals from sleep in a terrified state.

Nitrates
Vasodilator drugs used to treat *angina pectoris* and severe *heart failure*.

Nitrosamine
A substance formed in the stomach and intestine from some preservatives in food that may contribute to the development of cancer.

Nocturia
The disturbance of a person's sleep at night by the need to pass urine.

Nocturnal emission
Ejaculation during sleep, usually associated with an erotic dream.

Node
A small, rounded mass of tissue that may be normal or abnormal; the term usually refers to a *lymph node*.

Nodule
See illustration above.

Nondisjunction
A mistake of genetic information that occurs when too much or too little *DNA* gets into an egg or sperm during its formation; it is the cause of many serious *genetic disorders*.

Nongonococcal urethritis
Inflammation of the *urethra* caused by *organisms* other than the bacterium that causes *gonorrhea*.

Non-Hodgkin's lymphoma
Any cancer of *lymphoid tissue* other than *Hodgkin's disease*.

Non-insulin-dependent diabetes
A type of *diabetes mellitus* that occurs mainly in overweight people over 40 and is usually treated by diet and *hypoglycemic drugs*.

Noninvasive
Describes any medical procedure that does not involve penetration of the skin or entry into the body through one of the natural openings.

Nonnarcotic analgesic
A painkilling drug, such as aspirin, that works by blocking the production of the substances that stimulate pain-sensitive nerve endings.

Nonspecific urethritis
Nongonoccocal urethritis.

Nonsteroidal anti-inflammatory drug
A painkilling drug, such as aspirin, that also reduces inflammation in joints and soft tissues, such as muscle.

Norepinephrine
A hormone that helps maintain a constant blood pressure by stimulating blood vessels to constrict and heart rate to increase when blood pressure falls below the normal level.

Norwalk virus
A virus that causes *gastroenteritis*, especially in children.

Nosocomial infection
An infectious disease acquired in a hospital.

NSAID
Nonsteroidal anti-inflammatory drug.

Nucleic acid
DNA or *RNA*.

Nucleoside analogues
Chemicals that can be used as drugs to interfere with the replication of viruses.

Nucleotide bases
The chemicals that form the building blocks of *DNA* and *RNA*; their sequence spells out the *genetic code*.

Nucleus
The roughly spherical central unit of a living cell that contains the cell's genetic material; or a group of nerve cells that have a common function.

Numbness
Partial or total loss of sensation in part of the body that results from interference with the passage of impulses along *sensory nerves*.

Nurse-midwife
A registered nurse who has special training in caring for and educating women during pregnancy and *labor*, supervising delivery, and providing postnatal care.

Nutrient
A substance in food that can be used by the body to sustain life and health; *carbohydrates*, fats, *proteins*, *vitamins*, and *minerals* are examples of nutrients.

Nystagmus
Involuntary, usually synchronous up-and-down, side-to-side, or rotational movements of the eyes.

O

Oat cell carcinoma
Small-cell carcinoma.

Obesity
A condition in which a person weighs 20 percent or more over the maximum desirable weight for his or her height.

Obsessive-compulsive disorder
A *neurosis* characterized by persistent ideas (obsessions) that make a person carry out repetitive, ritualized acts (compulsions).

Obstructive sleep apnea
See illustrations above right.

Occlusion
Blockage of any channel or opening in the body, which can result in infection or tissue destruction.

OBSTRUCTIVE SLEEP APNEA

*A condition in which a person stops breathing periodically for a few seconds during sleep because of a blockage in the upper **airways**. The most common cause of the blockage is excessive relaxation (during sleep) of the muscles of the soft palate at the back of the throat.*

AWAKE – AIRWAY OPEN

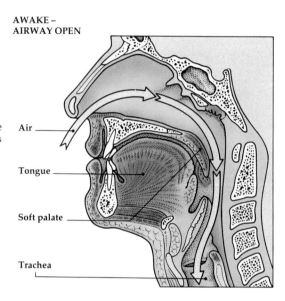

Air

Tongue

Soft palate

Trachea

ASLEEP – AIRWAY CLOSED

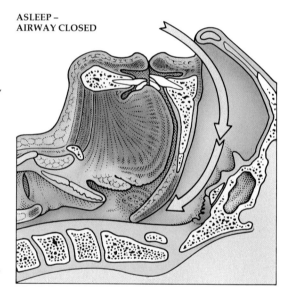

Occult blood
The presence of blood in body fluids or in feces that cannot be seen by the naked eye but can be detected by chemical tests; such tests are used to screen for cancer and as diagnostic aids.

Occupational disease
A disease caused by a particular job, usually resulting from the effects of long-term exposure to harmful substances in the workplace or of continuous or repetitive physical acts.

Occupational therapy
Treatment designed to help people disabled by an illness or accident to relearn physical skills and, when possible, to resume work.

Ocular
Relating to or affecting the eye and its structures.

Oculogyric crisis
A rare complication of a form of *Parkinson's disease*, in which the eyes are held fixed, usually up and sideways, for minutes or for hours.

Oculomotor nerves
The nerves that control most of the muscles that move the eyeball, the muscle that focuses the eye, the muscle that changes the *pupil* size, and the muscle that raises the upper eyelid.

Ohio bed
An open-sided bed for a baby in *intensive care* that provides ample space around the baby for life-support equipment and also maintains the baby's body temperature.

Olfactory nerves
A pair of nerves that convey smell sensations from the nose to the brain.

Oligodendroglioma
An uncommon, slow-growing brain tumor that primarily affects young or middle-aged adults.

Oligohydramnios
An abnormally small amount of *amniotic fluid* in the uterus during pregnancy, which can cause *miscarriage*, fetal deformities, or fetal death.

Oligospermia
A deficiency in the number of sperm in semen; it is a major cause of infertility.

Oncogenes
Altered *genes* that are responsible for the unregulated cell division characteristic of cancer.

Oocyte
An immature egg cell.

Oophorectomy
Surgical removal of one or both *ovaries*.

Open heart surgery
Any surgical procedure performed on the heart in which the heart is temporarily stopped and its function taken over by a mechanical pump.

Ophthalmia
Severe inflammation of the eye that can sometimes lead to blindness.

Ophthalmoplegia
Partial or total *paralysis* of the muscles that move the eyes.

Ophthalmoscopy
See illustration at top right.

Opportunistic infections
Infections caused by *organisms* that seldom produce disease in healthy people but frequently cause illness in people whose *immune systems* have been weakened by a disease such as *AIDS*, or as a result of *chemotherapy*.

Optic
Pertaining to the eyes or to sight.

Optician
A person who fits and supplies eyeglasses or contact lenses.

Optic nerves
See illustration below right.

Optic neuritis
Inflammation of an *optic nerve*, often affecting the field of vision.

Oral contraceptives
Pills containing a *progesterone*like drug, often combined with an *estrogen*like drug that women take to prevent pregnancy.

Orbit
Either of the two sockets in the skull that contain the eyeball, protective pads of fat, and various blood vessels, muscles, and nerves.

Orchiectomy
Surgical removal of one or both testicles.

Orchiopexy
An operation in which an *undescended testicle* is brought down into the *scrotum*.

Orchitis
Inflammation of a testicle.

Organ donation
Permission from a person (or from relatives after his or her death) for the surgical removal of one or more organs to be used in *transplant* surgery.

Organism
An individual, functioning life-form.

Orgasm
A series of involuntary contractions of the genital muscles, occurring at the peak of sexual excitement, that is experienced as an intensely pleasurable sensation.

Orphan drugs
Drugs used to treat rare diseases; because the market for these drugs is small, the government offers financial incentives to manufacturers.

Orthomyxoviruses
See illustration below.

Orthopnea
Breathing difficulty that occurs when a person is lying flat; it is a symptom of some heart and lung disorders, including *asthma*.

Orthotic
A device, such as a brace, that is used to control, correct, or compensate for deformities of bones, muscles, or joints.

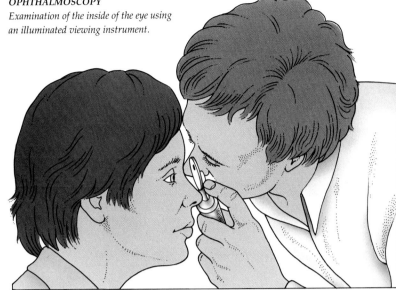

OPHTHALMOSCOPY
Examination of the inside of the eye using an illuminated viewing instrument.

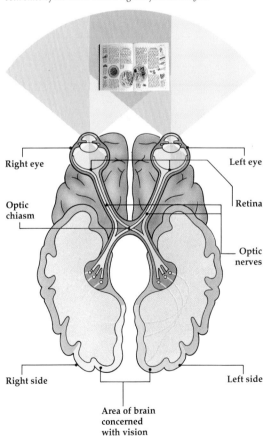

OPTIC NERVES
*A pair of nerves that transmit information about visual images received from the **retinas** of the eyes to the brain. Half the nerve fibers of each optic nerve cross over at the optic chiasm so that both sides of the brain receive signals from both eyes.*

Right eye — Left eye
Optic chiasm — Retina
— Optic nerves
Right side — Left side
Area of brain concerned with vision

BRAIN VIEWED FROM BELOW

ORTHOMYXOVIRUSES
*A family of large, spherical viruses that includes **influenza** viruses. The color-enhanced photograph above shows a single influenza virus (magnified 360,000 times).*

Osgood-Schlatter disease
Painful inflammation of the bony prominence just below the knee, usually occurring in adolescent boys.

Osmosis
The passage of a solvent (such as water) through a semipermeable membrane from a less concentrated solution to a more concentrated one.

Osmotic agent
A substance that is used to induce drainage of fluid from one side of a cell membrane to another.

Ossification
The process of bone formation.

Osteitis
Inflammation of bone, usually from infection.

Osteitis deformans
Paget's disease.

Osteoarthritis
See illustration below.

Osteoblast
A bone cell that builds new bone.

Osteochondritis dissecans
A disorder, thought to be caused by injury, in which small fragments of *cartilage* or bone are released into the interior of a joint (frequently the knee).

Osteochondritis juvenilis
Inflammation of a growing area of bone in a child or adolescent; it is thought to result from a disrupted blood supply.

Osteochondroma
A noncancerous tumor in children made up of bone capped with *cartilage*; it stops growing when the bone is fully developed.

Osteoclast
A bone cell that breaks down bone tissue; it plays a role in bone development, growth, and repair.

Osteodystrophy
Any generalized defect of bones caused by an abnormality of the body chemistry.

Osteogenesis imperfecta
A *genetic disorder* in which bones are abnormally *brittle* and easily broken.

Osteolysis
Degeneration of bone resulting from disease, infection, or lack of a blood supply; it can occur in disorders that involve blood vessels, such as *systemic lupus erythematosus, Raynaud's disease,* and *scleroderma.*

Osteoma
A noncancerous bone tumor that may occur on any bone, forming a rounded swelling.

Osteomalacia
Softening, weakening, and loss of minerals from adult bones caused by a deficiency of *vitamin D.*

Osteomyelitis
An infection of bones and *bone marrow,* usually caused by bacteria that have spread through the bloodstream or from an infection in the skin overlying the bone.

Osteopetrosis
A rare *genetic disorder* in which bone is abnormally dense.

Osteophyte
An outgrowth of bone that develops at the edge of a joint affected by *osteoarthritis.*

Osteoporosis
See illustrations below right.

Osteosarcoma
A cancerous bone tumor, occurring primarily in adolescents and older people, that spreads rapidly to other parts of the body, especially the lungs.

Osteosclerosis
An abnormal increase in bone density.

Osteotomy
A surgical procedure in which a bone is cut or fractured to change its length, to correct a deformity, or to improve the stability of a joint.

Otalgia
Earache.

OTC remedy
Over-the-counter remedy.

Otitis externa
Inflammation of the outer part of the ear, including the ear canal; it is usually caused by infection.

Otitis media
Inflammation of the *middle ear,* caused by an upper respiratory tract infection that has spread up the *eustachian tube.*

Otorrhea
A discharge from the ear.

Otosclerosis
An inherited disorder of the *middle ear* that causes progressive hearing loss; it can be treated with surgery.

Ototoxicity
Impaired hearing that results from the poisonous effects of certain drugs.

Outpatient treatment
Medical care given to a person in an office, clinic, or other facility that does not involve an overnight stay.

Ovaries
A pair of glands on either side of the uterus that produce eggs and the female sex hormones.

Overdose
A much-larger-than-recommended quantity of a drug.

Over-the-counter remedy
A medication available without a prescription.

Ovulation
See illustration above.

Ovum
An egg cell.

Oxidation
A damaging chemical reaction caused by the activity of *oxygen free radicals.*

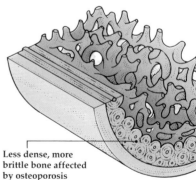

Egg   Ovary   Uterus

OVULATION
*The cyclic development and release of an egg from the **ovary**.*

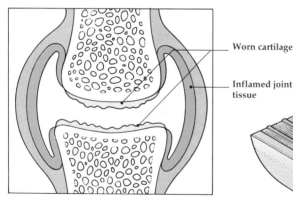

OSTEOARTHRITIS
*Progressive degeneration of the **cartilage** that lines joints, leading to inflammation, pain, stiffness, and restricted movement of the affected joint.*

Worn cartilage

Inflamed joint tissue

OSTEOPOROSIS
*A disorder in which bone density decreases, making bones thin, brittle, and more prone to fracture; it is most common in women after **menopause**.*

Normal dense bone

Less dense, more brittle bone affected by osteoporosis

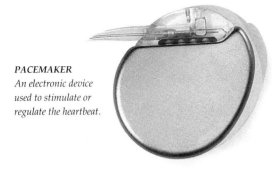

PACEMAKER
An electronic device used to stimulate or regulate the heartbeat.

Oximetry
Detection of the levels of oxygen in a person's blood using a device attached to the earlobe or fingertip.

Oxygen
A colorless, odorless, tasteless gas that is essential for breathing.

Oxygen concentrator
A device that separates oxygen from the air, used by people who need to breathe additional oxygen.

Oxygen free radicals
Active sources of oxygen – produced in the body by normal cell activity and by external agents such as radiation, pollution, and smoking – that damage cells; they are thought to play a role in cancer and aging.

Oxytocin
A hormone produced by the *pituitary gland* that causes contractions of the uterus during *labor* and stimulates the flow of milk for breast-feeding.

Ozone
A form of oxygen that occurs naturally in the upper atmosphere and protects the Earth from an excessive amount of the sun's harmful ultraviolet radiation.

Pacemaker
See illustration above.

Paget's disease
A disorder of unknown cause in which the normal process of bone formation is disrupted, causing the affected bones to weaken, thicken, and become deformed.

**Paget's disease
of the nipple**
A rare type of breast cancer in which a tumor starts in the milk ducts of the nipple.

Palate
The roof of the mouth.

Palliative treatment
Therapy that relieves the symptoms of a disorder but does not cure it.

Pallor
Abnormally pale skin, particularly of the face.

Palpation
Use of the hands during a physical examination to feel the consistency, size, and shape of parts of the body in order to find signs of disease.

Palpitation
An unusually rapid, strong heartbeat.

Palsy
Paralysis.

Pancreas
See illustration at right.

Pancreatitis
Inflammation of the *pancreas*, often caused by excessive alcohol use or overeating.

Pancreatography
Imaging of the *pancreas* and its network of ducts.

Pandemic
Describes a disease that occurs over a large geographical area and affects a large proportion of the population; a widespread *epidemic*.

Panic disorder
An emotional disturbance in which a person suffers from persistent anxiety that can bring on repeated panic reactions in stressful situations.

Pantothenic acid
A *vitamin*, widespread in foods, that aids the release of energy in cells.

Papilloma
A usually noncancerous tumor, often resembling a wart, that arises from *epithelium*.

Papillomaviruses
A family of viruses that cause *warts*; a woman's exposure to the strains that cause *genital warts* is thought to increase her risk of cervical cancer.

Pap smear
A diagnostic test in which cells are scraped from the surface of the *cervix* and examined under a microscope to detect abnormal cells that are or could become cancerous.

Paracentesis
A procedure in which a body cavity is punctured from the outside with a needle, usually to remove fluid for analysis.

Paralysis
The loss of nerve impulses to a muscle, resulting in an inability to use that muscle.

Paralytic ileus
A condition in which the muscle contractions that move food through the intestine slow down or stop.

Paramedic
A person trained to provide emergency medical care, such as resuscitation after an accident or heart attack.

Paramyxoviruses
A family of viruses that includes the organisms responsible for *measles*, *mumps*, and *rubella*.

Paranoia
A disorder characterized by the false belief that people or events are in some way related to oneself.

Paraphimosis
Constriction of the *glans penis* by a tight foreskin that has been pulled back, causing swelling and pain.

Paraplegia
Complete or incomplete *paralysis* of the legs.

Parasites
Organisms that live in or on (and derive nourishment from) other organisms; some cause disease in people.

**Parasympathetic
nervous system**
The part of the *autonomic nervous system* that predominates during times of relaxation; it conserves and restores energy.

Parathyroid glands
Two pairs of oval, pea-sized glands that are located next to the *thyroid gland* in the neck; they produce *parathyroid hormone*.

Parathyroid hormone
A hormone produced by the *parathyroid glands* that helps control the level of calcium in the blood.

Parathyroidectomy
The surgical removal of one or more *parathyroid glands*.

Parenteral
A term applied to the administration of drugs, nutrients, or other substances by any route other than the digestive tract.

Paresis
Partial *paralysis*.

Paresthesia
A tingling or prickly feeling in the skin; a "pins and needles" sensation.

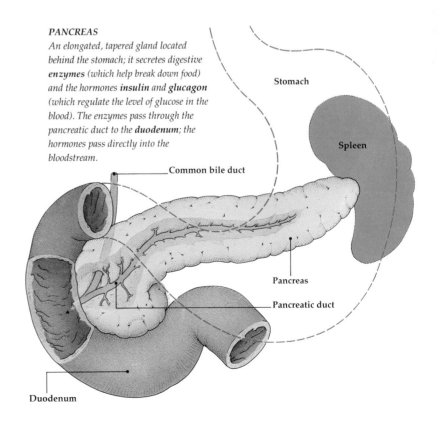

PANCREAS
An elongated, tapered gland located behind the stomach; it secretes digestive **enzymes** *(which help break down food) and the hormones* **insulin** *and* **glucagon** *(which regulate the level of glucose in the blood). The enzymes pass through the pancreatic duct to the* **duodenum***; the hormones pass directly into the bloodstream.*

Stomach

Spleen

Common bile duct

Pancreas

Pancreatic duct

Duodenum

Parietal lobes
Parts of each *cerebral hemisphere* that are involved in pain and touch sensations, speech, and control of spatial orientation.

Parkinson's disease
A degenerative brain disorder characterized by deficient secretion of *dopamine* by some brain cells, which leads to muscle rigidity, weakness, and tremor; it occurs most often in people older than 60.

Paronychia
An infection of the skin fold at the base of the nail.

Parotid glands
The largest pair of *salivary glands*, which lie on each side of the face, just below and in front of the ear.

Paroxysm
A sudden attack or a worsening or recurrence of symptoms or of a disease; or a *spasm* or *seizure*.

Partial mastectomy
Surgical removal of a cancerous tumor in the breast along with the overlying skin, a portion of the surrounding tissues, and some of the underlying muscles.

Partial seizure
A localized abnormal electrical discharge in the brain that affects isolated body or mental functions.

Passive exercise
Exercise using external force or other muscles in the body to restore muscle strength to an injured part of the body.

Passive smoking
Inhalation of smoke by nonsmokers from other people's cigarettes, cigars, or pipes; it increases the risk of respiratory disorders and cancer.

Patella
The kneecap.

Patent
Open or unobstructed.

Patent ductus arteriosus
A birth defect, occurring primarily in premature infants, in which the ductus arteriosus (a channel by which blood bypasses the lungs in the *fetus*) fails to close after birth.

Paternity testing
The use of tests such as *DNA fingerprints* to help determine whether or not a particular man is the father of a particular child.

PELVIC FLOOR EXERCISE
*Deliberate contraction of the muscles at the floor of the **pelvis** to strengthen and tone them. To do the exercise, sit as shown and tighten the muscles around the vagina (the muscles you use to stop the flow of urine) and anus. Hold for 8 to 10 seconds and relax. Repeat for several minutes two or three times a day.*

Pathogen
Any *microorganism* that causes disease.

Pathogenesis
The processes by which a disease (or disorder) originates and develops.

Pathological
Relating to disease or the study of disease.

Patient-controlled analgesia
A drug-delivery system that allows a person to control the amount of a painkilling drug he or she receives.

Peak flow measurement
The highest rate at which a person can exhale air; it is used to evaluate the severity of a person's *asthma*.

Pectoral muscles
Two muscles in the upper part of the chest that draw the arms across the body, move the shoulders, and raise some ribs.

Pellagra
A disorder caused by a deficiency of *niacin* and resulting in *dermatitis*, *diarrhea*, and *dementia*.

Pelvic examination
Examination of a woman's external and internal *genitals*, performed as part of a complete physical examination or to find the cause of pelvic pain or other symptoms.

Pelvic floor exercise
See illustration at left.

Pelvic inflammatory disease
See illustration at top right.

Pelvis
See illustrations above right.

Penile function tests
Tests used to find the cause of *impotence*; they include blood tests, studies of nerve function, and measurement of erections during sleep.

Penile implant
A silicone splint or an inflatable device inserted into the penis to enable a man who is impotent to have intercourse.

Penis
The external male reproductive organ.

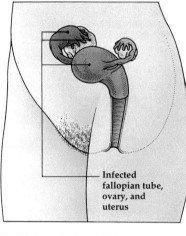

PELVIC INFLAMMATORY DISEASE
*Infection of the internal female reproductive organs, usually caused by a **chlamydia** infection; it is the most common cause of infertility in women.*

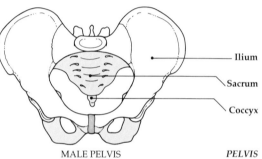

MALE PELVIS

FEMALE PELVIS

PELVIS
*The basin-shaped bony structure at the base of the spine, consisting of the **ilium** (hipbone), the **sacrum**, and the **coccyx**. A woman's pelvis is shallower and wider than a man's to facilitate childbirth.*

Pepsin
An *enzyme* secreted in the stomach that helps the body digest *protein*.

Peptic ulcer
A raw area in the *esophagus*, stomach, or *small intestine* that occurs as a result of erosion from stomach acid.

Percutaneous
Performed through the skin, such as an injection.

Perforation
A hole made in an organ or tissue by disease or injury.

Perianal abscess
A collection of pus beneath the skin around the *anus* that results from an infection.

Periarteritis nodosa
A disease in which segments of medium-sized arteries become inflamed, weakened, and prone to developing *aneurysms*.

Pericardial effusion
Fluid buildup inside the *pericardium*, which compresses the heart and interferes with its ability to pump blood.

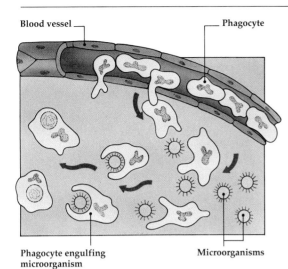

Blood vessel — — Phagocyte

Phagocyte engulfing microorganism — Microorganisms

PHAGOCYTE
*A cell of the **immune system** that can surround, engulf, and digest **microorganisms**, foreign particles, and cellular debris. The illustration above shows phagocytes squeezing through the walls of a blood vessel to engulf and destroy invading microorganisms.*

Pericarditis
Inflammation of the *pericardium*, which causes chest pain and fever.

Pericardium
See illustration below right.

Perinatal
Relating to the period just before or just after birth.

Perineum
The tissue between the external genital organs and the *anus* that extends internally up to the muscles at the base of the pelvis and the surrounding bony structures.

Periodic paralysis
A *genetic disorder* characterized by recurrent episodes of temporary weakness and paralysis of limb muscles.

Periosteum
A tough membrane containing blood vessels and nerves that covers all bone surfaces except those at the ends of bones inside joints.

Periostitis
Painful inflammation of the *periosteum*, usually resulting from injury or infection.

Peripheral nervous system
All the nerves that fan out from the *central nervous system* to the rest of the body.

Peripheral vascular disease
Narrowing of blood vessels outside the heart, which restricts blood flow and causes pain and numbness in the affected area.

Peristalsis
Wavelike muscle movement that moves food through the digestive tract and urine through the *ureters*.

Peritoneal dialysis
A method of *dialysis* that involves passing a special fluid into the abdomen through an incision and draining it out several hours later along with waste products and excess water.

Peritoneum
The two-layered membrane that lines the wall of the *abdominal cavity* and covers the abdominal organs.

Peritonitis
Inflammation of the *peritoneum* that can result when bacteria or other substances contaminate the *abdominal cavity*.

Pernicious anemia
A progressive type of *anemia* caused by an inability to absorb *vitamin B_{12}*, which is essential for the production of normal *red blood cells*; this type of anemia usually affects older people.

Perthes' disease
Painful degeneration of the growing area of the head of the thighbone in children; it may leave the hip permanently deformed.

Pertussis
A childhood bacterial infection (also called whooping cough) characterized by coughing fits that end in a peculiar "whoop" as breath is inhaled.

Petit mal
A type of *seizure* characterized by brief episodes of loss of awareness.

PET scanning
Positron emission tomography scanning.

Peutz-Jeghers syndrome
A *genetic disorder* characterized by small, usually noncancerous, *polyps* in the intestine and small, flat, brown spots on the lips.

pH
A measure of the acidity or alkalinity of a solution.

Phagocyte
See illustration above left.

Phantom limb
The perception that a limb is present after it has been amputated.

Pharyngitis
Inflammation of the *pharynx*, characterized by a sore throat and swollen glands.

Pharynx
The passage that connects the back of the mouth and nose to the *esophagus* and *trachea*; the throat.

Phenothiazines
A class of drugs used to treat *psychotic* illnesses; they are also used as *antiemetics*.

Phenotype
All the observable characteristics of an *organism* as determined by a combination of genetic and environmental factors.

Phenylketonuria
A *genetic disorder* in which the body cannot process the *amino acid* phenylalanine, which, unless excluded from the diet, builds up in the body, causing severe mental retardation; all newborns are screened for the disorder.

Pheochromocytoma
A noncancerous tumor that secretes the hormones *epinephrine* and *norepinephrine*, leading to intermittent, life-threatening elevations in blood pressure.

Pheromone
A substance secreted by animals that elicits a response from members of the same species, usually of the opposite sex.

Philadelphia chromosome
A defective *chromosome* present in most people with *myeloid leukemia*.

Phimosis
Tightness of the *foreskin*, preventing it from being drawn back over the head of the penis.

Phlebitis
Inflammation of a vein, which often leads to formation of a blood clot.

Phlebothrombosis
A condition in which a blood clot forms in a vein.

Phlegm
Sputum.

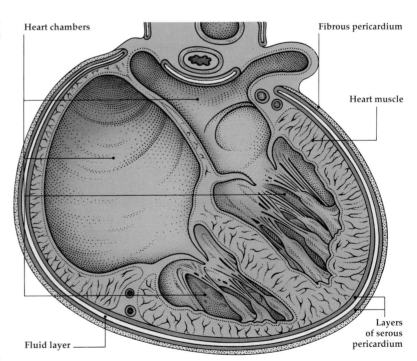

Heart chambers — — Fibrous pericardium

— Heart muscle

Fluid layer — — Layers of serous pericardium

PERICARDIUM
The membranous sac that encloses the heart and the roots of the major blood vessels that emerge from it. The pericardium has two parts – a tough outer bag (the fibrous pericardium) and an inner membrane (the serous pericardium). The serous pericardium has two layers separated by a thin film of lubricating fluid.

Phobia
A persistent, irrational fear of (and desire to avoid) a particular object, person, place, or situation.

Phosphates
Salts containing a *phosphorus* atom; they are an integral part of bones and teeth and they play a variety of other important roles in the body's chemistry.

Phospholipids
A group of fatty substances that are important components of the membranes that surround body cells.

Phosphorus
A *mineral* widely distributed in food that, in the form of *phosphates* and *phospholipids*, plays many important roles in the body.

Photocoagulation
Destruction of tissue by the heating effect of intensely focused light, such as that used in *laser treatment* for disorders of the *retina*.

Photophobia
Abnormal sensitivity of the eyes to sunlight.

Photosensitivity
Abnormal reaction to exposure to sunlight, usually in the form of a rash, that can result from some disorders or from the ingestion of particular drugs.

Phototherapy
Treatment using light.

Physical therapy
Treatment using physical methods (such as exercise) or agents (such as water, heat, or light).

Phytochemicals
Newly discovered nutrients in fruits and vegetables that may help protect against cancer and other disorders.

Pia mater
The innermost layer of the membranes covering the brain and *spinal cord*.

Pica
A craving to eat substances (such as dirt or coal) that are not food.

Pickwickian syndrome
A disorder of unknown cause characterized by obesity, shallow breathing, excessive daytime sleepiness, *sleep apnea*, and *heart failure*.

Picornaviruses
A group of viruses that cause *poliomyelitis*, viral *hepatitis*, *myocarditis*, *aseptic meningitis*, and the *common cold*.

PID
Pelvic inflammatory disease.

Pigmentation
Coloration of the skin and hair and the *irises* of the eyes by the pigment *melanin*.

Pilonidal sinus
A pit in the skin in the upper part of the cleft between the buttocks.

Pineal gland
A tiny region of the brain thought to be involved in daily biological cycles.

Pinealoma
A tumor arising from the *pineal gland*.

Pinkeye
Conjunctivitis.

Pinworm
A small parasitic worm that can infest the intestines; it occurs most frequently in children.

Pituitary adenoma
A noncancerous tumor of the *pituitary gland*.

Pituitary gland
A gland at the base of the brain that produces many hormones that influence the activity of other glands in the *endocrine system*.

Pituitary hormone
Any of various hormones that are produced by the *pituitary gland*.

Pityriasis alba
A common skin disorder of children and adolescents in which irregular, fine, scaly, pale patches appear on the face, usually the cheeks.

Pityriasis rosea
A common, mild, skin disorder of unknown cause in which flat, round, scaly-edged, dark pink spots appear over the trunk and upper parts of the arms.

Pivot joint
See illustrations at left.

PKU
Phenylketonuria.

Placebo
A chemically inactive substance given in place of a drug to test the effectiveness of that drug.

Placebo effect
A positive or negative response to a drug resulting from a person's expectations rather than from any real chemical effect.

Placenta
See illustration above.

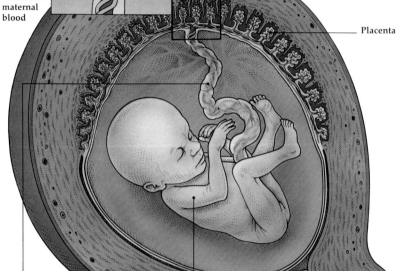

PLACENTA
An organ that develops in the uterus during pregnancy; it links the blood of the pregnant woman and the **fetus** *and allows nutrients and oxygen to pass through to the fetus and waste products to pass out into the maternal blood for removal.*

Maternal blood vessels

Fetal blood vessels

Pockets of maternal blood

Placenta

Umbilical cord

Fetus

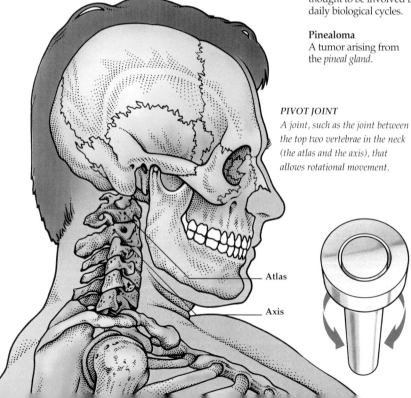

PIVOT JOINT
A joint, such as the joint between the top two vertebrae in the neck (the atlas and the axis), that allows rotational movement.

Atlas

Axis

Placental abruption
Premature detachment of the *placenta* from the wall of the uterus, which can cause severe bleeding that is life-threatening to both the pregnant woman and the *fetus.*

Placental insufficiency
An abnormal condition of pregnancy in which the *placenta* provides insufficient nutrition to the *fetus.*

Placenta previa
See middle illustration at right.

Plague
An infectious disease that mainly affects rats but can be transmitted to humans by the bites of rodent fleas.

Plantar reflex
The normal response of curling the toes downward when the sole of the foot is firmly stroked.

Plantar wart
A hard, horny, rough-surfaced area on the sole of the foot caused by a virus that is usually acquired from contaminated floors.

Plaque
A sticky coating consisting of saliva, bacteria, and food debris that forms on the teeth and is the major cause of tooth decay.

Plasma
The nutrient-filled, liquid part of blood that remains after the blood cells have been removed.

Plasma cell
A type of *lymphocyte* that manufactures *antibodies.*

Plasmapheresis
A procedure for removing unwanted substances from the blood by replacing some of a person's *plasma* with a plasma substitute; the technique is used to treat some *autoimmune diseases.*

Plasmid
A tiny package of *DNA* in a bacterium, separate from the bacterium's main DNA, that can transfer to other bacteria and change an organism's ability to adapt, such as making it resistant to *antibiotics*; plasmids are used in *genetic engineering* to produce large quantities of drugs.

Plasminogen
A *protein* naturally present in blood that, if activated, forms another substance, called plasmin, that can dissolve blood clots.

Platelet
A small blood cell that plays a role in blood clotting.

Pleura
The *pleural membranes.*

Pleural effusion
An accumulation of fluid between the *pleural membranes* that can cause difficulty breathing.

Pleural membranes
The two membrane layers that cover the lungs and line the chest cavity.

Pleural rub
A rubbing sound heard during breathing that occurs when the *pleural membranes* are inflamed.

Pleural space
The space between the *pleural membranes.*

Pleurisy
Inflammation of the *pleural membranes*, usually caused by a lung infection.

Pleurodynia
Pain in the chest caused by a viral infection.

Plummer-Vinson syndrome
Difficulty swallowing caused by webs of tissue across the upper *esophagus*, usually occurring in severe *iron-deficiency anemia.*

PMS
Premenstrual syndrome.

Pneumoconiosis
Any of a group of lung diseases caused by chronic, usually job-related, inhalation of dusts.

Pneumocystis pneumonia
An *opportunistic infection* of the lungs; a major cause of death in people with *AIDS.*

Pneumonectomy
Surgical removal of an entire lung.

Pneumonia
Inflammation of the lungs, causing coughing and fever; it is usually brought on by an infection.

Pneumothorax
See illustration at right.

Point mutation
An alteration in just a tiny piece of *DNA* in a *gene.*

Poliomyelitis
An infectious disease caused by a virus that usually produces only a mild illness but, in serious cases, can cause paralysis and death.

Polyarthritis
Arthritis that affects more than one joint.

Polycystic kidney disease
A disorder in which the kidneys are enlarged and contain many *cysts.*

Polycystic ovary syndrome
An inherited hormonal imbalance characterized by multiple *cysts* in the ovaries, infrequent or absent *ovulation*, scanty or absent *menstruation, infertility, obesity*, and *hirsutism.*

Polycythemia
A condition characterized by an abnormally large number of blood cells.

Polydactyly
A *birth defect* characterized by the presence of more than the normal number of fingers or toes.

Polydipsia
Excessive thirst; it is one of the first symptoms of *diabetes mellitus.*

Polymyalgia rheumatica
A disease of older people that is marked by aching pain and stiffness in the muscles of the hips, thighs, shoulders, and neck.

Polymyositis
An *autoimmune disease* characterized by muscle inflammation and weakness.

Polyp
A growth that projects, usually on a stalk, from a *mucous membrane* surface and can sometimes develop into cancer.

Polysaccharides
Carbohydrates, such as starch, that consist of three or more simple carbohydrate molecules; they are broken down into *glucose* to supply the body with energy.

Polyunsaturated fat
A type of fat found in most vegetable fats and oils that is thought to help reduce the risk of heart disease.

Polyuria
Excessive urination; it is one of the first symptoms of *diabetes mellitus.*

Popliteal artery
The continuation of the *femoral artery* behind the knee; it supplies blood to various muscles in the lower part of the leg and the foot.

Porphyria
See lower illustration below.

Portal hypertension
Increased blood pressure in the *portal vein*, usually as a result of *cirrhosis of the liver.*

Portal vein
A large blood vessel that carries blood from the stomach, intestine, and *spleen* to the liver.

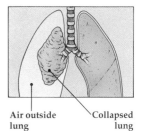

Air outside lung — Collapsed lung

PNEUMOTHORAX

A collection of air in the space between the chest wall and the lung. The air creates increased pressure on the outside of the lung, forcing it to collapse and causing chest pain and shortness of breath.

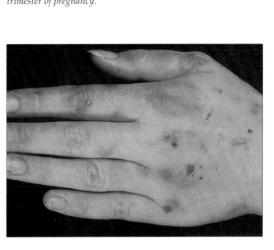

Uterus

Placenta

Cervix

PLACENTA PREVIA

*Abnormal implantation of the **placenta** in the lower part of the uterus, near or over the **cervix**; it is the most common cause of bleeding in the third trimester of pregnancy.*

PORPHYRIA

*Any of a group of **genetic disorders** caused by increased production of substances called porphyrins that can result in a skin reaction (shown above) to sunlight or in abdominal or nervous system disturbances from certain drugs.*

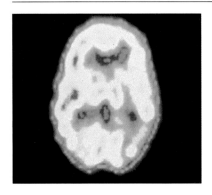 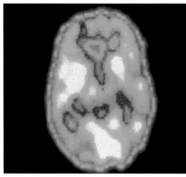

POSITRON EMISSION TOMOGRAPHY SCANNING
A computerized, diagnostic, imaging technique that produces two- or three-dimensional
images reflecting function of tissues such as those of the brain, heart, and blood vessels.
The color-enhanced scans above show a higher level of activity (yellow areas) in the
brain of a healthy person (left) than in the brain of a depressed person (right).

Positron emission tomography scanning
See illustrations above.

Postcoital contraception
The prevention of pregnancy after sexual intercourse has occurred, by taking hormonal drugs.

Posterior
Relating to or located in the back of the body.

Postmenopausal bleeding
Bleeding from the vagina after *menopause*.

Postmortem examination
Examination of a body after death to confirm or determine the cause.

Postmyocardial infarction syndrome
A condition that may occur after a heart attack or heart surgery, characterized by fever, chest pain, *pericarditis*, and *pleurisy*.

Postnatal
After birth; the term usually refers to the newborn.

Postpartum
After childbirth; the term usually refers to the mother.

Post-traumatic stress disorder
Emotional disturbance that comes on after a stressful or frightening experience, such as a natural disaster or military combat.

Postural drainage
Positioning the body to allow mucus to drain from the lungs.

Postural hypotension
Abnormally low blood pressure occurring when a person stands or sits up suddenly.

Potassium
A *mineral*, widely distributed in food, that is necessary for normal heart rhythm, the body's water balance, the conduction of nerve impulses, and the contraction of muscles.

Potassium-sparing diuretic drug
A *diuretic* drug given in conjunction with other diuretics to prevent excessive loss of *potassium* from the body.

Precancerous
Describes any condition in which cancer has a tendency to develop.

Preeclampsia
A serious condition in which high blood pressure and *edema* develop in a woman in the second half of pregnancy; untreated, it can lead to *eclampsia*.

Premature labor
Labor that begins before the 37th week of pregnancy.

Premature rupture of membranes
Rupture of the *amniotic sac* before the 37th week of pregnancy.

Premedication
Administration of drugs 1 to 2 hours before surgery to prepare a person for an operation.

Premenopausal
Describes the period of several years in a woman's life before *menopause*.

Premenstrual syndrome
A variety of emotional and physical changes that may affect a woman during the few days before *menstruation*; it is popularly referred to as PMS and is also called premenstrual tension.

Premotor cortex
The part of the *cerebral cortex* of the brain that coordinates complex, skilled movements, such as playing a musical instrument.

Prenatal care
Care of a pregnant woman and the developing *fetus* throughout pregnancy to make sure that both are healthy at delivery.

Prenatal diagnosis
Any of a number of techniques used to detect abnormalities in a *fetus*.

Prenatal testing
Tests performed on a woman or *fetus* during pregnancy to help prevent problems or detect them at a stage early enough for effective treatment.

Prepared childbirth
Techniques and training designed to enable a woman to give birth with a minimum of medical intervention; *natural childbirth*.

Prepatellar bursitis
Inflammation of the *bursa* just below the knee.

Prepuce
Foreskin.

Presbycusis
Progressive loss of hearing that occurs with aging.

Presbyopia
Progressive loss of the ability of the eyes to focus for near vision; it occurs with advancing age.

Pressure point
See illustration below.

Pressure sore
An ulcer that develops on the skin of a bedridden or immobile person as a result of sustained pressure; it is also called a bedsore.

Priapism
Persistent, painful erection of the penis without sexual arousal; it requires emergency treatment.

Prickly heat
An irritating rash associated with profuse sweating.

Primary
A term applied to a disease that has originated within the affected organ or tissue and is not derived from any other cause or source.

Prion
A very simple life-form that is thought to be the cause of *slow virus diseases*.

Procidentia
Severe *prolapse*, usually of the uterus.

Proctalgia
Pain in the *rectum*.

Proctitis
Inflammation of the *rectum*, causing soreness and bleeding.

PRESSURE POINT
One of the points on the body at which arteries lie near the surface, where the
pulse *can be felt and pressure applied to control bleeding. The illustration below*
shows the brachial artery pressure point, located on the inside of the upper arm.

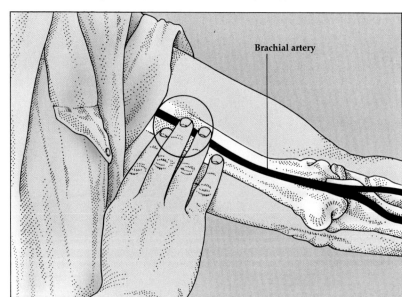

Brachial artery

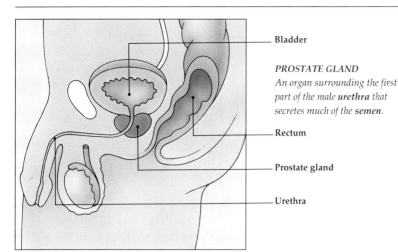

- Bladder

PROSTATE GLAND
*An organ surrounding the first part of the male **urethra** that secretes much of the **semen**.*

- Rectum
- Prostate gland
- Urethra

PROSTHESIS
*An artificial replacement for a missing or diseased part of the body. The illustration shows a prosthesis used to replace a hip joint damaged by **arthritis**.*

Proctoscopy
Examination of the anal canal and *rectum* using a viewing tube that is inserted through the *anus*.

Productive cough
A cough that brings up *sputum*; sputum that is clear is usually of no concern.

Progeria
Premature old age.

Progesterone
A female sex hormone produced by the *ovaries* that is essential for a healthy pregnancy; it ensures healthy development of the *fetus* by promoting normal growth and functioning of the *placenta*.

Progestin
Progesterone or progesterone-like hormones.

Prognosis
A medical assessment of the probable course and outcome of a disease.

Progressive muscular atrophy
A *motor neuron disease*.

Prolactin
A hormone produced by the *pituitary gland* that stimulates female breast development and milk production.

Prolactinoma
A noncancerous tumor of the *pituitary gland* that causes overproduction of *prolactin*.

Prolapse
Displacement of part or all of an organ or tissue from its normal position.

Prolapsed disc
Disc prolapse.

Prophylactic
A drug, procedure, or piece of equipment used to prevent disease; in popular usage the term also refers to a *condom*.

Proprioception
The body's system for collecting and analyzing information about its position relative to its surroundings and of body parts relative to each other.

Prostaglandin
Any of several hormonelike substances made in the body that produce a wide range of effects, including causing pain and inflammation in damaged tissue.

Prostaglandin analogue
A synthetic drug that acts like a naturally occurring *prostaglandin*.

Prostatectomy
Surgical removal of part or all of the *prostate gland*.

Prostate gland
See illustration above.

Prostatism
Symptoms (including a weak urinary stream and a frequent need to urinate) that result from enlargement of the *prostate gland*.

Prostatitis
Inflammation of the *prostate gland*, usually resulting from a bacterial infection.

Prosthesis
See illustration above right.

Proteins
Complex chemicals, made of *amino acids*, that form the structure of plants and animals and are vital for their growth and maintenance.

Prothrombin time
The time it takes for a blood sample to clot after adding clotting accelerators to it; the timing is done to check for a deficiency of blood-clotting factors or to determine the effectiveness of anti-clotting drugs.

Proton pump inhibitor
A drug that reduces the secretion of *gastric acid*; it is used to treat *peptic ulcers*.

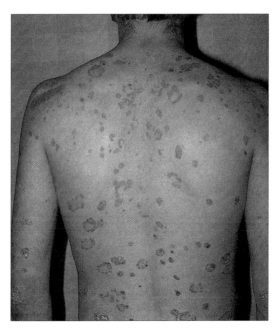

PSORIASIS
A common skin disease in which thickened patches of inflamed, red skin, often covered by silvery scales, appear on the body.

Proto-oncogene
A *gene* that is normally inactive in a cell but, if altered or "switched on," may become a cancer-causing *oncogene*.

Protozoan
The simplest, most primitive animal, consisting of a single cell, that is able to feed itself and reproduce.

Proximal
Describes a body part that is located closer to a point of reference than another body part.

Pruritus
Itching.

Pseudogout
A painful form of *arthritis* caused by deposits of calcium salts in a joint, usually the knee; it is most common in older people, especially after an illness.

Pseudomembranous enterocolitis
A severe, life-threatening, inflammatory condition of the *colon* that develops as a complication of the use of *antibiotics* by people whose immunity is weakened.

Psittacosis
A rare illness resembling *influenza* that can lead to *pneumonia*; people acquire it from exposure to the droppings of infected birds.

Psoralens
A group of drugs used along with ultraviolet light (in a technique called *PUVA*) to treat the skin disorders *psoriasis* and *vitiligo*.

Psoriasis
See illustration at left.

Psoriatic arthritis
A form of *arthritis*, usually affecting the finger joints, that develops in people with *psoriasis*; it can cause pitting of the fingernails.

Psychogenic
Originating from psychological or emotional problems rather than from a physical illness.

Psychosis
A severe mental disorder in which a person loses touch with reality.

81

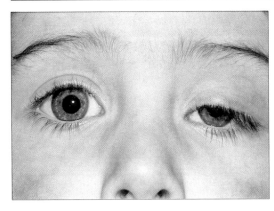

PTOSIS
A drooping of the upper eyelid.

Psychosomatic
Describes physical disorders that seem to have been caused, or worsened, by psychological factors.

Psychotherapy
A method of treating mental and emotional disorders using psychological techniques such as discussion, reinforcement, reassurance, and support.

Psychotic
Pertaining to *psychosis*.

Psychotropic drug
A drug that has an effect on the mind.

Ptosis
See illustration above.

Puberty
The period in a person's life when sexual characteristics develop, the sexual organs mature, and reproduction becomes possible.

Pubic louse
See illustration below.

Pudendal block
A type of localized *anesthesia* used to provide pain relief during childbirth.

Pudendum
The female *genitals*.

Puerperal sepsis
Infection that originates in the female *genital tract* within 10 days after childbirth, *miscarriage*, or *abortion*.

Puerperium
The period of time (about 6 weeks) following childbirth during which a woman's body returns to its prepregnant state.

Pulmonary artery
The artery that carries blood from the heart to the lungs.

Pulmonary stenosis
Narrowing of the *pulmonary artery* or *pulmonary valve*.

Pulmonary circulation
The route that blood travels from the heart, through the lungs, and back to the heart.

Pulmonary edema
A buildup of fluid in lung tissue, usually caused by *heart failure*.

Pulmonary embolism
See illustration at right.

Pulmonary fibrosis
Scarring and thickening of lung tissue, usually resulting from previous inflammation.

Pulmonary hypertension
Elevated blood pressure in the arteries that supply blood to the lungs.

Pulmonary insufficiency
A *pulmonary valve* defect that causes it to leak, thereby reducing the heart's pumping efficiency.

Pulmonary artery | Site of blockage
Heart | Lung
Route of embolus | Original site of embolus

PULMONARY EMBOLISM
*A life-threatening obstruction of the **pulmonary artery** or one of its branches. It usually occurs when a blood clot that has formed in a vein travels through the bloodstream to the lungs. A clot that travels from its site of origin is called an **embolus**.*

PUBIC LOUSE
A small, wingless insect (shown in the color-enhanced photograph below, magnified 45 times) that lives in the pubic hair and feeds on blood.

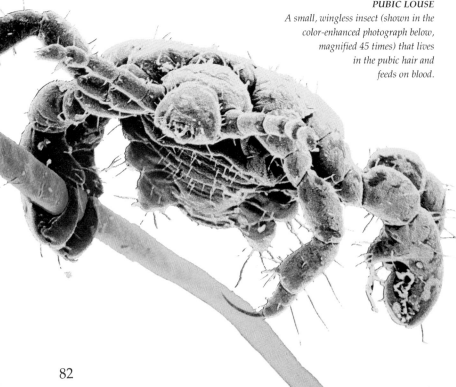

Pulmonary valve
The heart valve that prevents blood from flowing back into the right *ventricle* from the *pulmonary artery*.

Pulp
The soft tissue in the middle of each tooth that contains nerves and a rich supply of blood vessels.

Pulse
The rhythmic expansion and contraction of an artery as the heart pumps blood through it.

Pupil
The circular opening in the center of the *iris* through which light enters the eye.

Purpuric rash
A rash consisting of areas or spots of red, brown, or purple caused by bleeding in underlying tissues.

Pus
A pale yellow or green, creamy liquid made up of dead *white blood cells* and fluid that occurs at the site of a bacterial infection.

Pustule
A small skin blister containing *pus*.

PUVA
A treatment for skin disorders using a drug combined with controlled exposure to *ultraviolet light*; the letters stand for *psoralens* and ultraviolet A.

Pyelolithotomy
A surgical procedure to remove a *kidney stone*.

Pyelonephritis
Inflammation of the kidney, which is a common complication of *diabetes mellitus*.

Pyloric sphincter
A thickened, circular muscle in the stomach that controls the passage of food into the *small intestine*.

Pyloric stenosis
A narrowing of the muscle at the outlet from the stomach that slows the flow of food to the *small intestine*.

Pyloroplasty
A surgical procedure to widen the muscular outlet from the stomach.

Pyrexia
Fever.

Pyrogen
Any substance that produces fever.

Pyuria
The presence of *white blood cells* in the urine; it is usually a sign of a *urinary tract* infection.

Quadriceps muscle
The four-part muscle in the front of the thigh that straightens the knee.

Quadriplegia
Paralysis of the arms and legs, usually caused by damage to the *spinal cord* in the neck.

Quarantine
Isolation of a person who has a serious infectious disease or who has recently been exposed to one.

Rabies
A viral infection of the nervous system that is fatal if preventive treatment is not given; it mainly affects animals but can be transmitted to humans by the bite of an infected animal.

Radial keratotomy
A surgical procedure in which a series of tiny, shallow incisions are made on the *cornea* to correct mild or moderate nearsightedness.

Radiation
Any of a variety of types of energy in the form of waves or particles, including X-rays, radio waves, visible light, *ultraviolet light*, and gamma rays.

Radiation therapy
See illustration below.

Radical surgery
Extensive surgery aimed at eliminating a major disease (usually cancer) by removing all affected tissue and any surrounding tissue that might also be diseased.

Radioallergosorbent test
A test that detects the presence in blood of *antibodies* to various *allergens*; it is used to help find the cause of an allergy.

Radiography
The production of images of internal body structures by passing X-rays or gamma rays through the body and onto film; the image results from the varying amounts of *radiation* absorbed by tissues of different density.

Radioimmunoassay
A laboratory test that uses radioactive substances to measure the concentration of specific *antibodies* or *antigens* in the blood.

Radionuclide scanning
A diagnostic imaging technique based on the detection of *radiation* emitted by radioactive substances introduced into the body.

Radiopaque
Blocking the passage of X-rays or other forms of *radiation*; radiopaque substances such as barium are used to make organs stand out more clearly on X-ray images.

Radius
The larger of the two long bones of the forearm that runs down the thumb side of the arm.

Radon
A radioactive gas, formed in rocks such as granite, that may seep into houses from the ground; long-term exposure to radon may increase the risk of cancer.

Rales
Abnormal breathing sounds characterized by bubbling or crackling noises when a person inhales.

Rash
A group of spots or an area of red, inflamed skin.

Raynaud's disease
A disorder in which exposure to cold causes the small arteries that supply the fingers and toes to contract suddenly, cutting off blood flow and causing the digits to change color.

Receptor
A nerve cell that responds to a specific stimulus by producing nerve impulses; or an area on the surface of a cell to which a body chemical must bind to have its effect.

Receptor defect
A defect in a *receptor* that prevents the chemical that normally binds to it from having its effect.

RECONSTRUCTIVE SURGERY
Surgery to rebuild part of the body that has been damaged by injury, disease, some kinds of surgery, or the effects of aging, or that has been malformed since birth. The illustrations show reconstruction of a breast after surgery for cancer.

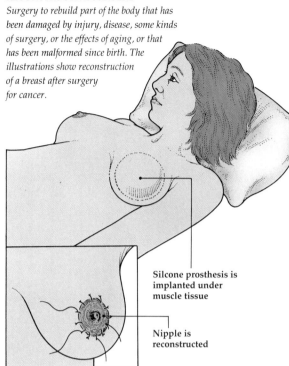

Silcone prosthesis is implanted under muscle tissue

Nipple is reconstructed

Recessive gene
A *gene* that produces an effect only when two copies of it are present or when a single copy of it is unopposed by a corresponding *dominant gene*.

Recessive inheritance
A pattern of inheritance that usually requires that a person inherit two copies of a particular recessive gene (one from each parent) to be affected by it; affected people have unaffected parents.

Recombinant DNA
Artificially produced *DNA*, formed by inserting a *gene* or part of a gene from one organism into the genetic material of another.

Reconstructive surgery
See illustration above.

Rectal prolapse
Protrusion through the *anus* of the membrane lining the *rectum*; it is usually brought on by straining during defecation.

Rectum
A short, muscular tube that forms the lowest part of the *large intestine*, where feces collect before being eliminated from the body.

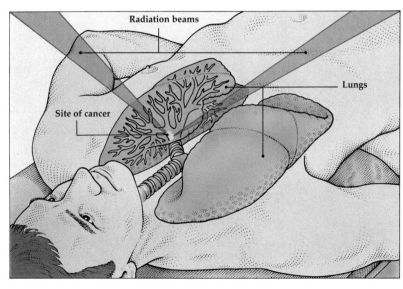

RADIATION THERAPY
*Treatment of cancer and occasionally other diseases by X-rays or other forms of **radiation**; as radiation passes through the diseased tissue, it destroys or slows the development of abnormal cells.*

Radiation beams

Lungs

Site of cancer

Red blood cell
See illustration at right.

Reduction of fracture
The technique of manipulating or surgically realigning displaced broken bone ends.

Referred pain
Pain felt in the body at a site other than its source.

Reflex
An action that occurs predictably and automatically in response to a specific stimulus.

Reflux esophagitis
A backflow of acid from the stomach into the lower part of the *esophagus* that is caused by inefficiency of the valve between the esophagus and stomach.

Regurgitation
The return of swallowed food or drink from the stomach back into the mouth; or the backflow of blood through a defective *heart valve*.

Rehabilitation
Treatment aimed at enabling a person to live an independent life after illness, injury, or drug or alcohol addiction.

Rehydration
Treatment of *dehydration* by the administration of fluids, sugar, and salts by mouth or by *infusion*.

Reiter's syndrome
A disorder in men characterized by *arthritis* and often *urethritis* and *conjunctivitis*; it usually follows a case of *nongonococcal urethritis*.

Relapse
The return of an illness after an apparent recovery or the return of symptoms after a *remission*.

REM (rapid eye movement) sleep
A phase of sleep during which the eye muscles contract rapidly and dreaming occurs.

Remission
A partial or complete disappearance of the symptoms of a disease.

Renal cell carcinoma
The most common type of kidney cancer.

Renal colic
Intermittent spasms of severe pain on one side of the back, usually caused by a *kidney stone*.

Renal tubular acidosis
A condition in which the kidneys are unable to excrete normal amounts of acid generated by the body's chemical processes.

Renin
An *enzyme* that helps to regulate blood pressure.

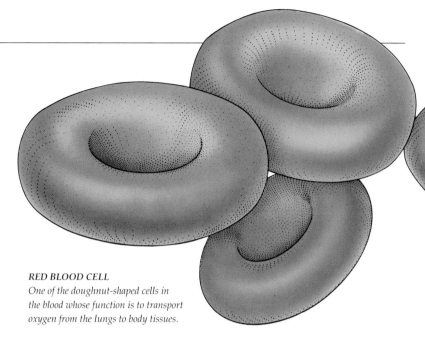

RED BLOOD CELL
One of the doughnut-shaped cells in the blood whose function is to transport oxygen from the lungs to body tissues.

Repetitive strain injury
See illustration below left.

Replication
The process of copying, duplicating, or reproducing.

Reproductive system
The male and female organs and connecting tubes and glands necessary for sexual intercourse and the production of offspring.

Resection
Surgical removal of all or part of a diseased or injured organ or structure.

Respiration
The processes by which *oxygen* and *carbon dioxide* are exchanged between body cells and the bloodstream and by which oxygen is used by cells to produce energy.

Respirator
Ventilator.

Respiratory arrest
Cessation of breathing.

Respiratory distress syndrome
A lung disorder caused by damage from illness or injury characterized by increasing difficulty breathing and resulting in a life-threatening oxygen deficiency in the blood.

Respiratory failure
A condition in which the *carbon dioxide* level in the blood increases and the *oxygen* level falls.

Respiratory system
The organs responsible for carrying *oxygen* from the air to the bloodstream and for expelling the waste product *carbon dioxide*.

Resting pulse
The *pulse* rate of a person who is at rest both physically and emotionally.

Restriction enzyme
A key chemical used in *genetic engineering* as biological scissors to cut *DNA* at specific points.

Reticulocyte count
The number of immature *red blood cells* in a blood sample; it is used to determine bone marrow activity and to help diagnose *anemia*.

Retina
See illustration above.

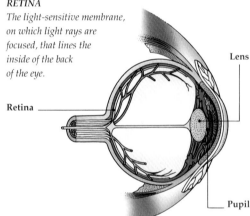

RETINA
The light-sensitive membrane, on which light rays are focused, that lines the inside of the back of the eye.

Lens

Retina

Pupil

Retinal artery occlusion
Blockage of an artery that supplies blood to the *retina*, causing loss of part of the *visual field* and blindness in that region; it can result from *arteriosclerosis* and *carotid artery* disease.

Retinitis pigmentosa
A *genetic disorder* in which nerve cells in the *retina* degenerate, causing a gradual loss of the *visual field*.

Retinoblastoma
An inherited cancer of the *retina* that affects infants and children.

Retinoid
A synthetic compound, similar to *vitamin A*, that is used to treat skin conditions such as *acne* and *psoriasis*; it may also help to eliminate fine wrinkles.

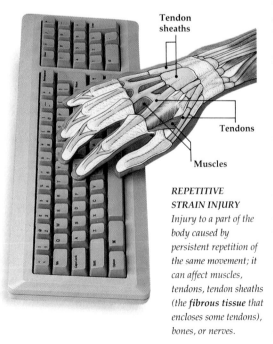

Tendon sheaths

Tendons

Muscles

REPETITIVE STRAIN INJURY

*Injury to a part of the body caused by persistent repetition of the same movement; it can affect muscles, tendons, tendon sheaths (the **fibrous tissue** that encloses some tendons), bones, or nerves.*

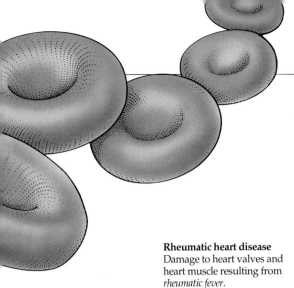

Retinopathy
Damage to or disease of the *retina* that often results from *diabetes mellitus* or persistent high blood pressure.

Retinoscopy
A test to assess nearsightedness or farsightedness by shining a beam of light into the eye and observing reflections of the beam back through the *pupil*.

Retroviruses
A large group of viruses whose genetic material is *RNA* instead of *DNA*; examples include the virus that causes *AIDS* and the virus that causes *T-cell leukemia*.

Reye's syndrome
A disorder primarily affecting children under 15 and characterized by brain and liver damage following a viral infection; it may be related to taking aspirin for the infection.

Rhabdoviruses
A group of viruses that includes the virus that causes rabies.

Rh blood group
A blood group classified by the presence or absence of a substance called Rhesus (Rh) factor on the surface of *red blood cells*; people with the substance are Rh positive, those without it are Rh negative.

Rheumatic fever
A disease that causes inflammation in various organs and tissues throughout the body following a throat infection with certain strains of *streptococci* bacteria.

Rheumatic heart disease
Damage to heart valves and heart muscle resulting from *rheumatic fever*.

Rheumatoid arthritis
See illustration below.

Rheumatoid factors
Specific *antibodies* found in the blood of 80 percent of people with *rheumatoid arthritis*; their measurement may help confirm a diagnosis of rheumatoid arthritis.

Rh immunoglobulin
A preparation given to prevent a pregnant woman with Rh-negative blood (whose fetus is Rh positive) from becoming *Rh sensitized*.

Rh incompatibility
A mismatch between the *Rh blood group* of a pregnant woman and that of the *fetus*.

Rhinitis
Inflammation of the *mucous membrane* that lines the nose, which causes sneezing, nasal discharge, and facial discomfort; when it occurs seasonally it is called *allergic rhinitis* (hay fever).

Rhinophyma
Bulbous deformity and redness of the nose, which is a complication of severe *rosacea*; it occurs primarily in older men.

Rhinoplasty
A surgical procedure to change the structure of the nose, either for cosmetic reasons or to correct an injury or deformity.

Rh sensitized
Describes a woman with Rh-negative blood who has developed permanent *antibodies* against Rh-positive blood as a result of exposure to Rh-positive blood from a *fetus* during pregnancy.

Eroded cartilage and bone ends

Painful, swollen joints

RHEUMATOID ARTHRITIS
*A chronic **autoimmune disease** in which joints become painful, swollen, and stiff. In severe cases, the cartilage (and eventually the bone underneath) is eroded and the joints become deformed.*

Rhythm method
A *natural method of family planning* based on avoiding sexual intercourse during the times when fertilization can occur.

Rib cage
The framework of bones attached to the spine and central breastbone that supports the chest wall and forms a protective shield around the heart, lungs, and other organs in the chest.

Riboflavin
A *vitamin* found in many foods that is essential for energy production and many other biochemical processes and helps to maintain healthy skin.

Ribonucleic acid
A substance that helps in various ways to decode the genetic instructions carried in the *deoxyribonucleic acid* (DNA) of cells.

Ribosome
A small structure found inside cells, composed of *RNA* and *protein*, that plays a part in protein production.

Any form of fungal skin infection marked by ring-shaped, reddened, scaly, or blistery patches.

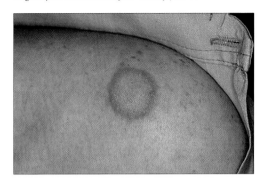

Rickets
A childhood disease, caused by a deficiency of *vitamin D* and other nutrients, that leads to bone deformities, usually in the legs.

Rickettsia
See illustration below.

Rigor mortis
The stiffening of muscles that occurs after death.

Ringworm
See illustration above.

Rinne's test
A test to diagnose *conductive hearing loss* using a vibrating tuning fork held near the outer-ear canal and against the *mastoid bone*.

RNA
Ribonucleic acid.

Rocky Mountain spotted fever
An infectious disease transmitted by ticks and characterized by small, pink spots on the wrists and ankles; the spots spread over the body, darken, enlarge, and bleed.

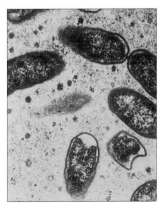

RICKETTSIA
A type of small bacterium, transmitted to people by insect bites, that has caused many of the world's worst epidemics. Rickettsia rickettsii, *shown in the color-enhanced photograph at left (magnified 18,000 times), causes **Rocky Mountain spotted fever**. Another species causes **typhus**.*

Rorschach (inkblot) test
A psychological test in which a person is asked to respond to a series of inkblots by saying what image or emotion each one evokes.

Rosacea
A chronic, *acne*like skin disorder of adults marked by an abnormally red nose and red cheeks; the cause is not known.

Roseola infantum
An infectious disease that primarily affects young children and is characterized by irritability, fever, and a rash.

Rotator cuff
A reinforcing structure around the shoulder joint that is composed of four muscle tendons that merge with the fibrous outer covering of the joint.

Rotavirus
A virus that causes *gastroenteritis* in infants.

Roundworm
Any of several types of long, cylindrical worms that are parasites of humans.

Rubella
A viral infection, also called German measles, that causes a mild illness with a rash and fever in children; if it affects a woman in early pregnancy it can cause harm to the *fetus* and lead to severe birth defects.

Rubeola
Measles.

Runners' knee
Pain on the outside of the knee, caused by a strain in the *fibrous tissue* that supports the knee joint; it occurs in long distance runners.

Rupture
A tear or a break in continuity of an organ or body tissue, such as occurs in the muscles of the groin in a *hernia*.

Saccharides
A large group of *carbohydrates* that includes sugars and starches.

SALIVARY GLANDS
The three pairs of glands – called the parotid, submandibular, and sublingual glands – that secrete saliva to aid digestion. The saliva travels from the glands through ducts into the mouth.

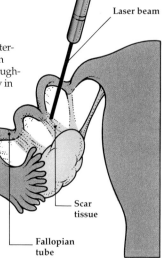

Parotid duct opens on the inside of the cheek

Tongue

Sublingual ducts release saliva under the tongue

Sublingual gland

Parotid gland

Submandibular duct opens on the underside of the tongue

Submandibular gland

Sacroiliac joints
A pair of rigid joints in the lower back that are located between each side of the *sacrum* and an *ilium*.

Sacroiliitis
Inflammation of the *sacroiliac joints*, usually caused by *ankylosing spondylitis* or *rheumatoid arthritis*, that produces aching pain in the lower back.

Sacrum
The large, triangular bone in the lower part of the spine that sits like a wedge between the hipbones.

Saddle joint
A joint, such as the joint at the base of the thumb, that has two interlocking, saddle-shaped surfaces.

SADS
Seasonal affective disorder syndrome.

Safe sex
A term used to describe preventive measures, such as using *condoms*, that can help reduce the risk of acquiring a *sexually transmitted disease*, such as *AIDS* or *gonorrhea*.

Saline
Salty, or containing salt; or a salt solution.

Salivary glands
See illustration above.

Salmonella
A group of bacteria including those that cause food poisoning and *typhoid fever*.

Salmonellosis
A form of *gastroenteritis* caused by ingestion of food or water contaminated with a type of *salmonella*.

Salpingectomy
Surgical removal of one or both *fallopian tubes*.

Salpingitis
Inflammation or infection of a *fallopian tube*.

Salpingography
X-ray examination of the *fallopian tubes* after injection of a *contrast medium*.

Salpingolysis
See illustration at right.

Salpingo-oophorectomy
Surgical removal of one or both of the *fallopian tubes* and *ovaries*.

Salpingostomy
A surgical procedure to make an opening in a blocked *fallopian tube*.

Saphenous vein
A long vein that runs just under the skin surface from the foot to the groin on the inside of the leg.

Sarcoidosis
A chronic disease of unknown cause characterized by inflammation in organs and tissues throughout the body, especially in the lungs, *lymph nodes*, liver, skin, and eyes.

Sarcoma
A cancer originating from any tissue – including muscle, bone, fat, or blood vessels – other than the skin or *mucous membranes*.

Saturated fat
A type of fat found in meats and dairy products; a high level in the diet may contribute to the development of heart disease and some cancers.

SALPINGOLYSIS
*Surgical removal of scar tissue that has formed between a **fallopian tube** and surrounding tissues. The scar tissue is either cut away with a scalpel or broken down with a laser beam.*

Laser beam

Scar tissue

Fallopian tube

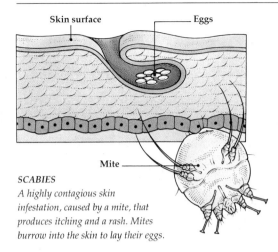

SCABIES
*A highly contagious skin
infestation, caused by a mite, that
produces itching and a rash. Mites
burrow into the skin to lay their eggs.*

Saturday night palsy
Temporary *paralysis* of
muscles in the forearm
caused by prolonged
pressure on a nerve in the
armpit; it can occur when
a person falls asleep with
an arm dangling over the
back of a chair.

Scabies
See illustrations above.

Scanning
Techniques used to record
and display an image of a
body organ or tissues for
careful study.

Scarlet fever
An infectious childhood
disease caused by a strain
of *streptococci* bacteria and
characterized by a sore
throat, fever, and rash.

Schistosomiasis
A parasitic disease, common
in tropical countries, that can
damage organs such as the
bladder or liver; it is caused
by a type of *fluke*.

Schizophrenia
Any of a group of serious
mental disorders characterized by disturbances in
thinking, emotional reac-
tion, and behavior; no single
cause for the disorder is
known, but inheritance is
thought to be a factor.

Schönlein-Henoch purpura
Inflammation of the blood
vessels, causing a *purpuric
rash* and leaking of blood
into the joints, kidneys,
and intestine; it occurs most
often in young children and
usually follows an infection
such as a sore throat.

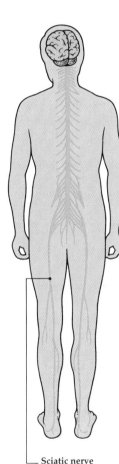

— Sciatic nerve

SCIATIC NERVE
*The body's longest
nerve, which extends
from the lower end
of the **spinal cord**
through the buttocks
and down the leg to
the foot.*

Sciatica
Pain that radiates along the
sciatic nerve down the leg,
caused by pressure on the
nerve that usually results
from a *disc prolapse*.

Sciatic nerve
See illustration below left.

Sclera
The tough, white, outer layer
of the eyeball that maintains
the eyeball's size and form
and is attached to muscles
that move it.

Scleroderma
An *autoimmune disease*, most
common in middle-aged
women, that can affect many
organs and tissues in the
body, particularly the skin,
arteries, kidneys, esophagus,
and lungs.

Sclerotherapy
A method of treating *varicose
veins* by injecting them with
a chemical solution that
eventually destroys them.

Scoliosis
See illustration below right.

Screening
The testing of apparently
healthy people to detect a
specific disease or disorder
at an early, treatable stage.

Scrotum
The pouch of skin and
muscular tissue that hangs
behind the penis and
contains the *testicles.*

Scurvy
A disease caused by inadequate intake of *vitamin C*
and characterized by
bleeding gums, weakness,
and bleeding into the skin,
joints, and muscles.

Seasonal affective
disorder syndrome
A form of depression that
seems to be related to the
shorter daylight hours of
the fall and winter months.

Sebaceous cyst
A large, smooth *nodule*
under the skin that contains
yellow, cheese-like material
consisting of skin debris and
sebum; it is usually noncancerous and harmless.

Seborrhea
Excessive secretion of *sebum*,
causing increased oiliness of
the face and a greasy scalp.

Sebum
An oily secretion produced
by glands in the skin; excess
production of sebum is
associated with the development of *acne*.

Secondary
Describes a disease,
disorder, or complication
that follows or results from
another disease.

Secretin
A hormone secreted by the
small intestine that stimulates
the *pancreas* to produce an
alkaline solution to aid
digestion.

Sedatives
A group of drugs that have a
calming effect; they are used
to reduce pain and anxiety,
induce sleep, and relax a
person before surgery.

Seizure
A sudden episode of uncontrolled electrical activity in
the brain, causing a temporary lapse in consciousness
or a series of involuntary
muscle contractions.

Selenium
A *mineral* needed by the
body in tiny amounts; it
is considered to be an
antioxidant.

Semen
The thick fluid mixed with
sperm that is secreted by the
male reproductive organs
and discharged from the
penis on *ejaculation*.

Semen analysis
A method of determining
the concentration, shape,
and mobility of sperm, usually to diagnose *infertility*.

Seminal vesicles
Two small pouchlike glands
located at the top of each *vas
deferens* that produce the
majority of the fluid in *semen*.

Seminiferous tubules
Tiny coiled tubes inside
the *testicles* in which sperm
are produced.

Seminoma
A type of testicular cancer
that can be treated effectively with *chemotherapy*.

SCOLIOSIS
*A common abnormality, usually starting in
childhood, in which the spine is bent to one side.*

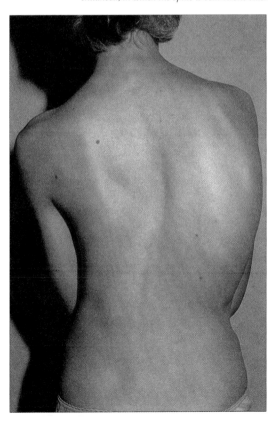

Sensate focus technique
A method taught to couples who are experiencing sexual problems that is aimed at making both partners more aware of pleasurable body sensations and reducing anxiety about performance.

Sensitization
The initial exposure of a person to an *allergen* or foreign *protein* that leads to a reaction by the *immune system*; on subsequent exposures the reaction is stronger and faster.

Sensorineural hearing loss
A type of deafness caused by damage to the inner ear or the *auditory nerve* that impairs the transmission of sounds from the inner ear to the brain.

Sensory cortex
The area of the brain in which sensory information is consciously perceived.

Sensory nerve
A nerve that carries information about bodily sensations to the brain or *spinal cord*.

Sensory organs
The specialized organs, such as the eyes and ears, that collect and relay information to the brain about the senses – sight, hearing, smell, taste, and balance.

Sensory receptor
See illustration above right.

Sepsis
Infection of a wound or tissues with bacteria, which leads to the formation of pus or to the multiplication of bacteria and accumulation of their *toxins* in the blood.

Septal defect
A birth defect characterized by a hole in the wall separating the two heart chambers.

Septic arthritis
A form of *arthritis* in which joint inflammation is caused by a bacterial infection that usually produces *pus*.

Septicemia
A life-threatening illness caused by the rapid multiplication of bacteria in the blood and the release of bacterial *toxins*.

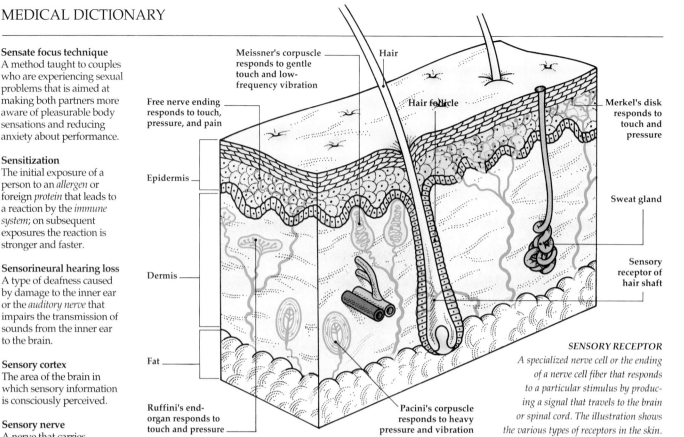

Meissner's corpuscle responds to gentle touch and low-frequency vibration

Hair

Free nerve ending responds to touch, pressure, and pain

Hair follicle

Merkel's disk responds to touch and pressure

Epidermis

Sweat gland

Dermis

Sensory receptor of hair shaft

Fat

SENSORY RECEPTOR
A specialized nerve cell or the ending of a nerve cell fiber that responds to a particular stimulus by producing a signal that travels to the brain or spinal cord. The illustration shows the various types of receptors in the skin.

Ruffini's end-organ responds to touch and pressure

Pacini's corpuscle responds to heavy pressure and vibration

Septic shock
A highly dangerous condition resulting from *septicemia* in which there is tissue damage and a dramatic drop in blood pressure.

Serotonin
A substance found in many body tissues that prompts small blood vessels to constrict at sites of bleeding, stimulates smooth muscle in the intestine to contract, and acts as a transmitter of nerve impulses between nerve cells in the brain.

Serum
The clear, thin, yellowish fluid that separates from blood when it clots.

Severe combined immunodeficiency
A usually fatal *genetic disorder* characterized by a deficiency of *immune system* cells that makes a person susceptible to infection.

Sex cell
Gamete.

Sex chromosomes
The *X* and *Y chromosomes* that determine sex; females have two X chromosomes, males have an X and a Y.

Sex gene
A *gene* on the *Y chromosome* whose presence determines that an *embryo* will develop into a male.

Sex hormones
Hormones that control the development of sexual characteristics and regulate various sex-related functions in the body.

Sex-linked disorder
A *genetic disorder* that is caused by a *gene* carried on a *sex chromosome* (usually the *X chromosome*); a male usually inherits it from his mother, who is unaffected.

Sexually transmitted diseases
Infections transmitted primarily by sexual intercourse or genital contact.

Sexual orientation
An individual's basic sexual attraction, either for members of the same or the opposite sex.

Shigellosis
A bacterial infection of the intestines that causes abdominal cramps, fever, and severe diarrhea, often with blood in the feces.

Shingles
An infection of the nerves that supply the skin, resulting in a painful rash of small, crusting blisters; it is caused by the same virus that causes *chickenpox*.

Shin splints
Pain in the lower part of the leg that worsens during exercise, caused by strain or damage to underlying structures.

Shock
A dangerous reduction in the flow of blood to body tissues that, if untreated, may lead to collapse, *coma*, and death.

Shock lung
Acute respiratory distress syndrome.

Shunt
An abnormal or surgically created passage between two usually unconnected body cavities or channels.

Sick building syndrome
A collection of symptoms (including loss of energy, headache, and dry, itchy eyes) sometimes reported by people who live or work in buildings served by closed ventilation systems.

Sickle cell anemia
A *genetic disorder*, occurring mainly in blacks, in which the structure of the *hemoglobin* in *red blood cells* is abnormal, causing the deformed red blood cells to plug blood vessels; it is characterized by chronic *anemia* and episodes of severe joint pain and fever.

Sickle cell trait
A less serious form of *sickle cell anemia*, in which only a small percentage of the *hemoglobin* is abnormal.

Sick sinus syndrome
Occurrences of abnormal heart rhythm caused by abnormal functioning of the heart's natural pacemaker, resulting in episodes of lightheadedness, dizziness, weakness, and fainting.

SIDS
Sudden infant death syndrome.

Sigmoid colon
The final, S-shaped section of the *colon*, which connects with the *rectum*.

Sigmoidoscopy
Examination of the *rectum* and *sigmoid colon* using a flexible viewing tube passed through the anal canal.

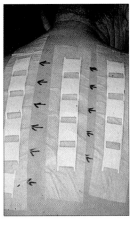

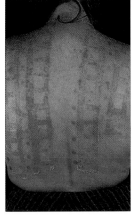

SKIN PATCH TEST
*A test in which patches of material containing suspected **allergens** are taped to a person's skin (left); doctors observe the skin (right) to determine which allergens cause a reaction.*

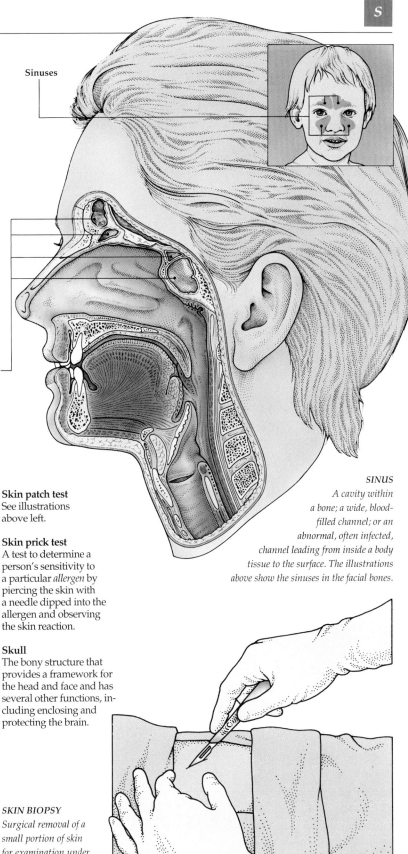

Sinuses

Sinuses

SINUS
A cavity within a bone; a wide, blood-filled channel; or an abnormal, often infected, channel leading from inside a body tissue to the surface. The illustrations above show the sinuses in the facial bones.

Silicone
Any of a group of synthetic substances that have been widely used as *implants* because they are resistant to body fluids and are not rejected by the body.

Silicosis
A lung disease caused by long-term inhalation of dust containing silica, a mineral (found in sand and rock) that is used in some manufacturing processes.

Single-gene disorder
A *genetic disorder* caused by a defect in a single *gene* or in a pair of genes.

Single photon emission computed tomography
An imaging procedure that uses technology similar to that of *computed tomography scanning* to produce cross-sectional images of tissues.

Sinoatrial node
The heart's natural pacemaker, consisting of a cluster of specialized muscle cells that emit electrical impulses that initiate heartbeats.

Sinus
See illustrations above right.

Sinus bradycardia
A slow, but regular, heart rate of less than 60 beats per minute caused by reduced electrical activity in the heart's pacemaker.

Sinusitis
Inflammation of the membrane lining the cavities (the sinuses) in the bones surrounding the nose, often caused by a bacterial infection after a cold.

Sinus tachycardia
A fast, but regular, heart rate of more than 100 beats per minute.

Sjögren's syndrome
A condition associated with some *autoimmune diseases* in which the eyes, mouth, nose, throat, and vagina become excessively dry.

Skin and muscle flap
A surgical technique in which a portion of skin and underlying muscle is removed and used to cover an area from which the skin and underlying tissue have been lost.

Skin biopsy
See illustration at right.

Skin graft
The transfer of a portion of skin from one part of the body to another to repair areas of lost or damaged skin.

Skin patch
An adhesive, drug-containing patch that, attached to the skin, slowly releases the drug into the bloodstream.

Skin patch test
See illustrations above left.

Skin prick test
A test to determine a person's sensitivity to a particular *allergen* by piercing the skin with a needle dipped into the allergen and observing the skin reaction.

Skull
The bony structure that provides a framework for the head and face and has several other functions, including enclosing and protecting the brain.

SKIN BIOPSY
Surgical removal of a small portion of skin for examination under a microscope.

89

MEDICAL DICTIONARY

Sleep apnea
Episodes of temporary cessation of breathing during sleep; it is most common in people who are overweight.

Sleeping sickness
A serious infectious disease of tropical Africa, spread by the bites of tsetse flies.

Sliding hiatal hernia
A type of *hiatal hernia* in which the stomach slides back and forth between the abdomen and the chest.

Slipped disc
Disc prolapse.

Slow virus diseases
A group of diseases that occur months or even years after a viral infection.

Small-cell carcinoma
The most dangerous and fastest spreading form of lung cancer; it is also called oat cell carcinoma.

Small intestine
The longest part of the *digestive tract*, beginning at the exit from the stomach and connected to the *large intestine*.

Smallpox
A highly contagious and often fatal viral infection that was common in the 19th century but has been totally eradicated by a worldwide *immunization* program.

Smear
A specimen for microscopic examination that is made by spreading a thin layer of cells onto a glass slide.

Smegma
A cheesy-white secretion that can accumulate under the *foreskin* of a man's uncircumcised penis or around a woman's *clitoris* if those areas are not kept clean.

Sodium
A *mineral* that is essential to maintenance of the body's water balance and blood pressure, the transmission of nerve impulses, and the contraction of muscles; it is present in table salt.

Sodium bicarbonate
An *antacid* used to treat digestive problems.

Solar plexus
A large network of nerves located behind the stomach.

Soluble fiber
A type of dietary *fiber* that is partially broken down by bacteria in the intestine.

Somatic
Of, relating to, or affecting the body.

Somatic cell
A general body cell as opposed to a *germ cell*.

Somatostatin
A hormone produced by the *hypothalamus* that inhibits the release of various other hormones.

Spasm
An involuntary muscle contraction.

Spasticity
Increased rigidity in a group of muscles that can lead to stiffness and restricted movement.

Spastic paralysis
An inability to move part of the body that is accompanied by involuntary muscle contractions.

SPECT
Single photon emission computed tomography.

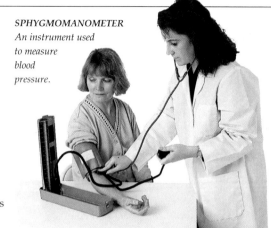

Speculum
A device for holding a body cavity open to enable a doctor to perform an examination or take a sample for study.

Speech therapy
Treatment to help people overcome problems with oral communication.

Sperm
The male sex cell that fertilizes the female egg.

Sperm antibody
An *antibody* produced by a woman's *immune system* that can destroy sperm.

Spermatocele
A harmless cyst in the *scrotum* that is filled with fluid and sperm; when small, it is usually painless and requires no treatment.

Sperm count
The number of normal, mobile sperm per unit of *semen*; the measurement is used to evaluate fertility.

Spermicide
A contraceptive preparation that kills sperm; spermicides containing nonoxynol 9 also help protect against *sexually transmitted diseases*.

Sphincter
A ring of muscle around a body passage or opening that acts as a valve.

Sphygmomanometer
See illustration above.

Spider nevus
A reddish-purple, raised dot on the skin from which small blood vessels radiate.

Spina bifida
A *neural tube defect* in which the spine fails to develop completely, leaving a portion of the *spinal cord* (usually in the lower back) exposed; it can be diagnosed in a *fetus* during pregnancy.

Spina bifida occulta
The most common and least serious form of *spina bifida*, in which there is little or no evidence of abnormality other than a hairy brown spot on the skin at the base of the spine.

Spinal anesthesia
Injection of a pain-killing drug into the area around the *spinal cord* to block pain sensation during surgery.

Spinal canal decompression
A surgical procedure to relieve pressure on the *spinal cord* or on a nerve root emerging from the cord.

Spinal cord
A cylinder of nerve tissue extending from the brain and running down the central canal in the spine.

Spinal fusion
A controversial surgical procedure to relieve back pain by joining two or more adjacent *vertebrae* with bone fragments obtained from the patient or from a bone bank.

Spinal nerve
A nerve that connects to the *spinal cord*.

Spinal tap
Lumbar puncture.

Spine
See illustration at left.

SPINE
*The column of 33 ringlike bones (**vertebrae**) that runs from the base of the skull to the **pelvis** and encloses the **spinal cord**. The spine is divided into the five regions indicated below.*

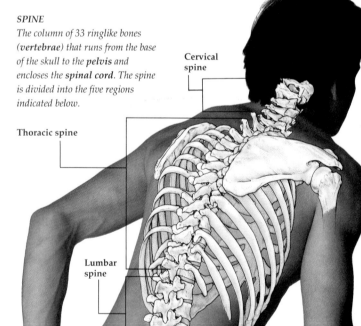

Cervical spine

Thoracic spine

Lumbar spine

Sacrum

Coccyx

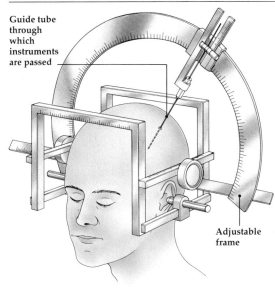

Guide tube through which instruments are passed

Adjustable frame

STEREOTAXIC SURGERY
*Brain surgery performed through a tiny hole in the skull and guided by X-rays or **computed tomography scanning**. A frame, shown above, is used to support the instruments used for surgery and ensure that they enter the brain at the correct angle.*

Spiral fracture
A corkscrew-shaped break in a long bone.

Spirochete
A spiral-shaped, mobile bacterium, such as the one that causes *syphilis*.

Spirometry
Tests performed using an instrument into which a person breathes to diagnose or monitor lung disorders.

Spleen
An organ in the upper part of the abdomen that removes and destroys worn-out *red blood cells* and helps to fight infection.

Splenectomy
Surgical removal of the *spleen*.

Splint
A device used to immobilize part of the body.

Splinter hemorrhage
A small, splinter-shaped bleeding spot under the nail; a feature of *endocarditis*.

Spondylitis
Inflammation of the joints between the *vertebrae* in the spine, resulting in backache and stiffness.

Spondylolisthesis
The slipping forward or backward of a *vertebra* over the one below, usually in the lower part of the back or in the neck.

Spondylolysis
A disorder of the spine in which parts of one of the lower *vertebrae* consist of relatively soft *fibrous tissue* that weakens the spine.

Sponge, contraceptive
Contraceptive sponge.

Spontaneous pneumothorax
A sudden accumulation of air in the space between the chest wall and the lung, causing the lung to collapse; it usually results from a ruptured blister on the surface of the lung.

Sporotrichosis
A chronic fungal infection acquired from plants and soil, usually through a skin wound; it occurs most often in gardeners and florists.

Sprain
See illustration below.

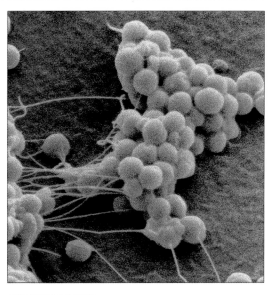

STAPHYLOCOCCUS
A common type of spherical bacterium that congregates in clusters like bunches of grapes. The color-enhanced photograph above shows a strain of staphylococcus known as Staphylococcus epidermidis *(magnified 22,000 times).*

Sprue
A chronic disorder caused by inability of the intestines to absorb nutrients from food, characterized by diarrhea and weakness.

Sputum
Mucus and other substances that are coughed up from the respiratory tract.

Squamous cell carcinoma
A slow-growing cancer of the skin, lung, and other sites including the *cervix* and *esophagus* that is derived from flat, platelike cells; on the skin it results from overexposure to the sun.

Stapedectomy
A surgical procedure to treat hearing loss caused by *otosclerosis*.

Staphylococcus
See illustration above.

Status asthmaticus
A life-threatening, prolonged attack of *asthma*, requiring emergency medical treatment.

Status epilepticus
Prolonged or repeated epileptic *seizures*, requiring emergency medical treatment.

STD
Sexually transmitted disease.

Stein-Leventhal syndrome
Polycystic ovary syndrome.

Stem cells
Cells, usually found in the bone marrow, that give rise to all the different types of blood cells in the body.

Stenosis
Narrowing of a duct, canal, passage, or tubular organ, such as a blood vessel.

Stent
A device that is used to hold a skin graft in place or to support tubular structures that have narrowed or are being joined.

Stereotaxic surgery
See illustration above left.

Sterilization
A surgical procedure to make a man or a woman incapable of reproducing.

Sternum
The breastbone.

Steroids
A group of chemically related natural or synthetic drugs and hormones that includes *corticosteroids*, *corticosteroid hormones*, and *anabolic steroids*.

Stillbirth
Birth of a dead *fetus* after the seventh month of pregnancy.

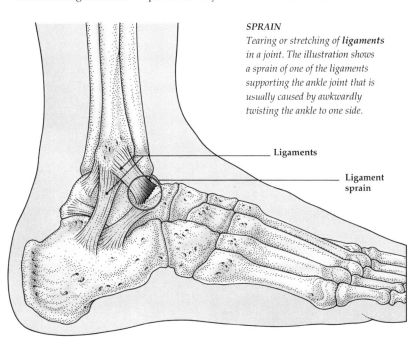

SPRAIN
*Tearing or stretching of **ligaments** in a joint. The illustration shows a sprain of one of the ligaments supporting the ankle joint that is usually caused by awkwardly twisting the ankle to one side.*

Ligaments

Ligament sprain

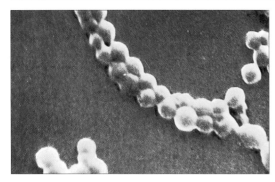

STREPTOCOCCUS
A common type of spherical bacterium that occurs in chains or pairs. The color-enhanced photograph above shows a strain of streptococcus known as Peptostreptococcus sp. *(magnified 7,000 times).*

Streptococcus
See illustration at left.

Stress fracture
A fracture that results from repetitive jarring of a bone.

Stress incontinence
Leakage of urine when coughing or laughing or while lifting heavy objects.

Stress ulcer
A *peptic ulcer* that may develop after shock, after serious injuries or burns, or during a major illness.

Stretch marks
Lines on the skin caused by thinning and loss of elasticity in the underlying layer; they often occur during pregnancy.

Stricture
Narrowing of a body passage.

Stroke
Damage to part of the brain caused by interruption of its blood supply or bleeding from a ruptured blood vessel, impairing sensation, movement, or function controlled by that area.

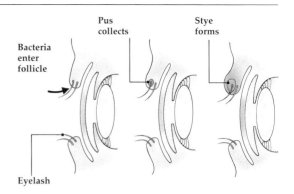

STYE
*A small, pus-filled **abscess** near the eyelashes that sometimes develops when bacteria invade the follicle of an eyelash and multiply, causing inflammation, swelling, and pain.*

Stokes-Adams syndrome
Adams-Stokes disease.

Stoma
A surgically formed opening – such as that created by a *colostomy* – to the surface of the body.

Stomach acid
Gastric acid.

Stomach bypass
A surgical procedure to divert food from the stomach into the *small intestine* when the stomach outlet is obstructed or to treat severe obesity.

Stomach stapling
A surgical procedure in which a small part of the stomach is partitioned off using metal staples instead of stitches; the operation is performed only as an extreme measure to try to treat severe obesity.

Stools
Feces.

Strabismus
An abnormal condition in which the eyes do not point in the same direction; examples include crosseye and *walleye.*

Strain
Muscle injury resulting from excessive physical force.

Strangulated hernia
A *hernia* in which the protruding organ or tissue becomes trapped, cutting off its blood supply; it often requires emergency surgery.

Strawberry nevus
A bright red, raised patch of skin that appears in early infancy and grows rapidly but, in most cases, eventually disappears.

Strep throat
A sore throat, caused by *streptococci* bacteria, that once commonly led to serious complications such as *rheumatic fever.*

Stye
See illustrations above.

Subarachnoid hemorrhage
See illustration below.

Subcutaneous
Beneath the skin.

Subcutaneous mastectomy
Surgical removal of all the tissue in a breast, leaving the overlying skin intact.

Subdural hematoma
A large blood clot between the outer and middle membranes surrounding the brain, usually following a head injury.

Subdural hemorrhage
See illustration below.

Submucosa
The layer of tissue that lies beneath a *mucous membrane.*

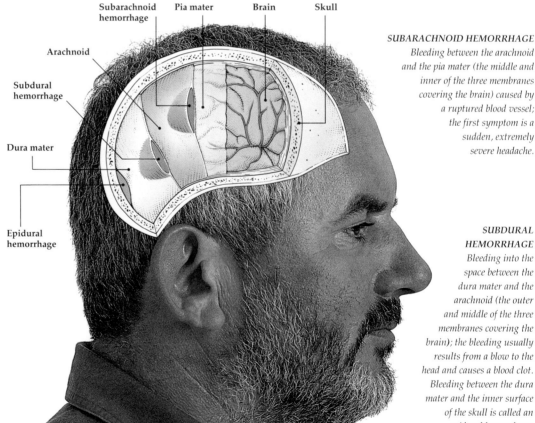

SUBARACHNOID HEMORRHAGE
Bleeding between the arachnoid and the pia mater (the middle and inner of the three membranes covering the brain) caused by a ruptured blood vessel; the first symptom is a sudden, extremely severe headache.

SUBDURAL HEMORRHAGE
Bleeding into the space between the dura mater and the arachnoid (the outer and middle of the three membranes covering the brain); the bleeding usually results from a blow to the head and causes a blood clot. Bleeding between the dura mater and the inner surface of the skull is called an epidural hemorrhage.

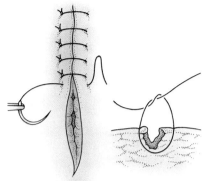

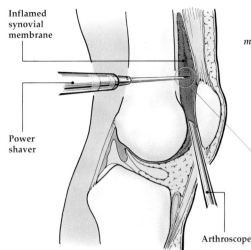

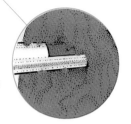

SYNOVECTOMY
*Surgical removal of the **synovial
membrane** to treat recurrent **synovitis**
(inflamed synovial membrane). The
inflamed membrane may be removed
using a viewing instrument called an
arthroscope and a power shaver
inserted through small incisions over
the joint (as shown at left for
the knee joint).*

Inflamed
synovial
membrane

Power
shaver

Arthroscope

SUTURE
*A surgical stitch used to close an incision or a wound. The type
of suture shown above, called an interrupted suture, is created by
passing a needle through both sides of a wound and knotting the
ends of the suture material together on one side.*

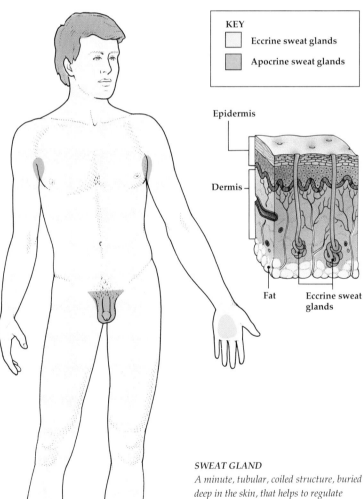

KEY

☐ Eccrine sweat glands

▨ Apocrine sweat glands

Epidermis

Dermis

Fat   Eccrine sweat
           glands

SWEAT GLAND
*A minute, tubular, coiled structure, buried
deep in the skin, that helps to regulate
body temperature by secreting sweat.
There are two types of sweat glands.
Eccrine sweat glands (shown in cross
section above) open directly onto the skin
and are found in most areas of the body.
Apocrine sweat glands open into hair
follicles and are concentrated in specific
areas, such as the armpits.*

Suction lipectomy
Liposuction.

**Sudden infant
death syndrome**
The abrupt, unexpected
death of an infant, which
cannot be explained even
after an *autopsy.*

Sunstroke
Heat stroke.

Suppository
A solid, cone-shaped,
medicated pellet made of
an inert substance, that is
inserted into the rectum or
vagina where it melts and
releases the drug.

Suppuration
The formation of *pus.*

**Supraventricular
tachycardia**
An abnormally fast heart-
beat caused by abnormal
electrical impulses in the
heart's upper chambers.

Surfactant
A mixture of substances
secreted by the tiny air sacs
of the lungs that prevents
the air sacs from collapsing.

Surgical drain
An appliance inserted into
a body cavity or wound to
permit drainage of fluid,
pus, or air.

Surrogate
A woman who agrees to
have a child that she will
give to someone else at birth;
this arrangement is controversial and now restricted
in some states.

Suture
See illustration above left.

Sweat gland
See illustration at left.

Sweat test
An evaluation of the
saltiness of sweat to help
determine if a person has
cystic fibrosis.

Swimmers' ear
An outer-ear infection
caused by germs that enter
the ear during swimming.

Sycosis barbae
Inflammation of the *hair
follicles* in the beard area,
resulting from infection
with bacteria.

**Sympathetic
nervous system**
The part of the *autonomic
nervous system* that predominates at times of stress; it
increases heart rate and
blood supply to muscles
and raises blood pressure.

Synapse
The junction between two
nerve cells across which
chemical messages pass.

Syndactyly
A *birth defect* in which two
or more fingers or toes are
fused together.

Syndrome
A group of signs and symptoms that, when they occur
together, constitute a particular disease or *genetic disorder.*

Synovectomy
See illustration above.

SYPHILIS

A sexually transmitted disease caused by a bacterium. Infection is initially characterized by painless sores on the genitals that, if untreated, are followed by a generalized illness and a rash (shown at right). If it remains untreated, syphilis can lead to widespread damage throughout the body and death.

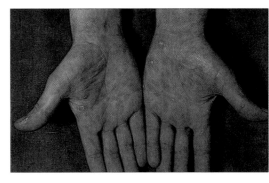

Synovial fluid
A clear, sticky liquid, resembling egg white, that lubricates joints.

Synovial membrane
A thin membrane lining the fibrous outer covering of a movable joint.

Synovitis
Inflammation of the *synovial membrane*, usually resulting from injury, that causes swelling, pain, and stiffness in the joint.

Syphilis
See illustration above.

Systemic
Affecting organs and tissues throughout the body rather than a specific part of it.

Systemic lupus erythematosus
An *autoimmune disease*, occurring predominantly in women, that affects many parts of the body including the skin, joints, heart, lungs, and kidneys.

Systole
The period during the cycle of the heartbeat in which the heart muscle is contracting and pumping blood.

Systolic pressure
Blood pressure measured while the heart is contracting; it is usually higher than *diastolic pressure*.

Tachycardia
An abnormally rapid heart rate of more than 100 beats per minute.

Tapeworm
See illustration below left.

Tar
A sticky brown substance that is inhaled in tobacco smoke and builds up in the lungs; it is a major cause of lung and other cancers.

Tarsal bone
One of the bones that make up the back part of the foot.

Tarsorrhaphy
A surgical procedure in which the eyelids are sewn together to protect the *cornea* from being scratched when people cannot close their eyelids because of nerve or muscle damage.

Tartar
A hard, crustlike deposit that can form on the crowns and roots of teeth and in the gums; excessive buildup causes gum disease and other dental problems.

Tay-Sachs disease
A *genetic disorder*, most common among Ashkenazi Jews, that causes severe nervous system disturbances and death, usually before the age of 3.

TB
Tuberculosis.

T cell
A *T lymphocyte.*

T-cell leukemia
A type of *leukemia* in which the abnormal *white blood cells* are T lymphocytes; it is caused by a virus similar to the one that causes *AIDS.*

Tear duct
A tiny channel that carries tears from the surface of the eye to the back of the nose.

Telangiectasia
A proliferation of small blood vessels in an area of skin, causing redness, usually on the nose or cheeks.

Temperature method
A *natural method of family planning* in which a woman seeks to determine the time of *ovulation* by taking her temperature daily; body temperature rises slightly at the time of ovulation.

Temporal arteritis
A disease in which arteries in the head, some of which pass over the temples in the scalp, become inflamed, causing a headache, weakness, and potential loss of vision.

Temporal lobes
The two lower, side lobes of the *cerebral hemisphere* that perceive sounds and smells and control some language functions.

Temporal lobe epilepsy
A form of *epilepsy* in which abnormal electrical discharges in the brain are confined to one of the *temporal lobes*; the person may have hallucinations and abnormal sensations of taste and smell. It can sometimes be corrected surgically.

Temporomandibular joint syndrome
A condition characterized by headache, facial pain, and restriction of jaw movement; it results when the jaw joints (the temporomandibular joints) and their supporting muscles and ligaments do not work together correctly.

Tendinitis
See illustration below.

Tendon
A strong fibrous cord, band, or sheet that joins a muscle to a bone.

Tendon transfer
A surgical procedure in which a tendon is repositioned to make a muscle perform a new function; it is used to restore function impaired by deformity or by permanent muscle injury or paralysis.

Tennis elbow
Painful inflammation of the outside of the elbow, resulting from overuse of muscles in the forearm.

Suckers for attaching
to intestinal wall

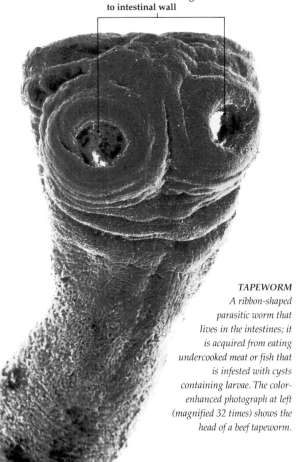

TAPEWORM

A ribbon-shaped parasitic worm that lives in the intestines; it is acquired from eating undercooked meat or fish that is infested with cysts containing larvae. The color-enhanced photograph at left (magnified 32 times) shows the head of a beef tapeworm.

Bony protrusion
from shoulder blade

Inflamed tendon

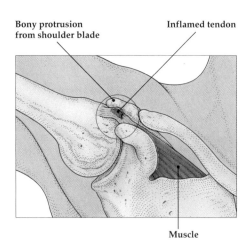

Muscle

TENDINITIS

Painful inflammation of a tendon, caused by injury, overuse, or prolonged pressure. The illustration shows tendinitis in the shoulder joint, which sometimes develops as a result of friction between the tendon and a bony protrusion from the shoulder blade when the arm is repeatedly raised above the head.

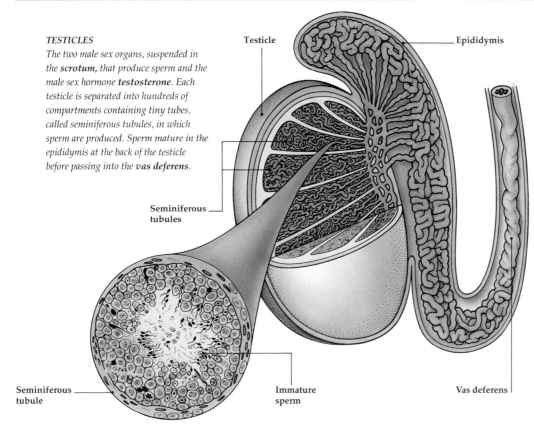

TESTICLES
*The two male sex organs, suspended in the **scrotum,** that produce sperm and the male sex hormone **testosterone**. Each testicle is separated into hundreds of compartments containing tiny tubes, called seminiferous tubules, in which sperm are produced. Sperm mature in the epididymis at the back of the testicle before passing into the **vas deferens**.*

Testicle

Epididymis

Seminiferous tubules

Seminiferous tubule

Immature sperm

Vas deferens

Tenosynovitis
Inflammation of the covering of a tendon, usually caused by increased pressure and friction from repeated movement of the affected part of the body.

Tenovaginitis
Inflammation or thickening of the fibrous wall of the sheath that surrounds a tendon.

TENS
Transcutaneous electrical nerve stimulation.

Tension headache
A headache associated with emotional strain or anxiety or with increased tightening of the muscles of the head and neck.

Teratogen
An agent, such as a drug or virus, that causes physical abnormalities in a developing *embryo* or *fetus*.

Teratoma
A tumor, usually found in an *ovary* or *testicle*, formed from tissues not normally found in that part of the body.

Termination of pregnancy
Abortion.

Testes determining factor
A *gene* on the Y *chromosome* that is thought to determine male sexual characteristics.

Testicles
See illustration above.

Testicular feminization syndrome
A rare *genetic disorder* in which a person who is genetically male develops female sex characteristics because the body's tissues do not respond to the male hormone *testosterone*.

Testosterone
A hormone produced by the *testicles* and in small amounts by the *ovaries*; it stimulates bone and muscle growth and the development of male sex characteristics.

Tetanus
A life-threatening disease of the nervous system caused by infection of a wound with a type of bacterium that is found in soil.

Tetracyclines
Antibiotics used to treat a wide range of infections, including many *sexually transmitted diseases*, *acne*, and *bronchitis*.

Tetralogy of Fallot
A form of *congenital heart disease* consisting of a collection of four heart defects and characterized by breathlessness and clubbing of the fingers and toes; surgery is required.

Thalamus
A structure deep within the brain that is an important relay center for sensory information coming into the brain; it may also play a part in long-term memory.

Thalassemia
An inherited blood disorder, characterized by defects in the production of *hemoglobin*, that results in *anemia* and irregular bone growth; it primarily affects people of Mediterranean origin.

Thallium scanning
A type of *radionuclide scanning* to assess heart function by determining how well different areas of heart muscle absorb a radioactive element called thallium, after it has been injected into the blood.

Therapeutic
Beneficial or relating to a treatment.

Therapeutic range
The dosage range over which a drug has a beneficial effect without producing side effects.

Thiamine
A *vitamin* – found in many foods including pork and green, leafy vegetables – that is essential for energy production and nerve and muscle function.

Thiazide diuretic
A type of *diuretic* that produces a moderate increase in urine production and is suitable for prolonged use under a doctor's supervision.

Thoracoscopy
Inspection of the membranes covering the lungs using a viewing instrument inserted through an incision in the side of the chest.

Thoracotomy
A surgical procedure in which the chest is opened to enable a surgeon to operate on a diseased heart, lung, or other organ that lies inside the chest cavity.

Thorax
The chest.

Thrill
A vibration caused by turbulent blood flow through a *heart valve* or an abnormal hole in the center wall of the heart that can be felt by placing a hand on the chest wall over the heart.

Thrombectomy
Removal of a blood clot (*thrombus*) from a blood vessel to restore circulation.

Thrombocytopenic purpura
A bleeding disorder that results from a deficiency of *platelets* in the blood; it is characterized by purple or reddish-brown discolored areas on the skin.

Thromboembolism
Blockage of a blood vessel by a fragment that has broken off from a blood clot elsewhere in the circulation.

Thrombophlebitis
Inflammation, often with formation of a blood clot, in part of a vein, usually one near the surface of the body.

Thrombosis
The formation of a *thrombus* inside a blood vessel.

Thrombus
A blood clot inside an intact blood vessel.

Thrush
Candidiasis.

Thymoma
A usually noncancerous tumor of the *thymus* gland.

Thymus
A gland, located in the upper part of the chest, that plays an important part in the *immune system*.

Thyroglossal cyst
A swelling in the neck that can occur when a duct that usually disappears during fetal development fails to do so; if the cyst becomes infected, it is usually removed surgically.

Thyroidectomy
Surgical removal of all or part of the *thyroid gland* to treat *goiter*, thyroid tumors, or *hyperthyroidism*.

Thyroid gland
A hormone-secreting gland in the neck that is essential for growth and *metabolism*.

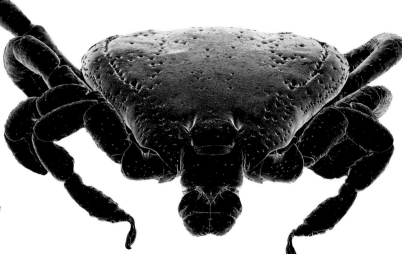

TICKS
*Small, eight-legged, blood-sucking creatures, some of which are capable of spreading infectious diseases such as **Lyme disease** and **Rocky Mountain spotted fever**. The color-enhanced photograph at right (magnified 23 times) shows a brown dog tick, which feeds on the blood of dogs.*

Thyroid hormones
The hormones secreted by the *thyroid gland*.

Thyroid-stimulating hormone
A hormone secreted by the *pituitary gland* that stimulates the *thyroid gland* to increase its secretion of hormones.

Thyroiditis
Inflammation of the *thyroid gland*.

Thyrotoxicosis
Various symptoms, such as a fast pulse and anxiety, that result from excessive secretion of *thyroid hormones* by the *thyroid gland*.

Thyrotropin-releasing factor
A hormone released by the *hypothalamus* that stimulates the *pituitary gland* to release *thyroid-stimulating hormone*.

Thyroxine
A *thyroid hormone* that helps control the rate of energy production in the body.

TIA
Transient ischemic attack.

Tibia
The inner and thicker of the two long bones in the lower leg; it is often referred to as the shinbone.

Tic
Involuntary, repetitive muscle movements, such as blinking or twitching, usually in the face.

Tic douloureux
Trigeminal neuralgia.

Ticks
See illustration above.

Tietze's syndrome
Pain in the chest similar to *angina pectoris* resulting from inflammation of the *cartilages* that attach the ribs to the breastbone.

Tinea
A group of fungal infections of the skin, hair, or nails; they are popularly referred to as *ringworm*.

Tinea versicolor
A rash consisting of discolored patches, caused by a fungal infection.

Tinnitus
A persistent ringing, hissing, or tinkling heard in the ear.

Tipped uterus
A condition in which the uterus inclines backward rather than slightly forward.

Tissue plasminogen activator
A substance produced in the body that dissolves blood clots; it is manufactured by *genetic engineering* as a drug to dissolve blood clots blocking *coronary arteries*.

Tissue typing
A series of tests performed to evaluate the compatibility of the tissues of a donor and a recipient before *transplant* surgery.

T lymphocyte
A type of *white blood cell* that acts to fight infections and cancer cells directly rather than by releasing *antibodies*.

T-lymphocyte killer cell
See illustration below.

TMJ syndrome
Temporomandibular joint syndrome.

Tolerance
The need to take increasingly higher doses of a drug in order for it to have the same effects.

Tomography
A diagnostic imaging technique that produces a cross-sectional image of an organ or part of the body; it is used with X-rays and *radionuclide scanning* to provide clearer images of organs or body parts.

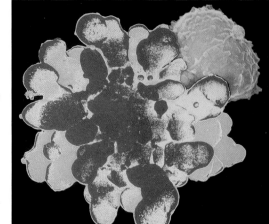

T-LYMPHOCYTE KILLER CELL
*A type of **T lymphocyte** that destroys invading germs and tumor cells. The color-enhanced photograph above (magnified 7,000 times) shows a T-lymphocyte killer cell (green) in the process of attacking a cancerous cell (pink and yellow).*

Tonometry
Measurement of the pressure of the fluid inside the eye, usually to detect and monitor *glaucoma*.

Tonsils
A pair of small oval masses of tissue at the back of the throat that helps fight upper respiratory tract infections.

Tonsillectomy
Surgical removal of the *tonsils*, usually performed in people with recurrent, severe *tonsillitis*.

Tonsillitis
Inflammation of the *tonsils*, frequently caused by a bacterial infection.

Torsion of a testicle
Twisting of the cord that is attached to a testicle, which cuts off the testicle's blood supply and may destroy it.

Total lung capacity
The volume of air that a person's lungs contain when he or she takes the deepest breath possible.

Tourette's syndrome
A disorder characterized by recurrent twitching, snorting, and sniffing noises, and involuntary shouting of obscenities.

Tourniquet
A device placed around an arm or leg to stop bleeding.

Toxemia
The presence of poisons in the bloodstream.

Toxemia of pregnancy
Preeclampsia or *eclampsia*.

Toxic epidermal necrolysis
A severe, blistering rash in which the surface layers of the skin peel off, exposing large areas of red, raw skin.

Toxicity
The degree to which a substance is poisonous.

Toxic shock syndrome
A life-threatening condition, caused by *toxins* produced by *staphylococci* bacteria, associated most often with the use of some highly absorbent tampons (now taken off the market).

Toxin
A poisonous substance.

Toxocariasis
Infestation (most often of children) with the *larvae* of a worm that normally lives in the intestines of dogs; it usually causes only a mild illness.

Toxoplasmosis
A common *protozoan* infection that is usually harmless; however, infection of a *fetus* during early pregnancy can result in miscarriage or stillbirth.

TPA
Tissue plasminogen activator.

Trace element
A *mineral* required by the body only in tiny amounts.

TRACHEA

*A thin-walled tube (also called the windpipe) composed of muscle, elastic **connective tissue**, and **cartilage**, that joins the **larynx** to the two main **bronchi**.*

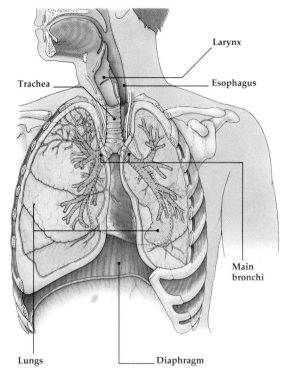

Larynx

Trachea — Esophagus

Main bronchi

Lungs — Diaphragm

TRACTION

A procedure in which part of the body is placed under tension to align two adjoining structures or to hold them in place. The illustration shows a traction technique used to align some types of fracture of the femur (thighbone).

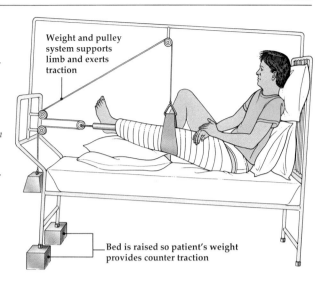

Weight and pulley system supports limb and exerts traction

Bed is raised so patient's weight provides counter traction

Trachea
See illustration above.

Tracheal breathing
The normal breath sound heard through a stethoscope from the area under the breastbone.

Tracheitis
Inflammation of the *trachea*, usually caused by infection.

Tracheoesophageal fistula
An abnormal passage that forms between the *trachea* and the *esophagus*; it may occur as a *birth defect* or as a result of surgery.

Tracheotomy
Nonemergency surgery in which a tube is inserted into the *trachea* to keep the airway open.

Trachoma
A persistent *chlamydia* infection of the *conjunctiva* and *cornea* that, if untreated, can lead to blindness.

Traction
See illustration above.

Trait
Any characteristic or condition that is determined by *genes*.

Transcription
The process by which the *genetic code* on a strand of DNA is converted into a matching code on an *RNA* strand during *protein* production.

Transcutaneous
Through the skin.

Transcutaneous electrical nerve stimulation
A method of relieving pain by applying minute electrical impulses to nerve endings beneath the skin.

Transferrin
A substance formed in the liver that transports iron throughout the body in the bloodstream.

Transfer RNA
A molecule of *RNA* that picks up a specific *amino acid* in a cell and lines it up with other amino acids in the correct order to make a particular *protein*.

Transient ischemic attack
A brief interruption in the brain's blood supply that results in temporarily impaired sensation, movement, vision, or speech.

Translation
The conversion of genetically coded instructions into a sequence of *amino acids* to make an essential *protein* inside a cell.

Translocation
The rearrangement of genetic information on a *chromosome*; or the transfer of a piece of one chromosome onto another.

Transmissible
Capable of being passed from one person or *organism* to another.

Transplant
To transfer an organ or tissue from one person to another or from one part of the body to another; or any organ or tissue that is transplanted.

Transurethral prostatectomy
See illustration at left.

Transverse myelitis
Inflammation of a localized area of the *spinal cord*, which can cause symptoms such as weakness or paralysis and numbness in the arms, lower part of the trunk, or legs.

Trapped nerve
Nerve compression.

Trauma
Physical injury or a severe emotional shock.

Traumatic arthritis
A form of *arthritis* that develops following an injury to a joint.

Travelers' diarrhea
Diarrhea – ranging from mild to debilitating, and lasting a few days – that can occur when a person visits a foreign country and ingests contaminated food or water; also called *amebic dysentery*.

Tremor
Involuntary, rhythmic, muscle movement caused by alternating contraction and relaxation of the muscles.

Triage
A system used to categorize injured people according to the severity of their injuries.

Triceps muscle
The muscle at the back of the upper part of the arm that straightens the elbow joint.

Trichiasis
An abnormal growing inward of the eyelashes that causes them to rub against the eyeball, which can result in loss of vision.

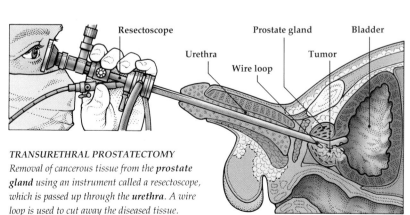

Resectoscope

Prostate gland   Bladder

Urethra   Tumor

Wire loop

TRANSURETHRAL PROSTATECTOMY
*Removal of cancerous tissue from the **prostate gland** using an instrument called a resectoscope, which is passed up through the **urethra**. A wire loop is used to cut away the diseased tissue.*

Trichinosis
An infestation with the *larvae* of a tiny worm, usually acquired by eating undercooked pork.

Trichomoniasis
See illustration at right.

Tricuspid insufficiency
Leaking of the *tricuspid valve*, which reduces the heart's pumping efficiency.

Tricuspid stenosis
Narrowing of the opening of the *tricuspid valve*, which puts a strain on the right side of the heart.

Tricuspid valve
The valve that guards the opening between the two chambers on the right side of the heart.

Tricyclic antidepressants
Drugs that are used to treat *depression*.

Trigeminal neuralgia
A disorder of the trigeminal facial nerve that causes bursts of excruciating facial pain in the area supplied by the nerve.

Triglyceride
The principal fat in the blood; measurement of its level can help in the diagnosis and treatment of many diseases, including diabetes, high blood pressure, and heart disease.

Trimester
See illustration above right.

Triple X syndrome
A *chromosome abnormality* in which a female has an extra *X chromosome*, which may cause a degree of mental retardation.

TRICHOMONIASIS
A sexually transmitted disease caused by a protozoan called Trichomonas vaginalis, illustrated below. In women, the infection causes an itchy, burning, vaginal discharge; infected men rarely have symptoms.

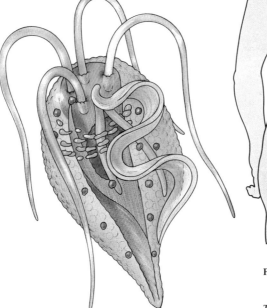

First trimester   Second trimester   Third trimester

TRIMESTER
One of the three periods of approximately 3 months each into which pregnancy is divided.

Trismus
Lockjaw.

Trisomy
The presence, in a person's cells, of three of a particular *chromosome* instead of the usual two; it is the cause of some severe *genetic disorders*.

Trisomy 21
Down's syndrome.

Trochlear nerve
A nerve that supplies a muscle that rotates the eye.

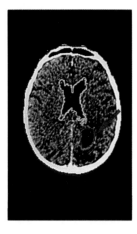

TUMOR
*An abnormal mass of tissue that forms when cells reproduce at an increased rate. In the color-enhanced image at left, produced by **computed tomography scanning**, a tumor is visible at the back of the right side of the brain (arrow). An untreated brain tumor can lead to brain damage and death.*

Trophoblast
The outer cell layer of a fertilized egg that develops into the *placenta* and *amniotic sac*.

Trophoblastic tumor
An abnormal growth that arises from the *trophoblast*.

Tropical sprue
A type of diarrhea of unknown cause that occurs in tropical regions.

Tubal ligation
A female sterilization procedure in which the *fallopian tubes* are surgically tied off and cut.

Tubal pregnancy
Implantation of a fertilized egg in a *fallopian tube*, causing severe abdominal pain and light vaginal bleeding; it can be fatal if not detected and treated.

Tubal reanastomosis
The surgical joining of the ends of a *fallopian tube* that has been severed in *tubal ligation* or from which a blocked section has been removed.

Tuberculin test
A skin test to determine if a person has been infected with *tuberculosis*.

Tuberculosis
An infectious disease caused by a bacterium that is usually transmitted by inhalation of infected airborne droplets; it primarily affects the lungs.

Tuberous sclerosis
A *genetic disorder* affecting the skin and nervous system characterized by an *acne*like skin condition, *epilepsy*, and mental retardation.

Tuboplasty
A surgical procedure to repair a narrowed or blocked *fallopian tube*.

Tumor
See illustration at left.

Tumor-specific antigen
A substance secreted by some tumors (or class of tumors) and in some conditions; its presence in the blood may be used to evaluate treatment.

Tunnel vision
A vision defect in which only objects that are straight ahead can be seen.

Turner's syndrome
A *genetic disorder* affecting females who have only one *X chromosome*.

Tympanic membrane
The *eardrum*.

Tympanoplasty
A surgical procedure to repair the eardrum and/or to reposition the tiny bones of the *middle ear* to treat hearing loss.

Typhoid fever
A serious infectious disease, with symptoms such as fever, headache, and digestive tract disturbances, caused by a *salmonella* bacterium transmitted in food or water.

Typhus
A group of infectious diseases caused by *rickettsia* bacteria that are spread by insects (such as lice and fleas) and mites.

Ulcer
An open sore on the skin or on a *mucous membrane* that is sometimes cancerous.

Ulcerative colitis
Chronic inflammation and ulceration of the *mucous membrane* lining of the *colon* and *rectum*.

Ulna
The long bone that runs down the forearm on the side of the little finger.

Ultrasound scanning
A diagnostic imaging procedure in which high-frequency sound waves are passed into the body and reflected back; a computer builds up an image of internal structures from the reflected waves.

Ultraviolet light
Invisible rays that produce the tanning and burning effects of sunlight.

Umbilical cord
The structure, consisting of two arteries and a vein embedded in a jellylike substance, that connects the *fetus* to the *placenta*; it supplies the fetus with oxygen and nutrients from the pregnant woman's blood and returns some waste products from the fetus.

Umbilical hernia
A condition present from birth in which a portion of intestine protrudes through a weakness in the abdominal wall, producing a swelling around the navel.

Unconsciousness
A state of loss of awareness from which a person can be aroused only with difficulty, if at all.

Undescended testicle
A *testicle* that has not descended into the *scrotum* from the abdomen, where it develops before birth.

Unsaturated fat
A type of fat or oil derived mainly from vegetable products that is thought to help reduce the risk of *coronary heart disease*.

Urea
A waste product of the breakdown of *proteins* and the main nitrogen-containing component of urine.

Uremia
The presence of excess *urea* and other waste products in the blood as a result of kidney failure.

Ureter
One of the two tubes that carry urine from the kidneys to the bladder.

Ureteral colic
Excruciating pain in the loin, resulting when a *kidney stone* gets trapped in a *ureter*.

Urethra
The channel by which urine passes from the bladder.

URINARY TRACT
The parts of the body – mainly the kidneys, ureters, bladder, and urethra – that are involved in the formation, storage, and excretion of urine. The urethra is much shorter in females than in males.

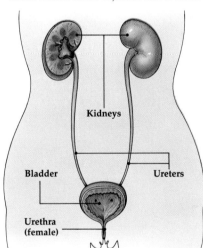

Kidneys

Bladder   Ureters

Urethra (female)

Urethral syndrome
Symptoms – including lower abdominal pain and frequent urges to urinate – of unknown cause that often intensify under stress.

Urethritis
Inflammation of the *urethra*, usually caused by infection, that results in a burning sensation and pain when urinating.

Urethrocele
Bulging of the *urethra* into the vagina, caused by a weakness in the muscles of the front wall of the vagina; it can be repaired surgically.

Urethrocystitis
Inflammation of the *urethra* and bladder, usually resulting from infection.

Uric acid
A waste product of the breakdown of *protein* in body cells; it is present in the blood and excreted from the kidneys in the urine.

Urinalysis
Chemical analysis, microscopic examinations, and other tests that can be performed on a sample of urine for diagnostic purposes.

Urinary antiseptic
An *antibacterial* drug that is used to treat recurrent infections of the *urinary tract*.

Urinary diversion
A surgical procedure to allow urine to pass out of the body through a channel other than the *urethra*.

Urinary incontinence
Involuntary urination with lack of control over bladder muscles; it is usually caused by injury, aging, or disease.

Urinary tract
See illustration at left.

Urine retention
Inability to empty the bladder completely.

Urticaria
A skin condition, commonly known as hives, that is characterized by itchy bumps surrounded by areas of inflammation.

Uterine inertia
Failure of the uterus to produce sufficiently strong contractions during *labor* to move the *fetus* through the birth canal.

Uterine prolapse
Descending of the uterus from its normal position, usually caused by stretching of supporting *ligaments* during childbirth.

Uterus
The hollow, muscular, female reproductive organ that sheds its lining each month during *menstruation* and in which a fertilized egg becomes embedded and a *fetus* develops.

Uveitis
Inflammation of the *iris* and the middle, blood vessel-containing layer in the wall of the eye (the choroid), which may lead to *glaucoma*.

Vaccination
Immunization.

Vaccine
A preparation that is given to induce *immunity* to a particular infectious disease.

Vacuum aspiration
A method of early (up to the 14th week) abortion in which the *fetus* and *placenta* are removed using a suction device.

Vacuum extraction
See illustration below.

Vagina
The muscular canal between the uterus and the external *genitals*; part of the female *reproductive system*.

VACUUM EXTRACTION
A procedure that helps to ease delivery by using a suction device attached to the baby's head; it is an alternative to forceps delivery. Suction created by a vacuum pump holds a cup in place on the baby's head while the obstetrician draws the baby through the birth canal by gently pulling on the device with each uterine contraction.

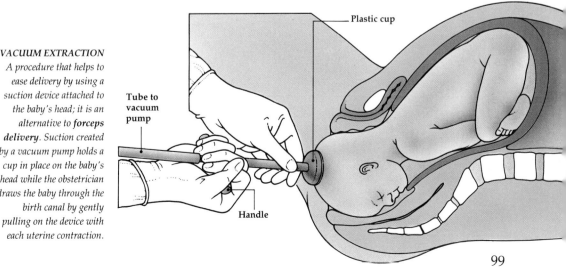

Plastic cup

Tube to vacuum pump

Handle

Vaginal ring
A flexible ring of silicone or other material that is inserted into the vagina to support the uterus following *uterine prolapse*.

Vaginismus
A painful, involuntary spasm of the muscles at the vaginal opening, making sexual intercourse difficult or impossible.

Vaginitis
Inflammation of the vagina, which can be caused by infection, *allergic reaction*, or an *estrogen* deficiency.

Vagus nerves
A pair of *cranial nerves* that regulate various functions, such as swallowing, speech, heart rate, and digestion.

Valve
A structure in a vessel or passage that allows fluid to flow in one direction, but closes to prevent it from flowing back.

Valvotomy
A surgical procedure performed to open up a narrowed *heart valve*.

Valvular heart disease
A defect in one or more *heart valves* that is present in *congenital heart disease* or produced by infection.

Valvuloplasty
Reconstructive surgery to repair a defective *heart valve*.

Varicella
Chickenpox.

Varicella-zoster virus
A type of *herpesvirus* that is the cause of both *chickenpox* and *shingles*.

Varices
Enlarged, twisted veins that occur in the legs as *varicose veins* and in the *esophagus* as *esophageal varices*.

Varicocele
A common condition in which *varicose veins* surround a testicle.

Varicose veins
See illustration above.

Variola
Smallpox.

Vascular
Relating to blood vessels.

Vascular headache
A headache that is caused by spasm and/or widening of the blood vessels in the brain and scalp.

Vasculitis
Inflammation of blood vessels caused by *allergic reaction* or occurring as a result of some diseases.

Vas deferens
One of a pair of narrow tubes that store sperm and carry it from the *testicles* to the *urethra*; both are severed in a *vasectomy*.

Vasectomy
See illustration below left.

Vasoconstriction
Narrowing of blood vessels.

Vasodilation
Widening of blood vessels.

Vasodilators
Drugs that widen blood vessels; they are used to treat disorders such as *angina pectoris* and *heart failure*.

Vasopressin
Antidiuretic hormone.

Vasovagal attack
Sudden slowing of the heartbeat brought on by pain, stress, shock, or fear, causing temporary loss of consciousness.

VD
Venereal disease.

Vegetative state
A term used to describe a type of deep *coma* in which only the basic body functions (such as breathing and heartbeat) are maintained.

Vein
A vessel that returns blood from the various organs and tissues of the body to the heart; by comparison, an *artery* carries blood away from the heart.

Vena cava
One of two major veins that drain deoxygenated blood from the body into the right side of the heart.

VARICOSE VEINS
Enlarged, twisting veins just beneath the skin, usually in the legs (shown at left) and occurring mostly in women.

Venereal disease
Any *sexually transmitted disease*.

Venipuncture
Piercing of a *vein* with a needle to withdraw blood or to inject drugs or fluid.

Venography
See illustration below.

Venom
Poison excreted by a snake, insect, or other animal in its sting or bite.

Venous thrombosis
A condition characterized by a clot in a vein.

Ventilation
The exchange of gases between the lungs and the surrounding air; or the use of a machine (a *ventilator*) to take over the breathing of a person who is unable to breathe on his or her own.

Ventilation scan
An image produced by a type of *radionuclide scanning* of the lungs in which a person inhales a radioactive gas.

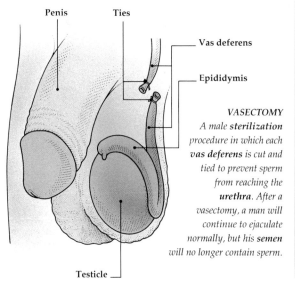

VASECTOMY
*A male **sterilization** procedure in which each **vas deferens** is cut and tied to prevent sperm from reaching the **urethra**. After a vasectomy, a man will continue to ejaculate normally, but his **semen** will no longer contain sperm.*

Penis Ties
Vas deferens
Epididymis
Testicle

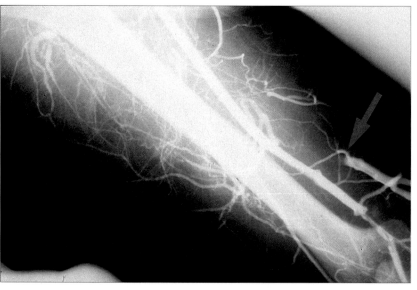

VENOGRAPHY
*A diagnostic imaging procedure used to examine veins after injection of a **contrast medium**. The venogram below shows a vein, just above the elbow, blocked by a blood clot (arrow). No blood flow is visible above the clot.*

Ventilator
See illustration at right.

Ventricle
A small cavity in the brain filled with *cerebrospinal fluid*; or either of the two lower, stronger, thicker-walled chambers of the heart.

Ventricular fibrillation
Rapid, ineffective, uncoordinated contractions of the *ventricles* of the heart that, if not treated immediately, can be fatal.

Ventricular septal defect
A hole in the wall (septum) between the *ventricles* of the heart; the most common *congenital* heart defect.

Ventricular tachycardia
An abnormally fast heartbeat of between 140 and 220 beats per minute that is initiated in the *ventricles* rather than by the heart's natural pacemaker.

Vernix
A pale, greasy, cheeselike substance that covers the skin of a newborn.

Version
Manipulation of a *fetus* in the uterus to change its position, usually to facilitate delivery.

Vertebra
See illustration below right.

Vertebral artery
One of the pair of arteries passing up the neck to supply blood to the brain.

Vertebrobasilar insufficiency
Intermittent episodes of dizziness, difficulty speaking, double vision, and weakness caused by reduced blood flow to the brain.

Vertex presentation
The usual, head-down position of a *fetus* at the time of delivery.

Vertigo
A feeling of faintness or dizziness.

Very low-density lipoprotein
A blood protein that transports *triglycerides* to tissues to be used for energy or stored as fat; a high level in the blood is associated with *coronary heart disease*.

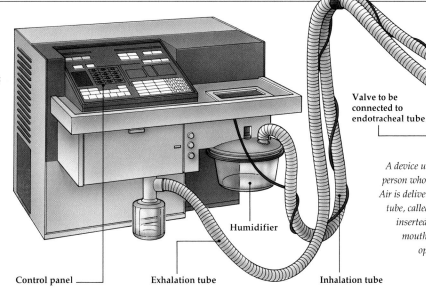

Valve to be connected to endotracheal tube

Humidifier

Control panel

Exhalation tube

Inhalation tube

VENTILATOR
*A device used to take over breathing in a person who has lost the ability to breathe. Air is delivered to the person's lungs via a tube, called an endotracheal tube, that is inserted into the **trachea** through the mouth or nose or through a surgical opening in the front of the neck.*

Vesicle
A small blister, usually filled with clear fluid, that forms at the site of skin damage; or any small saclike structure in the body.

Vestibular glands
Two small glands located on each side of the opening of the vagina that secrete a clear, lubricating mucus during sexual stimulation.

Villus
One of the millions of tiny, hollow, hairlike projections from the surface of the *mucous membrane* lining of the *small intestine*; the villi contain lymph vessels, blood vessels, and cells that absorb digested nutrients.

Vincent's gingivitis
Painful bacterial infection and ulceration of the gums, usually associated with poor oral hygiene; it is also known as trench mouth.

Viral
Of, relating to, or caused by a virus.

Viremia
The presence of viruses in the blood.

Virilization
The development in a woman of masculine characteristics as a result of overproduction of male sex hormones.

Virulence
The ability of a *microorganism* to overcome body defenses and cause disease.

Virus
A simple, tiny infectious agent that can multiply only by invading the cells of other *organisms*; more than 200 disease-causing viruses have been identified.

Visual acuity
Sharpness of vision.

Visual field
The total area on all sides that can be seen while looking straight ahead.

Visualization
The act of forming a mental image, used as a self-help technique to aid relaxation and concentration or to learn to cope with fear.

Vital sign
An indication – such as a *pulse*, a heartbeat, constriction of the *pupil* when exposed to light, or chest movements caused by breathing – that a person is still alive.

Vitamin
A complex chemical essential in small amounts for normal functioning of the body; vitamins must be obtained from the diet or from supplements.

Vitamin A
A *vitamin* – found in foods such as liver, eggs, and various vegetables and fruits – that is essential for formation of strong bones and teeth, for protecting the *mucous membranes* from infection, and for healthy skin, hair, and eyes.

Vitamin B complex
A group of closely related *vitamins* – including *thiamine, riboflavin, niacin, vitamin B₆, vitamin B₁₂, folic acid, pantothenic acid,* and *biotin* – that play an essential role in the body's chemical processing.

Vitamin B₆
A *vitamin* found in many foods that is essential for making *hemoglobin*, maintaining healthy skin, and regulating the functioning of the nervous system.

Vitamin B₁₂
A *vitamin*, found only in foods of animal origin, that is essential for the formation of *red blood cells* and the genetic material in cells and for the healthy functioning of the nervous system.

Vitamin C
A *vitamin* found in citrus fruits and vegetables that is essential for healthy bones, teeth, gums, and blood vessels and may also strengthen the body's defenses against infection; it is an *antioxidant*.

Vitamin D
A *vitamin* produced by the action of sunlight on the skin and found in oily fish, liver, eggs, and fortified milk and other dairy products; the vitamin enhances the absorption of calcium by the intestine and is essential for strong bones and teeth.

Vitamin D-resistant rickets
An inherited form of *rickets* in which the body is unable to use *vitamin D*.

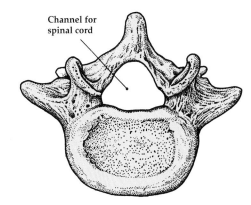

Channel for spinal cord

VERTEBRA
*Any of the 33 bones that form the **spine**. Vertebrae vary in structure depending on the part of the spine in which they are located. The vertebra shown in cross section above is from the lower (lumbar) region of the spine.*

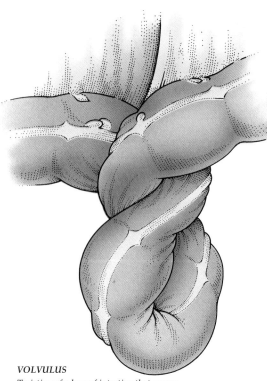

VOLVULUS

Twisting of a loop of intestine that causes intestinal obstruction. Surgery is usually necessary to treat the condition.

Vitamin E
A *vitamin* – found in foods such as vegetable oils, eggs, fish, and whole-grain products – that protects cells from damage caused by *oxygen free radicals*; it is an important *antioxidant*.

Vitamin K
A *vitamin* – found in foods such as leafy green vegetables and yogurt – that is essential for normal blood clotting and the body's use of calcium.

Vitiligo
A skin disorder – thought to be an *autoimmune disease* – in which patches of skin lose their color.

Vitreous hemorrhage
Bleeding into the *vitreous humor*, usually caused by diabetic *retinopathy*, that can lead to blindness.

Vitreous humor
The transparent gel that fills the large main cavity of the eye behind the *lens*.

VLDL
Very low-density lipoprotein.

Vocal cords
Two fibrous sheets of tissue in the *larynx* that vibrate as air is breathed out and that are responsible for voice production.

Volvulus
See illustration at left.

Von Willebrand's disease
A *genetic disorder*, similar to *hemophilia*, that is characterized by excessive bleeding after injury or surgery.

V/Q lung scans
Images produced by a type of *radionuclide scanning* of the lungs and the blood vessels in the lungs; the scans are used to diagnose a *pulmonary embolism*.

Vulva
The external, visible part of the female *genitals*, consisting of the *clitoris* and the *labia*.

Vulvitis
Inflammation of the *vulva*, caused by infection, aging, or an *allergic reaction*.

Vulvovaginitis
Inflammation of the *vulva* and *vagina*, usually caused by an infection.

WART

*A contagious, harmless growth on the skin or **mucous membrane**, caused by a **papillomavirus**. The size and appearance of a wart and the part of the body affected depend on which strain of the virus is involved. The warts on the thumb shown at right are known as common warts.*

Walleye
Strabismus in which the affected eye turns outward.

Wart
See illustration below right.

Weber's test
See illustration below left.

Wegener's granulomatosis
A rare disorder, of unknown cause, in which *granulomas* associated with areas of persistent tissue inflammation develop in the nasal passages, lungs, and kidneys.

Weight-bearing exercise
Exercise, such as walking, done against gravity to stimulate bone growth and build up bone density; it can help prevent *osteoporosis*.

Wernicke's encephalopathy
A brain disorder – characterized by confusion, unsteady gait, and abnormal eye movements – that primarily affects chronic alcoholics as a result of *thiamine* deficiency.

Western blot test
A blood test to detect the presence of *antibodies* to specific *antigens*, such as those on the *AIDS* virus.

Wheeze
A high-pitched, whistling sound produced in the chest during breathing; it is caused by narrowing of the airways, as in asthma.

Whiplash injury
An injury to the joints and/or soft tissues of the neck that is caused by sudden jerking of the head backward or forward; it often occurs in traffic accidents.

Whipple's disease
A rare intestinal disease, probably caused by a bacterial infection, that has many effects throughout the body, including *malabsorption*, weight loss, joint pains, swollen *lymph nodes*, fever, abnormal skin pigmentation, and *anemia*.

Whipworm
A large *roundworm* that infests the intestine, sometimes causing diarrhea and vomiting.

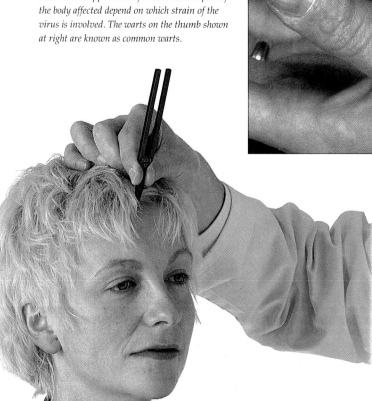

WEBER'S TEST

A test, used to help determine the cause of hearing loss, in which a vibrating tuning fork is placed against the forehead.

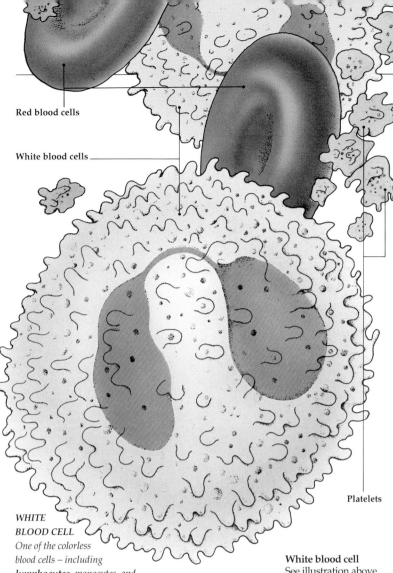

Red blood cells

White blood cells

WHITE BLOOD CELL
One of the colorless blood cells – including **lymphocytes,** *monocytes, and* **granulocytes** *– that play a central role in the body's* **immune system.** *White blood cells,* **red blood cells**, *and* **platelets** *(illustrated above at 6,000 times actual size) can be seen under a light microscope.*

Platelets

WILSON'S DISEASE
A **genetic disorder** *in which copper accumulates in the liver and is slowly released into other parts of the body, eventually causing severe damage to the liver and brain. A ring of golden-brown pigment around the outer edge of the* **cornea**, *caused by deposits of copper, is one of the characteristic signs of the disease.*

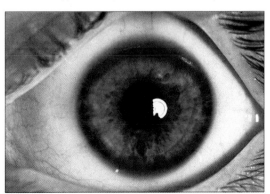

White blood cell
See illustration above.

White blood cell count
A count of the number of *white blood cells* in a blood sample; it is used to evaluate infection and diseases of the blood-forming organs.

Whitehead
A tiny, hard, painless, white blemish that may occur, usually in clusters, on the cheeks, nose, and around the eyes; it is common in babies and young adults.

Whitlow
A painful *abscess* on the fingertip or toe, caused by infection with the *herpes simplex* virus or with a bacterium.

Whooping cough
Pertussis.

Wilms' tumor
A type of kidney cancer that mainly affects children, usually before age 5.

Wilson's disease
See illustration at left.

Withdrawal bleeding
Vaginal bleeding associated with discontinuation of hormonal medication, such as occurs at the end of each cycle of the combined *oral contraceptive* pill.

Withdrawal method
An extremely unreliable form of contraception in which the male partner withdraws his penis before *ejaculation* occurs.

Xanthelasma
A condition characterized by yellowish deposits of fatty material in the eyelids, which is often associated with a raised level of fat in the blood.

Xanthine
A type of *bronchodilator* drug used to treat *asthma*.

Xanthomatosis
A condition in which fatty deposits accumulate in the internal organs, the brain, tendons, and the skin; if it occurs in the linings of blood vessels it can lead to *atherosclerosis*.

X chromosome
One of the two *sex chromosomes*; females have two, males have one.

Xeroderma pigmentosum
An inherited skin disease in which extreme sensitivity to light causes premature aging of the skin and an increased risk of skin cancer.

Xerophthalmia
An abnormal dryness of the *cornea* and *conjunctiva* of the eyes caused by a deficiency of *vitamin A*.

X-linked disorder
A *genetic disorder* determined by a *gene* located on the *X chromosome*; almost all those affected are males.

X-linked inheritance
The pattern of inheritance of a trait or disorder determined by a *gene* located on the *X chromosome*.

XYY syndrome
A group of characteristics – including unusual tallness, a slightly lowered intelligence, and behavior disorders – that occur in men who have an extra *Y chromosome*.

Y chromosome
One of the two *sex chromosomes*; it provides male characteristics.

Yeast infection
A term that usually refers to the infection *candidiasis*.

Yellow fever
A life-threatening viral disease transmitted by mosquitoes and characterized by fever, headache, nausea, jaundice, and nose bleeding.

ZIFT
Zygote intrafallopian transfer.

Zinc
A mineral essential in tiny amounts for normal growth and development and for wound healing.

Zinc chloride
A white, odorless powder used as an *antiseptic* and antiperspirant.

Zollinger-Ellison syndrome
A disorder in which *gastrin*-secreting tumors stimulate excess production of *gastric acid*, which causes recurrent *peptic ulcers*.

Zoonosis
Any infectious or parasitic disease of animals that can be transmitted to people.

Zygote
A fertilized egg produced by the union of an egg and a sperm; it is the first cell of a new person.

Zygote intrafallopian transfer
A method of treating *infertility* by artificially placing an egg (that has been fertilized in a test tube) into a woman's *fallopian tube*.

AMA HOME MEDICAL LIBRARY INDEX

The code letter that precedes each page number in the index indicates the volume of the AMA Home Medical Library in which to look. Page numbers in *italics* refer to illustrations and captions. A key to the volumes and their code letters is given here.

Diet and Nutrition D	The Brain and Nervous System J	Accidents and Emergencies P
Fighting Cancer E	Women's Health K	The Respiratory System Q

Practical Family Health A	Exercise, Fitness, and Health F	Bones, Muscles, and Joints L	Genes and Inheritance R
Diagnosing Disease B	Monitoring Your Health G	A Healthy Digestion M	Pregnancy and Childbirth S
Your Heart C	Know Your Drugs and Medications H	The Battle Against Infection N	Your Child's Health T

Photograph sources:
Audio Visual Services, St Mary's Hospital Medical School **29** (top right); **54**; **55**
Barts Medical Picture Library **49** (bottom right); **94** (top left); **69**
Biophoto Associates **52** (top left); **69**
Institute of Dermatology **89**
National Blood Transfusion Service **38**
National Medical Slide Bank **26** (top right); **52** (center); **63** (bottom); **72**; **79**; **87**; **100** (top); **103**
Moorfields Eye Hospital **82** (top left)
Quantum Medical Systems **42** (top)
Science Photo Library **2** (center left); **22**; **23**; **25** (top); **26** (top left); **29** (top left); **31**; **33**; **34**; **39**; **40**; **41**; **42** (bottom); **43**; **57**; **58**; **60**; **63** (top); **65**; **66**; **71**; **73**; **80**; **82** (bottom); **85** (bottom right); **91**; **92**; **94** (bottom left); **96**; **98**; **100** (bottom); **102** (right)
Tony Stone Worldwide **46** (right)
John Watney Photo Library **21** (bottom right)
Dr Ian Williams **47**; **68**; **81**; **85** (top right)

The joint prosthesis on page 81 appears courtesy of:
Smith & Nephew Richards Ltd, UK

Commissioned photography:
Steve Bartholomew
Jim Forrest
Yaël Freudmann
Stephan Oliver
Susanna Price
Barry Richards
Clive Streeter
Paul Venner

Airbrushing:
Paul Desmond
Roy Flooks
Trevor Hill
Imago
Richard Manning
Janos Marffy
Roger Stewart

Leader lines:
Graham James

Index:
Sue Bosanko

Illustrators:
David Ashby
Paul Bailey
Russell Barnet
Tony Bellue
Andrew Bezear
Russell Birkett
Peter Bull
Joanna Cameron
Karen Cochrane
Graham Corbett
Peter Cox
Paul Desmond
Sean Edwards
David Fathers
Bill le Fever
Evelina Frescura
Tony Graham
Andrew Green
Grundy & Northedge Designers
Trevor Hill
Chris Jenkins
Kevin Jones Associates
Lindum Artists
Janos Marffy
Marks Illustration and Design
Annabel Milne
Coral Mula
Karin Murray
Gilly Newman
Gillian Oliver
Lynda Payne
Howard Pemberton
Andrew Popkiewicz
James Robbins
Guy Smith
Lydia Umney
Philip Wilson
John Woodcock

La Dolce Vita

Michele Scicolone

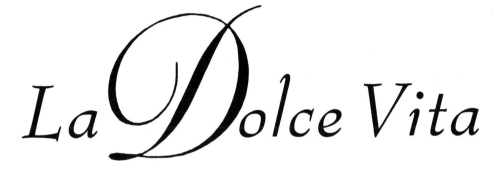

La Dolce Vita

Enjoy Life's Sweet Pleasures with
170 Recipes for Biscotti, Torte, Crostate, Gelati,
and Other Italian Desserts

Photographs by Susan Goldman

William Morrow and Company, Inc.

N e w   Y o r k

Library of Congress Cataloging-in-Publication Data

Scicolone, Michele.
    La dolce vita / by Michele Scicolone.
        p. cm.
    Includes index.
    ISBN 0-688-11149-1
    1. Desserts—Italy.   2. Cookery, Italian.   I. Title.
    TX773.S334   1993
    641.8'6'0945—dc20   92-2339
                                                     CIP

Printed in the United States of America

First Edition

1 2 3 4 5 6 7 8 9 10

BOOK DESIGN BY RICHARD ORIOLO

To Charles

Acknowledgments

The inspiration for this book came from the many marvelous Italian-style desserts I have tasted throughout my life. Friends, family members, and acquaintances encouraged me and contributed suggestions, recipes, and information. A heartfelt thank you to them all, especially my mother, Louise Tumminia, who first taught me to cook and bake, my aunt Loretta Balsamo, and my friends Kathie Devine, Henry Penas, and Carla and Bud Simons.

Thank you to my husband, Charles, who contributed the chapter on wines, digestives, and liqueurs and many other aspects of this book, and to Michelle Jones of Winebow, Inc., who supplied a great deal of information.

Just as important as the recipes and other material in a cookbook is the way they are put together. Thank you to my editor, Harriet Bell, for her vision of the book and invaluable input, to her assistant, Valerie Cimino, who is always helpful, photographer Susan Goldman for the luscious photos, Rick Ellis for styling the food so beautifully, Richard Oriolo for the overall design, and Judith Sutton for the sensitive copyediting.

A special thank you to my agent, Judith Weber, for her insight and unflagging interest.

Contents

Introduction

It always amuses me when someone says that Italians don't eat desserts. While it's true that they do not usually indulge in rich desserts as the last course of a meal, Italians eat sweets all day long. What with the thick fruit preserves slathered on morning toast, mid-morning *cornetti* (sweet croissants) with cappuccino, afternoon tea or coffee break with biscotti, after-dinner liqueur- or wine-spiked fruits and a late-evening gelato, Italy can certainly be described as a nation with a sweet tooth. Perhaps that is why they coined the phrase *la dolce vita*—life in Italy is sweet indeed.

Italians make many kinds of terrific sweets. Of course, there are the well-known creations such as cassata, sfogliatelle, and cannoli, but these are not the kind that I like best, nor are they the sort of thing most Italians would attempt to make at home. Ultrarich desserts such as these are reserved for special occasions and are usually purchased from the local *pasticceria*, or bakery shop.

My favorite Italian desserts are the simple sweets served at home or in informal trattorias that may not always look picture perfect, but are invariably delicious, satisfying, and easy to make. Thick-crusted *crostate*, or tarts, filled with fresh or dried fruit or pastry cream, colorful fruit compotes, ice cream and ice cream and fruit combinations, ices, semifreddi, puddings, plain cakes, and biscotti are the kinds of sweets I prefer. While I do serve many of these desserts to guests in my own home, sometimes I also serve cheese after a meal, often with fruit or a fruit sauce and a dessert wine. Then there are the marvelous *digestivi*, liqueurs and brandies that Italians typically drink at the end of a meal, either instead of or with dessert.

In an Italian-American household, such as the one in which I grew up, holiday desserts were always a multi-course affair. Immediately after dinner, we would dismantle the gorgeous fruit centerpiece that my father spent an hour or more assembling. With the skill of an architect, he constructed his masterpiece, polishing each pear and apple and balancing the pieces for color, shape, and size. My father delicately layered colored grapes, tangerines and clementines, bananas, and oranges. Wedges of fennel, which of course is not a fruit but a vegetable, were an important part of the assortment because Italians believe that fennel's soothing anise flavor aids digestion. Admirers and curious children were not allowed near the fruit sculpture until it was time for the fruit to be eaten. Then we would all dig in and demolish it.

In winter, baskets of hot roasted chestnuts were passed along with an assortment of almonds, hazelnuts, and walnuts to crack and munch with the fruit and the last of the dinner wine. Then the table was cleared. While some of the guests took a walk or a nap, the dishes were washed, the crumbs swept away, and the table reset.

Later we returned to the table for the "real" desserts—my mother's home-baked cakes and biscotti, often augmented by store-bought pastry.

Often, my father would choose a sweet wine to go with dessert. My favorite was always Asti Spumante, to which we sometimes added a few drops of Grand Marnier. There was always an assortment of liqueurs, brandy, and digestivi on hand. I was fascinated by the bright green, gold, and yellow bottles that my father offered guests from a silver tray. In addition to after-dinner drinks, most digestivi were also used for other purposes. There was blackberry brandy to cure stomachaches and bitter Fernet Branca for serious indigestion. Maraschino was used to flavor the *macedonia*, or fruit salad, and Marsala added to zabaglione. Anisette or sambuca spiked our after-dinner coffee, while grappa warmed us on a frosty day.

Last, but not least, was the coffee—always strong and black, made in our enormous old Napoletana-style coffee pot and served in my mother's beautiful demitasse cups that she had collected from all over the world.

Elaborate desserts such as these were reserved for holiday meals, however. On most days, our meals ended with fruit, perhaps some plain biscotti, or a simple spoon dessert.

This book is filled with sweets for every occasion from holiday dinners to family meals, from afternoon tea to an elegant dinner party. Many of these recipes are old family favorites, or were given to me by friends from their families' recipe files. Others are my interpretation of some of the contemporary desserts I have sampled while traveling in Italy. Even calorie counters will find many delicious choices among the fruit desserts and ices that are satisfying yet surprisingly low in calories and fat.

Most of these sweets are easy to make and many of them can be prepared in minutes. No special equipment is necessary and the techniques are as simple as can be.

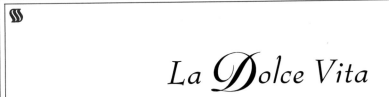

La Dolce Vita

Ingredients

Farina ✑ Flour

Gluten is a protein found in wheat flour. Flour with a high gluten content will result in a tougher or more chewy cake than a cake baked with a low-gluten flour. Bleached all-purpose flour has a protein content of about 11 grams per ounce, which is right for just about all but the most delicate cakes and pastries. All the baked goods in this book were tested with bleached all-purpose flour. Note that unbleached all-purpose flour has a slightly higher gluten content. Information on the protein content of flour is given on the side of the package.

The most commonly made mistake in baking is not measuring the ingredients properly. It is essential to use dry measuring cups for dry ingredients and a liquid measure for liquid ingredients. Dry ingredients should be spooned into the cup and heaped above the rim. Then the excess should be swept away and the contents of the cup leveled with a spatula.

Uova ✑ Eggs

Large eggs are used in all the recipes in this book. Using small or extra-large eggs may affect the results.

Eggs should be kept refrigerated with the pointed ends down. Crack eggs one at a time into a small cup and inspect them before adding them to the rest of the ingredients.

In many recipes, the egg whites are separated from the yolks so that they can be beaten to incorporate air. Added to a cake batter or mousse mixture, the beaten whites lighten the texture considerably. To beat egg whites, it is essential that the bowl and beaters be completely free of oil or fat and that the whites not have even a fleck of yolk, since the yolk contains fat. When separating egg whites and yolks, use three bowls, separating the eggs over one bowl to catch drips, then placing the whites and yolks in the other two bowls. That way, if you break a yolk, the entire batch of whites and yolks is not wasted.

Egg yolks are less likely to break when eggs are cold. However, for baking purposes or for beating egg whites, it is best to have the eggs at room temperature since they will blend more easily and whip up to a greater volume. You can either take them out of the refrigerator an hour or so before using, or simply place them in a bowl of warm water for five minutes. Dry the shells before cracking.

Noci e Semi ❧ Nuts and Seeds

Italians use mainly walnuts, hazelnuts, almonds, pistachios, chestnuts, and pine nuts in desserts, and they use quite a lot of them. Sesame and poppy seeds are used frequently, the sesame seeds in the South, where they were introduced by the Arabs, and poppy seeds in the North, probably because of the Austrian influence.

I generally buy nuts and sesame seeds in bulk at my local health food store. Since the store has a good turnover, these items are always fresh. They also have a large selection in different forms, including shelled, sliced, and blanched nuts.

Like all foods that contain oil, nuts and seeds can become rancid if they are kept for too long a period of time. Always taste and smell nuts and seeds before using them. If they do not smell sweet and fresh, they should be discarded or your dessert will have an off taste and smell.

Store nuts and seeds in airtight containers in the refrigerator or freezer so that they do not pick up flavors from other foods.

Unless they will be toasted during the cooking process, most nuts and seeds taste better if they are toasted before cooking. A light toasting brings out the flavor.

To toast shelled walnuts, hazelnuts, almonds, pine nuts, sesame seeds or poppy seeds, spread them in a single layer in a shallow pan. Place in a preheated 350°F. oven and bake, stirring occasionally, for 5 to 10 minutes. The nuts or seeds are done when they darken slightly. Let the nuts cool before chopping or grinding.

To chop nuts, place them on a cutting board and chop with a large knife. Nuts can also be chopped in a food processor, but be careful not to overprocess them or they will become pasty.

Mandorle / Almonds.

Almonds are sold either in the shell, shelled but with the skin on (unblanched), shelled with the skin off (blanched), sliced, or slivered. Blanched almonds are slightly sweeter than almonds with the skin on.

To blanch almonds, place them in a pan with water to cover. Bring to a boil, remove from the heat, and let stand for 1 minute. Drain and peel off the skins.

Nocciole / Hazelnuts or Filberts.

Hazelnuts are sold in the shell or shelled with the skin on. To remove the skin, toast the shelled nuts in the oven as directed above. When the skins begin to split, remove the nuts from the oven and wrap them in a towel. Rub the nuts with the towel to loosen the skins and then remove them.

Noci / Walnuts.

Walnuts are sold in the shell or shelled. To remove the skins, use the method described above for hazelnuts.

Pignoli / Pine Nuts.

Pine nuts are the seeds of certain pine trees extracted from the pine cones. Since harvesting them is a difficult process, these nuts can be very expensive. Pine nuts have a tendency to turn rancid quickly, so be sure they are very fresh when you buy them (return them to the store if they are not). Health food stores and many ethnic markets sell pine nuts in bulk as opposed to those available at the supermarket in high-priced little jars.

Castagne / Chestnuts.

Fresh chestnuts are sold in the shell during the winter months. Unlike other nuts, chestnuts must be cooked before they are eaten. Generally, they are roasted, but they can also be boiled or cooked in the microwave oven. Instructions for cooking and peeling chestnuts are given in the individual recipes.

Since peeling chestnuts is tedious, you may prefer to buy them already cooked and peeled. They come vacuum sealed in jars. Chestnuts are also available as a sweetened purée, good for ice creams and puddings.

Store fresh chestnuts in the refrigerator.

Burro & Butter

Whenever butter is called for, it means unsalted butter. Unsalted butter has a sweet fresh flavor, and using unsalted butter allows you to add salt to foods to your own taste. I do not like the taste of margarine and never use it. For baking purposes, butter will blend better with other ingredients if it is first softened to cool room temperature. You can either remove the butter from the refrigerator half an hour to an hour ahead of time or microwave it for a few seconds on low power. Be careful not to overdo it as the butter melts easily and in most cases melted butter will not give the same results as softened butter.

Cioccolata & Chocolate

There is nothing like good-quality chocolate. When you bite into it, it breaks with a snap. The pieces melt smoothly on your tongue. The flavor is rich and mellow, sometimes with a hint of coffee or spice.

Most of the recipes in this book call for semisweet chocolate, though bittersweet or sweet chocolate can be used. Do not substitute milk chocolate for semisweet, as the results will be quite different. My favorite brands include Callebaut, Perugina, Tobler, Lindt, and Maillard.

Chocolate chips are formulated to retain their shape in baking so they are not a good choice for melting.

There are several ways to melt chocolate, but never use high heat or the chocolate will scorch and become grainy. The simplest method is to break the chocolate up into a bowl and set the bowl over, not in, hot water. When the chocolate is softened, remove it from the heat and stir until it is completely smooth. Chocolate can also be melted in the microwave oven. Check the instructions given by your oven's manufacturer and use low or moderate power.

No matter which method you choose, always be sure that there is no water in the bowl with the chocolate or it may "seize." If this should happen, you may be able to restore the texture by stirring in a teaspoon of solid vegetable shortening for each ounce of chocolate.

Cacao ❦ Cocoa

Dutch-process cocoa is less bitter and has better chocolate flavor than ordinary cocoa. Dröste is the most commonly available brand of Dutch-process cocoa.

Farina di Granturco ❦ Cornmeal

Cornmeal adds a pleasant crunch and sweet flavor to a number of biscotti and cakes that are specialties of Northern Italy. For best flavor and fine texture, use fine yellow cornmeal, preferably stone-ground.

Olio d'Oliva ❦ Olive Oil

A number of the recipes in this book call for olive oil. For baking, a mild-tasting olive oil is preferable so that it will not interfere with the delicate flavors of cakes and cookies. Some extra-virgin olive oils are too rich for this purpose. I generally use a pure grade of oil or a mild-tasting extra-virgin oil.

Biscotti

〰〰〰

COOKIES

Nutty biscotti have recently become the rage in this country, but Italians have been enjoying them for ages. Historians trace their origins to little cakes made with honey and nuts that were eaten by the Romans on festive occasions. Later, sailors found that bread baked twice so it was hard and dry would keep better on long sea voyages. Somehow the two ideas were joined and the name biscotti, meaning "twice-baked," came to be applied to all kinds of cookies and crackers.

Italians eat biscotti for breakfast, as a snack with coffee or milk, or after a meal with wine. Since Italian biscotti are often hard, they are usually dunked or, as the Italians say, inzuppato ("soaked"), before eating. Real Italian biscotti tend to be far less rich than some of the biscotti that have become popular here, and many are low in sugar and fat.

There are all kinds of biscotti in this chapter. Some are authentically Italian, like the classic Biscotti di Prato, worthy enough to be dunked in your finest vin santo or Marsala. Others are pure fantasy, inspired by the Italian originals but nowhere to be found in Italy. Some are delicate and some are hearty, but all are delicious and fun to make and eat.

Tips for Making Biscotti

- Heavy-duty baking sheets are essential to prevent cookies and other baked foods from sticking or scorching on the bottom. Look for baking sheets that have only one turned-up end. These make it easier to slide logs of biscotti off the sheet.

- Unless a recipe recommends otherwise, buttering and flouring baking sheets helps to prevent the cookies from sticking as they bake. To do so, lightly butter the baking sheet. Sprinkle all-purpose flour over the pan and tilt it to spread the flour evenly. Then tap the pan on a countertop and tilt the pan to remove excess flour. A large salt shaker filled with all-purpose flour is handy for dusting pans.

- When baking biscotti of any kind, it is best to bake only one sheet at a time. The pan can be placed in the center of the oven where the air can circulate around it and the cookies will bake evenly. If you must put two pans in the oven at one time, be sure to rotate them halfway through the baking time.

- Some biscotti doughs are quite sticky. For easier handling, dampen your hands before shaping the dough into logs. Another technique is to use two spoons to drop the dough into a row of closely spaced mounds onto the baking sheet. With a rubber spatula, connect the mounds and smooth the sides.

- If the weather is hot and humid, you may need to chill the dough for easier handling before baking it.

- To cut a log of baked dough into even slices for biscotti, let the log cool on the baking sheet for at least ten minutes, or until it is firm enough to move. Use a long metal spatula to slide the log onto a cutting board. Position a large heavy chef's knife at an angle across the log, placing the tip on the board. Then press down firmly to cut through the log.

- Store baked cookies in a tightly sealed tin once they are thoroughly cooled. Most will keep for at least three weeks, though some will last much longer.

$\mathcal{B}$iscotti di Noci

ALMOND AND HAZELNUT BISCOTTI

Makes 8 dozen

If I had to trace the origin of the idea for this book, it would lead me to this recipe. I began developing it a number of years ago, adjusting and reworking it until it suited my taste exactly. Along the way, I collected numerous other biscotti recipes, though these are still my favorite. They are just rich and sweet enough and are always a pleasure to have on hand.

1½ cups toasted almonds

½ cup hazelnuts, toasted and skinned (page 3)

4 cups all-purpose flour

2 teaspoons baking powder

1 teaspoon ground cinnamon

5 large eggs, at room temperature

8 tablespoons (1 stick) unsalted butter, melted and cooled

2 cups sugar

1½ teaspoons grated lemon zest

1. Preheat the oven to 350°F. Butter two large baking sheets.
2. In a food processor or blender, finely grind ½ cup of the almonds. Coarsely chop the remaining 1 cup almonds and the hazelnuts.
3. Combine the flour, baking powder and cinnamon. Stir in the ground and chopped nuts.
4. In a large bowl, whisk the eggs until frothy. Stir in the melted butter, sugar, and lemon zest just until combined. With a wooden spoon, stir in the dry ingredients until blended. The dough will be sticky.
5. Drop the dough by large spoonfuls onto the baking sheets to form four 12-inch strips spaced about 4 inches apart. Smooth the tops and sides of each strip with a rubber spatula. Bake for 25 minutes, or until the strips are firm when pressed in the center. Remove from the oven but do not turn it off. Let the strips cool for 10 minutes.

continued

6. Slide the strips onto a cutting board and, with a heavy knife, cut them diagonally into ½-inch slices. Place the slices upright on the baking sheets. Bake for 20 minutes, or until crisp. Transfer to wire racks to cool.

$\mathscr{B}$iscotti di Prato
TUSCAN ALMOND BISCOTTI
Makes 4½ dozen

The medieval town of Prato, near Florence, is credited with making the best almond biscuits, sometimes called *cantucci*, in all of Tuscany. These hard, crunchy cookies are meant to be dunked in vin santo, an amber-colored dessert wine. This "holy" wine gets its name from a Greek bishop who attended a church conference in Florence in 1439. When he tasted the wine, he exclaimed, "This is the wine of Xantos!" referring to the good wine from his homeland. But his colleagues understood him to be calling the wine *santo*, meaning "holy," and the name stuck.

The plain, simple flavor of these cookies is classically Tuscan. They never compete with wine, but when enjoyed together the result can only be described as ambrosial.

2½ **cups all-purpose flour**

1 **teaspoon baking powder**

½ **teaspoon baking soda**

1 **teaspoon salt**

4 **large eggs**

¾ **cup sugar**

1 **teaspoon grated orange zest**

1½ **teaspoons vanilla extract**

1 **cup toasted almonds, coarsely chopped**

1. Preheat the oven to 325°F. Butter and flour a large baking sheet.
2. Sift together the flour, baking powder, baking soda, and salt.

3. In a large bowl, beat the eggs and sugar until light and foamy. Beat in the orange zest and vanilla. Stir in the dry ingredients, then stir in the almonds.

4. Shape the dough into two 14- by 2-inch logs about 4 inches apart on the prepared baking sheet. Smooth the tops and sides with a rubber spatula. Bake for 30 minutes, or until firm and golden. Remove the baking sheet from the oven and reduce the oven heat to 275°F. Let the logs cool for 10 minutes.

5. Transfer the logs to a cutting board. With a large heavy chef's knife, cut the logs diagonally into ½-inch slices. Stand the slices about ½ inch apart on the baking sheet. Bake for 30 minutes, or until lightly toasted. Transfer to wire racks to cool.

Henry's Biscotti

Makes 8 dozen

〽 My friend Henry Penas makes tender yet crisp biscotti that everyone seems to love. They are made with olive oil, and they are more tender than some of the other variations.

Chopped dried fruits such as figs or prunes can be substitued for the candied cherries.

2¾ cups all-purpose flour
1 teaspoon baking powder
1 teaspoon ground cinnamon
1 teaspoon salt
3 large eggs
1 cup sugar
1 cup olive oil
1 teaspoon vanilla extract
½ teaspoon lemon extract
1 cup chopped toasted walnuts
1½ cups candied cherries

1. Preheat the oven to 325°F. Butter two large baking sheets.

2. Combine the flour, baking powder, salt, and cinnamon.

3. In a large bowl, beat the eggs, sugar, olive oil, and the extracts until well blended. Stir in the dry ingredients. Then stir in the walnuts and cherries. The dough will be very soft.

4. Divide the dough in quarters. Shape the dough into four 12- by 2-inch logs about 4 inches apart on the prepared baking sheets. Bake for 20 to 25 minutes, or until lightly browned. Remove from the oven but do not turn it off. Let the logs cool for 10 minutes.

5. Slide the logs onto a cutting board. With a large heavy knife, cut the logs diagonally into ½-inch slices. Lay the slices on the baking sheets and return the sheets to the oven. Turn off the heat, and leave the cookies in the oven for 30 minutes. Transfer to wire racks to cool.

Kathie's Anise Walnut Biscotti

Makes 4 dozen

Kathie Devine is an old friend from high school days. She provided me with this recipe for tender, buttery biscotti with a subtle anise flavor.

1½ cups all-purpose flour

½ teaspoon baking powder

¼ teaspoon salt

8 tablespoons (1 stick) unsalted butter, softened

½ cup sugar

2 large eggs, at room temperature

2 teaspoons anise extract

1 cup lightly toasted walnuts, coarsely chopped

1. Preheat the oven to 350°F. Butter and flour a large baking sheet.

2. Combine the flour, baking powder, and salt.

3. In the large bowl of an electric mixer, beat the butter until light and creamy. Beat in the sugar until fluffy. Beat in the eggs one at a time. Beat in the anise extract. On low speed, beat in the flour mixture just until combined. Stir in the nuts.

4. Shape the dough into two 12- by 1½-inch logs on the prepared baking sheet. Smooth the sides with a rubber spatula. Bake for 20 minutes, or until the logs are lightly browned and firm when pressed lightly in the center. Remove from the oven but do not turn it off. Let the logs cool for 10 minutes.

5. Slide the logs onto a cutting board and cut diagonally into ½-inch-thick slices. Stand the biscotti on the baking sheet. Bake for 10 minutes, or until the cookies are lightly toasted. Transfer to wire racks to cool.

Union Square Cafe's Almond Hazelnut Biscotti

Makes 6 dozen

New York's Union Square Cafe serves these satisfying biscotti. Explaining why people love them, owner Danny Meyer says that "everyone can relate to cookies, but nobody likes to admit to dunking Oreos in milk. Biscotti are more romantic . . . a mature treat."

5 cups all-purpose flour

1 teaspoon baking powder

1 teaspoon salt

5 large eggs, at room temperature

2 cups sugar

1 teaspoon vanilla extract

1 teaspoon anise extract

1 teaspoon almond extract

⅔ cup toasted almonds

⅔ cup hazelnuts, toasted and skinned (page 3)

1. Preheat the oven to 325°F. Butter and flour a large baking sheet.

2. Combine the flour, baking powder, and salt.

3. In the large bowl of an electric mixer, beat 4 of the eggs, the sugar, and the extracts on high speed until the mixture forms a smooth ribbon when the beaters are lifted, about 10 minutes. On low speed, beat in the dry ingredients. Stir in the nuts.

4. Divide the dough into 3 pieces and shape each piece into a 9- by 2¼-inch log. Place the logs about 2 inches apart on the prepared baking sheet. Beat the remaining egg and brush it over the logs. Bake for 40 minutes, or until golden.

5. Remove the baking sheet from the oven, and reduce the heat to 275°F. Let the logs cool for 10 minutes. Slide the logs onto a cutting board and cut into ¼-inch-thick slices. Arrange the slices cut sides up on a baking sheet. Bake the slices for 15 to 20 minutes, or until lightly toasted. Transfer to wire racks to cool.

Biscotti Glassata con Cioccolata

CHOCOLATE-GLAZED CHOCOLATE BISCOTTI

Makes 4 dozen

6 ounces semisweet chocolate

5 tablespoons plus 1 teaspoon unsalted butter

2⅓ cups all-purpose flour

2 teaspoons baking powder

3 large eggs, at room temperature

⅔ cup sugar

1 teaspoon vanilla extract

2 cups toasted walnuts

GLAZE

6 ounces semisweet chocolate

2 tablespoons unsalted butter

1. Preheat the oven to 300°F. Butter and flour a large baking sheet.

2. Place the chocolate and butter in a small bowl set over a saucepan of warm water, and heat over low heat until softened. Remove from the heat and stir until smooth. Let cool.

3. Combine the flour and baking powder.

4. In a large bowl, beat the eggs, sugar, and vanilla until light. Stir in the cooled chocolate mixture. Stir in the flour mixture and the nuts.

5. Divide the dough in half. Shape the dough into two 14- by 2-inch logs on the prepared baking sheet, spacing the logs 4 inches apart. Smooth the tops and sides with a rubber spatula. Bake for 35 minutes, or until the logs are firm when pressed in the center. Let cool for 10 minutes. Do not turn off the oven.

6. Slide the logs onto a cutting board. With a large heavy knife, cut each log diagonally into ½-inch slices. Stand the slices on the baking sheet. Bake for 15 minutes, or until crisp. Transfer to wire racks to cool completely.

continued

7. To make the glaze: Place the chocolate and butter in a small saucepan set over warm water, and heat over low heat until softened. Remove from the heat and stir until smooth. With a small knife, spread the glaze thinly over one side of each cookie. Place on a rack and let stand until the chocolate is set. Store in a cool place.

Ecce Panis's Chocolate Macadamia Nut Biscotti

Makes 8 dozen

Ecce panis means "behold the bread" in Latin. It is also the name of one of New York City's best bakeries. In addition to terrific bread, Chef Craig Kominiak makes these sensational biscotti. Of course, they are totally unlike anything you will ever find in Italy, but I think it is interesting to see what a creative chef has done with a good idea. Besides, they are irresistible. Since they are packed with nuts and coconut, they tend to crumble easily, so handle them with special care.

5 ounces semisweet chocolate

6 tablespoons unsalted butter

2 cups all-purpose flour

1 cup Dutch-process cocoa powder, sifted

2 teaspoons baking powder

1 teaspoon salt

4 large eggs, at room temperature

½ cup granulated sugar

½ cup dark brown sugar

¼ cup coffee liqueur

1 tablespoon dark rum

1 teaspoon vanilla extract

1 cup lightly packed flaked coconut

1 cup unsalted macadamia nuts, coarsely chopped

1 egg white, lightly beaten

1. Place the chocolate and butter in a small heatproof bowl. Set the bowl over a small saucepan partially filled with simmering water and heat over low heat until softened. Remove from the heat and stir until smooth. Let cool.

2. Sift together the flour, cocoa powder, baking powder, and salt.

3. In the large bowl of an electric mixer, beat the eggs until foamy. Add the sugars, liqueur, rum, and vanilla and beat until smooth. Stir in the cooled chocolate mixture. Add the dry ingredients and stir until well combined. Stir in the coconut and nuts. Cover and refrigerate for 1 hour.

4. Preheat the oven to 300°F. Butter and flour a large baking sheet.

5. Divide the dough into 4 pieces. With lightly dampened hands, shape each piece into a 10-inch log. Place the logs about 2 inches apart on the prepared baking sheet. Brush with the beaten egg white. Bake for 45 minutes, or until the logs spring back when pressed in the center. Slide the logs onto a rack and let cool for 1 hour. Reduce the oven temperature to 250°F.

6. Cut the logs diagonally into ½-inch slices. Place the slices cut sides up on ungreased baking sheets. Bake the biscotti, turning once, for 15 to 20 minutes, or until lightly toasted. Transfer to wire racks to cool.

Biscotti di Uva, Noci, e Cioccolata

RAISIN, NUT, AND CHOCOLATE BISCOTTI

Makes 4 dozen

1⅔ cups all-purpose flour

1 teaspoon baking powder

½ teaspoon salt

2 large eggs

⅔ cup sugar

½ cup walnuts, coarsely chopped

½ cup semisweet chocolate chips

½ cup dark raisins

1 egg yolk beaten with 1 teaspoon water, for egg wash

1. Preheat the oven to 350°F. Butter and flour a large baking sheet.

2. Combine the flour, baking powder, and salt.

3. In the large bowl of an electric mixer, beat the eggs and sugar until very pale and thick. Stir in the dry ingredients. Stir in the nuts, chocolate chips and raisins.

4. Divide the dough in half. With dampened hands shape each half into a 12-inch log. Place the logs about 4 inches apart on the prepared baking sheet, and brush with the egg wash. Bake for 20 to 25 minutes, or until firm and golden brown. Let cool on the baking sheet for 10 minutes. Do not turn off the oven.

5. Carefully slide the logs onto a cutting board. With a sharp knife, cut each log diagonally into ½-inch slices. Stand the slices ½ inch apart on the baking sheet. Bake for 10 minutes or until dry and lightly toasted. Transfer to wire racks to cool.

Rhode Island Biscotti di Vino

WINE BISCUITS

Makes 4 dozen

Southwestern Rhode Island has a large Italian-American population. These cookies, a Southern Italian import, are popular there.

2½ **cups all-purpose flour**

2½ **teaspoons baking powder**

1 **teaspoon salt**

2 **large eggs, at room temperature**

1 **cup sugar**

½ **cup dry Marsala**

¼ **cup olive oil**

½ **teaspoon vanilla extract**

1. Preheat the oven to 375°F. Butter two large baking sheets.

2. Combine the flour, baking powder, and salt.

3. In a large bowl, beat the eggs and ½ cup of the sugar until well blended. Beat in ¼ cup of the Marsala, the oil, and vanilla extract. Stir in the dry ingredients.

4. Divide the dough into 6 pieces and cut each one into 8 pieces. Roll each piece between your palms into a 4-inch log and shape it into a ring, pinching the edges together to seal.

5. Place the remaining ½ cup sugar and remaining ¼ cup Marsala in two small bowls. Dip one side of each cookie first in the wine, then in the sugar. Place the cookies sugar side up 1 inch apart on the prepared baking sheets. Bake for 18 to 20 minutes, or until golden brown. Transfer to wire racks to cool.

Biscotti di Vino Rosso

RED WINE BISCUITS

Makes 2 dozen

🌀 A nice way to finish a meal is to serve these not too sweet cookies with a wedge of Parmigiano-Reggiano and a glass of red wine.

2½ cups all-purpose flour

½ cup sugar

1½ teaspoons baking powder

1 teaspoon salt

1 teaspoon freshly ground black pepper

½ cup dry red wine or Marsala

½ cup olive oil

1 egg white, beaten until foamy

2 tablespoons lightly toasted sesame seeds

1. Preheat the oven to 350°F.

2. In a large bowl, stir together the flour, sugar, baking powder, salt, and pepper. Add the wine and olive oil and stir with a wooden spoon just until smooth.

3. Divide the dough into 4 pieces, and shape each piece into a 10-inch log. Flatten the logs slightly. Brush with the egg white and sprinkle with the sesame seeds.

4. Cut the logs into ¾-inch slices. Place the slices 1 inch apart on ungreased baking sheets. Bake for 25 minutes, or until lightly browned. Transfer to wire racks to cool.

Biscotti di Mondo X

CHOCOLATE GRANOLA COOKIES

Makes 5 dozen

At Mondo X, a rehabilitation center for drug addicts in Cetona in Tuscany, the members work restoring and maintaining a beautiful restaurant, inn, and working farm called La Frateria di Padre Eligio. The food can be quite good, especially the desserts. I loved these chewy cookies, something like chocolate granola bars. The dough is a bit tricky to work with, so I find it best to roll it out between sheets of wax paper.

1 cup all-purpose flour

¾ cup wheat bran

½ cup rolled oats (not instant)

¼ cup Dutch-process cocoa powder

12 tablespoons (1½ sticks) unsalted butter, softened

4 ounces semisweet chocolate, melted and cooled

¾ cup sugar

1 teaspoon salt

Confectioners' sugar

1. Preheat the oven to 350°F. Butter and flour two large baking sheets.
2. Combine the flour, bran, oats, and cocoa powder.
3. In the large bowl of an electric mixer, beat the butter and melted chocolate until well blended. Beat in the sugar and salt. Add the dry ingredients and stir until a firm dough forms.
4. Divide the dough in half. Place one piece between two sheets of wax paper and roll out, turning and lifting the paper often, to a ⅛-inch thickness. With a fluted 2-inch round cookie cutter, cut the dough into circles. Place the circles 1 inch apart on the prepared baking sheets. Repeat with the remaining dough, rerolling the scraps and cutting out more cookies.
5. Bake for 12 minutes. Let cool on the baking sheets for about 10 minutes, then transfer to wire racks to cool completely. Sprinkle with confectioners' sugar before serving.

Ossa da Mordere

BONE COOKIES

Makes 4 dozen

⑂ Borgomanero is a sleepy little town where I often stop when visiting Lake Orta in Northern Italy. One of the local specialties is *tapulon*, a stew made with donkey meat which I haven't been able to bring myself to taste. I have no problem with the cookies called *ossa da mordere* ("bones to chew"), however.

The only thing these hard, crunchy cookies have in common with bones is their appearance, which is dry and somewhat bone-shaped. They keep forever and taste great dipped into a glass of sweet wine. I always bring a sack of them home with me along with another local favorite, *brutti ma buoni*, "ugly but good" cookies.

Ossa da mordere are made in practically every region of Italy and there are many variations. Some are called *ossa di morte*, "bones of the dead," and are served on November 1, the Feast of All Saints.

3 large egg whites, at room temperature

1½ cups sugar

1 teaspoon ground cinnamon

1 teaspoon grated lemon zest

½ teaspoon baking powder

¼ teaspoon grated nutmeg

¼ teaspoon ground cloves

1¾ cups all-purpose flour

1½ cups chopped blanched almonds

¼ cup milk

1. Preheat the oven to 350°F. Butter two large baking sheets.

2. In the large bowl of an electric mixer, beat the egg whites until foamy. Add the sugar, cinnamon, lemon zest, baking powder, nutmeg, and cloves and beat until well blended. Stir in the flour and almonds.

3. Gather about 2½ tablespoons of dough in the palm of your hand

and roll it into a 2½- by ½-inch log. Repeat with remaining dough, placing the logs 1 inch apart on the prepared baking sheets.

4. Brush the tops with the milk. Bake for 20 minutes, or until lightly browned. Transfer to wire racks to cool.

$\mathcal{B}$ussolai

VENETIAN BUTTER RINGS

Makes 40

8 tablespoons (1 stick) unsalted butter, softened

⅔ cup sugar

3 large egg yolks

1½ teaspoons grated lemon zest

1 teaspoon vanilla extract

2 cups all-purpose flour

½ teaspoon salt

1 egg white, beaten until foamy

1. In the large bowl of an electric mixer, beat the butter and sugar at medium speed until light and fluffy. Beat in the egg yolks one at a time. Beat in the lemon zest and vanilla extract. On low speed, beat in the flour and salt.

2. Turn the dough out onto a sheet of plastic wrap, shape it into a ball, and flatten it slightly. Wrap tightly and refrigerate for at least 1 hour, or overnight.

3. Preheat the oven to 325°F. Butter and flour two large baking sheets.

4. Cut the dough into quarters, and cut each quarter into 10 pieces. Roll each piece between your fingers into a 4-inch rope, shape into a ring, and pinch the ends together to seal. Place the rings 1 inch apart on the prepared baking sheets. Brush lightly with the beaten egg white.

5. Bake the cookies for 15 minutes or until lightly browned. Transfer to wire racks to cool.

Biscotti Regina
SESAME COOKIES
Makes 3½ dozen

Sesame seeds were brought to Sicily by the Arabs, who ruled there for centuries. Unhulled sesame seeds, available in health food stores, give the cookies an authentic flavor.

1 cup (4 ounces) unhulled sesame seeds

2 cups all-purpose flour

⅔ cup sugar

1 teaspoon baking powder

½ teaspoon salt

½ cup solid vegetable shortening

2 large eggs, at room temperature

1 teaspoon vanilla extract

1 teaspoon grated lemon zest

1. Preheat the oven to 350°F. Grease two large baking sheets.

2. Spread the sesame seeds in a large roasting pan and bake, shaking the pan occasionally, for 15 to 20 minutes, or until golden brown. Let cool.

3. In a large bowl, combine the flour, sugar, baking powder, and salt. Cut in the shortening until the mixture resembles fine crumbs.

4. In a small bowl, beat together the eggs, vanilla, and lemon zest. Stir into the dry ingredients.

5. Pick up about 3 tablespoons of dough, and shape it into a 2½- by ¾-inch log with your fingertips. Repeat with the remaining dough. Roll the logs in the sesame seeds, pressing the seeds into the dough, and place 1 inch apart on the prepared baking sheets.

6. Bake for 30 minutes, or until golden brown. Transfer to wire racks to cool.

Palline di Limone

GLAZED LEMON COOKIES

Makes 80

4 cups all-purpose flour

1 tablespoon baking powder

½ teaspoon salt

8 tablespoons (1 stick) unsalted butter, at room temperature

¾ cup sugar

3 large eggs, at room temperature

1 tablespoon lemon extract

2 teaspoons grated lemon zest

⅓ cup milk

ICING

1½ cups confectioners' sugar

3 tablespoons fresh lemon juice

1. Combine the flour, baking powder, and salt.

2. In the large bowl of an electric mixer, beat the butter and sugar at medium speed until light and fluffy. Beat in the eggs one at a time, scraping the sides of the bowl as necessary, and beat until well blended. Beat in the lemon extract and lemon zest.

3. Stir in half of the flour mixture and then the milk. Add the remaining flour and stir until thoroughly incorporated. Cover and chill for at least 1 hour, or overnight.

4. Preheat the oven to 350°F.

5. Pinch off 1-inch pieces of the dough and shape them into balls. Place the balls 2 inches apart on ungreased baking sheets. Bake for 15 to 18 minutes, or until puffed but not browned. Transfer to wire racks to cool.

6. To make the icing: In a bowl, combine all of the confectioners' sugar and lemon juice. Stir in a few drops of water, or just enough to make the icing easy to spread. Brush the cookies generously with the icing. Let dry on wire racks.

Biscotti di Pignoli

PINE NUT MACAROONS

Makes 70

§ Scottsdale, Arizona is a beautiful city, but good Italian bakeries are scarce there. My sister Annette always asks me to bring some of her favorite pine nut macaroon cookies from Brooklyn's Court Pastry Shop whenever I come to visit.

One day a student from one of my cooking classes gave me a recipe for macaroons made with almond paste that tasted a lot like my sister's favorite. I made a few adjustments, added the pine nuts, and they were perfect. Now Annette can make her own pignoli cookies.

The almond paste sold in cans is a little more expensive but of much better quality than the kind sold in a box. Solo is the most commonly available canned brand in my area. If you can't find it, ask at your local bakery if they will sell you almond paste by the pound. Bakeries generally buy it in big commercial-size cans.

These cookies tend to stick: For best results, line the baking sheets with parchment paper. The cookies will stick to the paper, but will be easily released when water is applied to the back of the paper as described. Parchment is available in most supermarkets and housewares stores.

1 pound almond paste (2 8-ounce cans)

1 cup sugar

3 large egg whites, lightly beaten, at room temperature

1 cup pine nuts

Confectioners' sugar

1. Preheat the oven to 300°F. Line two large baking sheets with parchment paper.

2. Crumble the almond paste into the large bowl of an electric mixer. Add the sugar and beat until well blended. Add the egg whites gradually and beat until smooth.

3. Drop the dough by rounded teaspoonfuls 1½ inches apart onto the prepared baking sheets. Sprinkle the cookies with the pine nuts, patting the nuts lightly into the surface of the dough so that they will adhere.

4. Bake for 25 to 30 minutes, or until the cookies are golden brown. Let the cookies cool on the baking sheets.

5. Gently turn the parchment paper over onto a work surface and brush the bottom lightly with cool water. Let stand briefly until the cookies are released from the paper. If necessary, brush again with water.

6. Just before serving, sprinkle the macaroons with confectioners' sugar. If not eaten the same day, freeze the cookies in plastic bags to maintain their texture. Thaw at room temperature.

Torcetti

BUTTER COOKIE TWISTS

Makes 32

3¼ cups all-purpose flour

1 teaspoon baking powder

¼ teaspoon salt

12 tablespoons (1½ sticks) unsalted butter, softened

1 cup sugar

2 large eggs

1 teaspoon vanilla extract

1 egg yolk beaten with 1 tablespoon water, for egg wash

1. Combine the flour, baking powder, and salt.

2. In the large bowl of an electric mixer, beat the butter until creamy. Add the sugar and beat until light and fluffy. Beat in the eggs one at a time. Beat in the vanilla. Stir in the dry ingredients. Shape the dough into a disk and wrap it in plastic wrap. Chill for several hours, or overnight.

3. Preheat the oven to 375°F. Butter and flour two large baking sheets.

4. Divide the dough in quarters. Cut each into 8 pieces. Roll each piece into an 8-inch rope, then fold the rope in half, twist it twice, and pinch the ends together. Arrange the cookies 1 inch apart on the prepared baking sheets.

5. Brush the egg wash over the cookies. Bake for 12 to 15 minutes, or until lightly browned. Transfer to wire racks to cool.

Zaletti

CORNMEAL DIAMONDS

Makes about 6 dozen

In Venetian dialect, *zaletti* means "little yellow things." These cookies are flavored with grappa, an Italian brandy distilled from grape skins and seeds after they have been pressed to make wine.

> ¾ cup golden raisins
>
> ¼ cup grappa or brandy
>
> 1½ cups all-purpose flour
>
> 1 cup fine yellow cornmeal
>
> ½ teaspoon salt
>
> 12 tablespoons (1½ sticks) unsalted butter, softened
>
> ⅔ cup sugar
>
> 1 large egg
>
> 1½ teaspoons grated lemon zest
>
> 1 teaspoon vanilla extract

1. In a small bowl, soak the raisins in the grappa until plump, at least 1 hour.

2. Preheat the oven to 375°F. Butter and flour two large baking sheets.

3. Combine the flour, cornmeal, and salt.

4. In a large bowl, beat together the butter and sugar. Beat in the egg, lemon zest, and vanilla until well blended. Stir in the dry ingredients. Add the raisins and grappa, and stir until combined. Cover and chill for 1 hour.

5. On a lightly floured surface, roll out the dough to a ¼-inch thickness. Cut the dough into 1-inch-long diamond shapes. Place the cookies about ½ inch apart on the prepared baking sheets. Bake for 12 to 15 minutes, or until lightly browned around the edges. Transfer to wire racks to cool.

orti

CHOCOLATE SPICE RINGS

Makes 4 dozen

🍥 A 3-inch doughnut cutter is the perfect tool for cutting out these long-keeping biscotti from Venice. I often serve them with a dry red wine, but they are also good with Marsala.

> 3 cups all-purpose flour
>
> ¾ cup Dutch-process cocoa powder, sifted
>
> 1½ teaspoons baking powder
>
> 1 teaspoon ground cinnamon
>
> ¼ teaspoon ground cloves
>
> ½ teaspoon ground ginger
>
> ½ teaspoon salt
>
> ½ teaspoon freshly ground white pepper
>
> ¾ cup sugar
>
> ⅓ cup molasses
>
> 4 tablespoons unsalted butter, softened
>
> 2 large eggs
>
> ⅓ cup dry red wine
>
> 1 cup toasted almonds, finely chopped

GLAZE

> 1 egg white
>
> ¼ cup sugar
>
> ¼ cup toasted almonds, chopped

1. Sift together the flour, cocoa, baking powder, cinnamon, cloves, ginger, salt, and pepper.

2. In the large bowl of an electric mixer, beat the sugar, molasses, and butter until light and fluffy. Beat in the eggs and wine. Stir in the dry ingredients and the chopped almonds. Divide the dough in half and shape each piece into a disk. Wrap each piece in plastic wrap and refrigerate for at least 8 hours, or overnight.

3. Preheat the oven to 350°F. Butter two large baking sheets.

4. On a lightly floured surface, roll out one piece of dough to a ¼-inch thickness. With a 3-inch doughnut cutter, cut out rings; or, with a 3-inch round cutter, cut out circles, then use a 1-inch round cutter to cut out the centers of the circles. Place the rings about 1 inch apart on the prepared cookie sheets. Repeat with the remaining dough. Reroll the scraps and cut out more rings.

5. To make the glaze: In a small bowl, beat the egg white with a wire whisk until frothy. Beat in the sugar and almonds. Brush the glaze over the dough rings.

6. Bake for 20 minutes, or until the cookies are firm and lightly browned. Transfer to wire racks to cool.

$\mathcal{B}icciolani$

CORNMEAL SPICE COOKIES

Makes 4 dozen

The flavor of these spicy cookies improves on standing a day.

1¼ cups all-purpose flour
1 cup fine yellow cornmeal
1 teaspoon ground cinnamon
¼ teaspoon grated nutmeg
⅛ teaspoon ground cloves
½ pound (2 sticks) unsalted butter, softened
1 cup sugar
2 large egg yolks

1. Combine the flour, cornmeal, and spices.

2. In the large bowl of an electric mixer beat the butter and sugar until light and fluffy. Beat in the egg yolks until well blended. Stir in the dry ingredients, scraping the sides of the bowl as necessary, until well blended. Divide the dough in half and shape into two 9- by 1½-inch logs. Wrap in plastic wrap and chill for several hours, or until very firm.

3. Preheat the oven to 400°F. Butter two large baking sheets.

4. Cut the logs of dough into ¼-inch slices. Place the slices 1 inch apart on the prepared baking sheets. Bake for 10 to 12 minutes, or until lightly browned around the edges. Transfer to wire racks to cool.

Crumiri

CORNMEAL COOKIES

Makes 4 dozen

Delicate and buttery, these cookies come from Piedmont, where cornmeal is usually eaten in the form of polenta. They make a lovely dessert with strawberries and a glass of Moscato d'Asti or Asti Spumante.

1¾ cups all-purpose flour

¾ cups fine yellow cornmeal

1 teaspoon salt

½ pound (2 sticks) unsalted butter, softened

¾ cup sugar

1 large egg, at room temperature

1 teaspoon vanilla extract

1. Preheat the oven to 375°F. Butter and flour two large baking sheets.
2. Combine the flour, cornmeal, and salt.
3. In the large bowl of an electric mixer, beat the butter and sugar until light and fluffy. Beat in the egg and vanilla. Stir in the dry ingredients until well blended. Cover and chill for 1 hour.
4. Spoon the dough into a piping bag or cookie press fitted with a large star tip. Pipe out 2½-inch-long crescents 1 inch apart on the prepared baking sheets.
5. Bake for 15 to 20 minutes, or until golden brown. Transfer to wire racks to cool.

Tegoline

ALMOND AND ORANGE TILES
Makes 24

Shaped like curved roof tiles, these fragile wafers from the Val d'Aosta crumble easily, so handle with care. They also can be shaped into small cups to hold ice cream or ices or rolled into cigarette shapes. They tend to become limp in damp weather, so store them in airtight containers and use them as soon as possible after they are made.

1 cup sliced blanched almonds

½ cup sugar

4 tablespoons unsalted butter, at room temperature

2 teaspoons grated orange zest

2 large egg whites, at room temperature

⅓ cup all-purpose flour

1. Preheat the oven to 400°F. Butter and flour two large baking sheets. Have ready two rolling pins or wine bottles for molding the cookies.

2. In a food processor or blender, combine ½ cup of the almonds and 2 tablespoons of the sugar. Process until finely ground.

3. In the large bowl of an electric mixer, beat the butter until light. Add the remaining sugar and beat until fluffy. Beat in the orange zest and egg whites until well blended. Beat in the ground almonds. Stir in the flour just until combined.

4. Drop the batter by level tablespoons 6 inches apart onto the prepared baking sheets. With a spatula, spread each mound of batter evenly into a 3½-inch circle. Sprinkle each round with some of the remaining ½ cup almonds.

5. Bake the cookies one sheet at a time, for 5 to 6 minutes, or until the centers are lightly browned and the edges are a darker brown. Remove the baking sheet from the oven and let it rest on the open oven door for 30 seconds, or until the cookies are just firm enough to handle. With a metal spatula, remove the cookies from the sheet and drape them over the rolling pin. Work quickly or the cookies will become too brittle. If this happens, return them to the oven briefly until they are warm and soft. Let the cookies cool on the rolling pin until set.

6. Bake and form the remaining cookies in the same way. Let cool completely, then store the cookies in airtight containers.

Cookie Cups for Ice Cream or Ices. Omit the ½ cup almonds used for sprinkling. As the cookies are removed from the sheets, gently mold each one over an inverted custard cup.

Cigarettes. Omit the ½ cup almonds used for sprinkling. As the cookies are removed from the sheets, immediately roll each one up around the handle of a wooden spoon.

*C*roccantini

CHOCOLATE HAZELNUT MERINGUES

Makes 4 dozen

1½ cups hazelnuts, toasted and skinned (page 3)

3 large egg whites, at room temperature

½ cup sugar

1 teaspoon ground cinnamon

6 ounces semisweet chocolate, melted and cooled

1. Preheat the oven to 325°F. Butter two large baking sheets.

2. Finely chop ½ cup of the hazelnuts. Coarsely chop the remaining 1 cup nuts.

3. In the small bowl of an electric mixer, beat the egg whites until soft peaks form. Add the sugar 1 tablespoon at a time, beating constantly at high speed, and beat until the whites are thick and glossy and the sugar is dissolved. Beat in the cinnamon. Fold in the melted chocolate and the nuts.

4. Drop the butter by rounded tablespoonfuls onto the prepared baking sheets. Bake for 18 minutes, or until the meringues are firm. Remove to wire racks to cool.

Parma Chocolate Cookies

Makes 40

❧ I spotted these plump chocolate cookies with a dollop of raspberry jam in the center in a wonderful bakery in Parma. They reminded me of old-fashioned thumbprint cookies, but the combination of chocolate, raspberry, and hazelnuts is much more sophisticated.

12 tablespoons (1½ sticks) unsalted butter, softened

½ cup sugar

½ teaspoon salt

3 ounces semisweet chocolate, melted and cooled

2 cups all-purpose flour

¾ cup hazelnuts, toasted, skinned (page 000), and finely chopped

About ⅓ cup seedless raspberry jam

1. Preheat the oven to 350°F. Butter two large baking sheets.

2. In the large bowl of an electric mixer, beat the butter, sugar, and salt until light and fluffy. Add the melted chocolate and beat until well blended, scraping the sides of the bowl as necessary. Stir in the flour until well blended.

3. Shape the dough into 1-inch balls. Roll the balls in the chopped nuts, pressing lightly so they will adhere. Place the balls about 1½ inches apart on the prepared baking sheets.

4. With the handle of a wooden spoon, poke a deep hole in each ball of dough, shaping the dough around the handle to retain the round shape. Place about ¼ teaspoon jam in each hole. (Do not add more jam or it may run out as the cookies bake.)

5. Bake the cookies for 18 to 20 minutes, or until the jam is bubbling and the cookies are lightly browned. Transfer to wire racks to cool.

Ciambelline Glassate
GLAZED RING COOKIES
Makes 32

The unusual baked-on glaze on these cookies dries to a high gloss that looks very professional. The glaze can be tinted with food coloring or sprinkled with multicolored candy beads before baking—nice for a festive occasion. Brush the glaze on lightly or it will be too thick where it collects in the ridges of the cookies.

3 cups all-purpose flour

1½ teaspoons baking powder

1 teaspoon ground cinnamon

8 tablespoons (1 stick) unsalted butter, softened

¾ cups sugar

1 teaspoon grated lemon zest

2 large eggs

1 large egg white

GLAZE

1 cup confectioners' sugar

1 large egg white

1. Preheat the oven to 350°F. Butter and flour two large baking sheets.
2. Combine the flour, baking powder, and cinnamon.
3. In the large bowl of an electric mixer, beat the butter and sugar until light and fluffy. Beat in the lemon zest.
4. Beat in the eggs one at a time, beating well after each addition, then beat in the egg white. Stir in the dry ingredients until smooth.
5. Divide the dough into quarters and cut each quarter into 16 pieces. Roll each piece of dough into a 4-inch rope. Twist 2 ropes together to form a braid, and shape into a ring, pinching the ends together to seal. Repeat with the remaining ropes, and place the rings 1 inch apart on the prepared baking sheets.

continued

6. Bake the cookies for 15 to 20 minutes, or until lightly browned.

7. Meanwhile, make the glaze: Whisk together the confectioners' sugar and egg white until smooth.

8. Remove the cookies from the oven and brush the tops lightly with the glaze. Return to the oven and bake for 5 minutes more. Transfer to wire racks to cool.

Baci di Giulietta

JULIET'S KISSES

Makes 4 dozen

Verona is the setting for Shakespeare's great tragedy *Romeo and Juliet*. After a visit to the house that supposedly belonged to Juliet's family, you can stop at one of the local bakeries for some delicious cookie kisses named for the heroine and the hero (page 40). Outside of Verona, these delicate cookies are called Baci di Dama, or Lady's Kisses.

½ *pound (2 sticks) unsalted butter, softened*

½ *cup confectioners' sugar*

¼ *teaspoon salt*

1 *teaspoon vanilla extract*

1⅔ *cups all-purpose flour*

⅓ *cup Dutch-process cocoa powder, sifted*

½ *cup finely chopped toasted almonds*

FILLING

2 *ounces semisweet chocolate*

2 *tablespoons unsalted butter*

⅓ *cup blanched almonds, toasted and finely chopped*

1. Preheat the oven to 350°F.

2. In the large bowl of an electric mixer, beat the butter and sugar on high speed until light and fluffy. Beat in the salt and vanilla. On low speed, beat in the flour, cocoa, and almonds just until blended.

3. Roll teaspoonfuls of the dough into ¾-inch balls. Place about 1 inch apart on ungreased baking sheets. Bake the cookies until firm but not browned, 10 to 12 minutes. Transfer to wire racks to cool.

4. To make the filling: In a small heatproof bowl placed over a saucepan of simmering water, combine the chocolate and butter, and heat until softened. Remove from the heat and stir until smooth. Stir in the almonds.

5. Spread about 1 teaspoon of the chocolate mixture on the bottom of one cookie. Place a second cookie bottom side down on the filling and press together lightly. Place on a wire rack until the filling is set, and repeat with the remaining cookies and filling.

Baci di Romeo

ROMEO'S KISSES

Makes 3½ dozen

½ pound (2 sticks) unsalted butter, softened
½ cup confectioners' sugar
¼ teaspoon salt
½ teaspoon almond extract
2 cups all-purpose flour

FILLING
2 ounces semisweet chocolate
2 tablespoons unsalted butter
⅓ cup blanched almonds, toasted and finely chopped

1. Preheat the oven to 350°F.

2. In the large bowl of an electric mixer, beat the butter and sugar on high speed until light and fluffy. Beat in the salt and almond extract. On low speed, beat in the flour just until blended.

3. Roll teaspoonfuls of the dough into ¾-inch balls. Place about 1 inch apart on ungreased baking sheets. Bake the cookies until firm but not browned, 10 to 12 minutes. Transfer to wire racks to cool.

4. To make the filling: In a small heatproof bowl set over a saucepan of simmering water, combine the chocolate and butter, and heat until softened. Remove from the heat and stir until smooth. Stir in the almonds.

5. Spread about 1 teaspoon of the chocolate mixture on the bottom of one cookie. Place a second cookie bottom side down on the filling and press together lightly. Place on a wire rack until the filling is set, and repeat with the remaining cookies and filling.

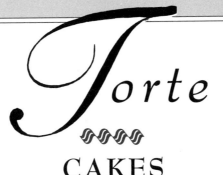

Torte

CAKES

Italian pastry shops always have fabulous displays. Lavish layer cakes oozing rich cream fillings, deep tortes topped with perfect fruit glistening under jewellike glazes, and beautifully sculpted and colored marzipan fruits, nuts, and vegetables are among the temptations that cry out for a taste. The selection varies according to the season and the region. In fall and winter, especially in Piedmont, chestnuts seem to be in and on top of cakes everywhere. In Parma and Bologna the specialty is torta ricciolina topped with crunchy golden strands of fresh egg pasta. In Sicily, gorgeous cassatas soaked in liqueur and layered with ricotta have pride of place.

Though Italian cakes run the gamut from plain and simple to elaborate and ornate, most cooks leave the fancy cakes to pastry chefs and concentrate on simpler creations at home. Cheesecakes, nut and fruit cakes, and simple sweetened yeast breads are typically made at home.

Preparing Pans for Baking

Many cakes will be easier to remove from their baking pans if the pan has first been buttered and floured. To do so, crumple a small piece of paper and use it to pick up a small amount of butter or vegetable shortening. Spread the butter in a thin even layer over the surface of the pan. Sprinkle with flour. Tap the pan gently to distribute the flour evenly and remove the excess.

Delicate cakes sometimes need extra help in the form of a paper pan liner. Cut off a length of wax paper slightly longer than the diameter of the pan. Fold the paper in half, then in quarters, then in eighths. You will have a wedge-shaped piece of folded paper. Hold the point of the wedge at the center of the pan and, with scissors, trim off the wide end just short of the pan rim. Open up the paper and you will have a round disk that will fit perfectly in the bottom of the pan. Butter the pan but do not flour it. Insert the paper disk and butter it also, smoothing out any wrinkles. Sprinkle with flour and knock out the excess.

Torta Rovesciata alle Pesche

UPSIDE-DOWN PEACH POPPY SEED CAKE

Serves 8

This beautiful cake looks as if it took great skill to make but it is no trouble at all. Tiny blue-black poppy seeds add a nutty flavor and crunchy texture. Since poppy seeds have a tendency to turn rancid, always store them in the refrigerator or freezer to keep them fresh. Smell and taste them before using, just to be sure.

2 large peaches, thinly sliced

1½ cups all-purpose flour

2 teaspoons baking powder

8 tablespoons (1 stick) unsalted butter, softened

¾ cup sugar

2 large eggs, at room temperature

1 teaspoon vanilla extract

1 tablespoon poppy seeds

½ cup milk

GLAZE

¾ cup apricot jam

2 tablespoons sugar

½ cup chopped toasted walnuts

1. Preheat the oven to 350°F. Butter a 9-inch springform pan. Line the bottom of the pan with a circle of wax paper and butter the paper.

2. Arrange the peach slices pinwheel fashion in the bottom of the pan.

3. Combine the flour and baking powder.

4. In the large bowl of an electric mixer, beat the butter and sugar until light and fluffy. Beat in the eggs one at a time and beat until smooth. Stir in the vanilla and poppy seeds. Stir in half the flour mixture. Stir in the milk and the remaining flour just until blended.

5. Spread the batter over the peaches. Tap the pan on the countertop to settle the batter. Bake for 40 to 45 minutes, or until the cake is golden and a cake tester inserted in the center comes out clean.

6. Run a thin spatula around the edge of the cake and remove the rim of the pan. Invert the cake onto a rack. Remove the bottom of the pan and carefully peel off the wax paper. Let cool.

7. To make the glaze: In a small saucepan, combine the jam and sugar and heat, stirring, until the sugar is dissolved and the glaze is thick.

8. Brush the warm glaze over the top and sides of the cake. Sprinkle a ½-inch border of chopped walnuts around the top edge of the cake, and pat the remaining nuts around the sides. Let set for at least 15 minutes before serving.

Torta di Susine

PLUM TORTE

Serves 8

On an autumn trip to Parma, all of the bakeries—and there are many—seemed to be featuring thick, juicy, plum-filled tortes like this one. It can be made throughout the year, substituting apples, pears, or peaches in their season.

DOUGH

3 cups all-purpose flour

¾ cup sugar

2 teaspoons baking powder

1 teaspoon grated lemon zest

½ teaspoon salt

12 tablespoons (1½ sticks) unsalted butter, softened and cut into bits

1 large egg

1 large egg yolk

1½ teaspoons vanilla extract

FILLING

2½ pounds firm ripe plums, thinly sliced

½ cup sugar

½ teaspoon ground cinnamon

1 tablespoon fresh lemon juice

½ cup toasted pine nuts

1 tablespoon unsalted butter, cut into bits

1 large egg yolk, lightly beaten

2 tablespoons sugar

1. To make the dough: In a large bowl, combine the flour, sugar, baking powder, lemon zest, and salt. With a pastry blender, cut in the butter until the mixture resembles coarse crumbs. In a small bowl, beat the whole egg, egg yolk, and vanilla together. Stir into the flour mixture just until a dough forms.

2. Divide the dough into two pieces, one twice as large as the other. Shape each piece into a flat disk. Wrap each one in plastic wrap and chill for at least 1 hour, or overnight.

3. Preheat the oven to 350°F.

4. On a lightly floured surface, roll out the larger piece of dough to a 12-inch circle. Place the dough in a 9-inch springform pan, pressing it up against the sides of the pan.

5. To make the filling: In a large bowl, toss together the plums, sugar, cinnamon, and lemon juice.

6. Pour the filling into the prepared pastry shell. Sprinkle with the pine nuts. Dot with the butter.

7. Roll out the remaining dough to a 10-inch circle. With a pastry cutter, cut the dough into ½-inch-wide strips. Arrange most of the strips lattice-fashion over the plums. Press the ends of the strips onto the bottom pastry to seal. Place the remaining strips around the edge of the dough to cover the ends of the lattice strips, and press to adhere.

8. Brush the beaten egg yolk over the pastry. Sprinkle with the sugar. Bake for 1 hour, or until the pastry is golden brown and the plum juices are bubbling. Transfer the torte to a rack and let cool for 10 minutes. Remove the rim of the pan and let cool completely.

Torciglione
UMBRIAN FRUIT CAKE
Serves 10

I can't tell you why, but this fruit-filled cake is made to resemble a snake—though a very benevolent one with coffee bean eyes and an almond tongue. Kids love it.

PASTRY

1½ cups all-purpose flour

3 tablespoons sugar

½ teaspoon salt

3 tablespoons unsalted butter, cut into bits

2 tablespoons olive oil

6 tablespoons ice water

FILLING

5 dried figs

5 pitted prunes

⅓ cup dark raisins

½ cup toasted walnuts, chopped

⅓ cup toasted almonds, chopped

2 tablespoons sugar

1 teaspoon grated lemon zest

¼ cup dry Marsala

2 teaspoons olive oil

DECORATION

2 coffee beans

1 almond

1 egg yolk beaten with 1 tablespoon water, for egg wash

1. To make the pastry: In a large bowl, combine the flour, sugar, and salt. With a pastry blender, blend the butter and oil into the dry ingredients until the mixture resembles coarse crumbs. Add the water and stir gently until the mixture begins to hold together. Shape the dough into a log. Wrap in plastic wrap and refrigerate for at least 1 hour.

2. In a small bowl, combine the figs, prunes, and raisins and add enough hot water to cover them by 1 inch. Set aside until the fruit is softened, 20 to 30 minutes.

3. Preheat the oven to 375°F. Butter and flour a large baking sheet.

4. To make the filling: Drain the fruit and pat dry. Chop coarsely. Combine the fruits, nuts, and remaining filling ingredients in a bowl and stir to mix.

5. On a lightly floured surface roll out the pastry to a 22- by 6-inch rectangle. Spoon the filling lengthwise down the center, leaving a 2-inch border on the long sides and a ½-inch border on the short sides. Fold the long sides over the filling and pinch the seam and ends closed.

6. Transfer the cake to the baking sheet. Slightly taper one end to form a tail. Flatten the other end to form a head, and narrow the neck slightly. With the tail end at the center, loosely coil up the snake. Press the coffee beans into the head to make eyes and poke the almond into the tip to form the tongue. Brush the pastry with the egg wash. Bake until golden, about 35 minutes.

7. Cool the cake on the baking sheet for 10 minutes. Then slide onto a rack to cool completely.

Torta di Arancia

ORANGE CAKE

Serves 8

As light as a cloud, this sponge cake is always nice to have on hand. Serve it plain with a glass of dessert wine, or with berries and cream.

1⅓ cups all-purpose flour

1 cup sugar

2 teaspoons baking powder

½ teaspoon salt

4 large eggs, separated

½ cup orange juice

⅓ cup olive oil

2 teaspoons orange zest

1 teaspoon vanilla extract

1. Preheat the oven to 325°F.

2. Combine the flour, ⅔ cup of the sugar, the baking powder, and salt.

3. In the large bowl of an electric mixer, beat the egg yolks, orange juice, oil, zest, and vanilla at medium speed until smooth. Stir in the flour mixture just until combined.

4. In a large bowl, beat the egg whites on medium speed until foamy. Gradually beat in the remaining ⅓ cup sugar and beat on high speed until soft peaks form. With a large rubber spatula, gently fold the whites into the yolk mixture, a little at a time.

5. Pour the batter into an ungreased 9-inch springform pan. Bake for 45 minutes, or until a cake tester inserted in the center comes out clean. Cool completely in the pan on a wire rack.

6. When cool, run a thin spatula around the side of the pan, and remove the rim. Invert the cake onto a rack and remove the base of the pan. Invert the cake onto a serving plate.

Focaccia all'Uva

GRAPE FOCACCIA

Serves 8

Focaccia is a flat bread that resembles pizza. Its name comes from *focus*, the Latin word for "hearth," where the bread originally was baked. Though focaccia is usually savory, this version from Tuscany, traditionally made during the harvest season with freshly picked grapes, is slightly sweet.

⅓ cup extra-virgin olive oil

2 tablespoons fresh rosemary leaves

1 package quick-rise active dry yeast

1 cup warm (105° to 115°F.) water

3 to 3½ cups all-purpose flour

¼ cup sugar

1 teaspoon salt

2½ cups red grapes (about 12 ounces), washed and thoroughly dried

1 cup walnuts

1. In a small saucepan, warm the oil over medium heat. Add the rosemary leaves and remove from the heat. Let cool.

2. In a large bowl, sprinkle the yeast over the warm water. Let stand until the yeast is foamy, about 5 minutes. Stir until dissolved.

3. Add the olive oil and rosemary, 3 cups of the flour, 2 tablespoons of the sugar, and the salt to the yeast mixture, and stir until a soft dough forms.

4. Turn the dough out onto a floured surface and knead until smooth and elastic, about 10 minutes, adding more flour if the dough feels sticky. Oil a large bowl and place the dough in it, turning once to oil the top. Cover with a towel and let rise in a warm place until doubled in bulk, about 45 minutes.

5. Preheat the oven to 375°F. Flour a 15- by 10- by 1-inch jelly-roll pan.

6. Punch the dough down to eliminate air bubbles. Stretch the dough out with your hands to fit the prepared pan. Scatter the grapes and nuts evenly over the dough, pressing them in lightly. Sprinkle with the remaining 2

tablespoons sugar. Bake for 30 to 35 minutes or until the dough is lightly browned and crisp.

7. Slide the focaccia out of the pan and onto a rack. Serve warm or at room temperature, cut into squares.

Torta di Mela

WARM APPLE CAKE

Serves 6 to 8

A very satisfying cake to serve with Mascarpone Custard Sauce (page 226).

1⅓ *cups all-purpose flour*

1 *teaspoon baking powder*

6 *tablespoons unsalted butter, at room temperature*

¾ *cup sugar*

2 *large eggs*

½ *cup milk*

1 *large Granny Smith or other tart apple, peeled and cut into ½-inch chunks (about 1½ cups)*

½ *cup dark raisins*

¼ *cup pine nuts*

1. Preheat the oven to 375°F. Butter and flour a 9-inch round cake pan.
2. Combine the flour and baking powder.
3. In a large bowl, beat the butter and sugar until light and fluffy. Add the eggs one at a time, beating well after each addition. Stir in the dry ingredients in three additions alternately with the milk in two additions. Stir in the apple chunks and raisins.
4. Spoon the mixture into the prepared pan and level the top. Sprinkle with the pine nuts.
5. Bake for 30 to 35 minutes, or until a cake tester inserted in the center comes out clean. Let cool in the pan for 10 minutes.
6. Unmold the cake onto a wire rack, then invert onto a serving plate. Serve warm or at room temperature.

Pane coi Santi

BREAD WITH SAINTS

Serves 8 to 10

The "saints" in this Tuscan sweet bread are the dried fruits, nuts, and spices mixed into the dough. It is usually made for the Feast of All Saints on November 1, and served with a glass of the season's newly made wine. Once it hardens, the bread is toasted and accompanied by *caffè latte* for dunking.

I adapted the recipe from one given to me by Donatella Cinelli, whose family owns the Fattoria dei Barbi winery in Montalcino. Donatella is passionate about preserving the traditional foods of her region and gives courses on cooking and related subjects on the winery grounds. There is also a charming restaurant on the property, called the Taverna Barbi, where good rustic cooking is served.

1 package active dry yeast

1 cup warm (105° to 115°F.) water

¼ cup olive oil

3 to 3½ cups all-purpose flour

¼ cup sugar

1 teaspoon anise seeds

½ teaspoon salt

¼ teaspoon freshly ground black pepper

1 cup dried figs, coarsely chopped

1 cup chopped walnuts, lightly toasted

½ cup golden raisins

1. In a large bowl, sprinkle the yeast over the warm water. Let stand until the yeast is foamy, about 5 minutes. Stir until dissolved.

2. Add the olive oil, 3 cups of the flour, the sugar, anise seeds, salt, and pepper to the yeast mixture, and stir until a soft dough forms.

3. Turn the dough out onto a floured surface and knead until smooth and elastic, about 10 minutes, adding more flour if the dough feels sticky. Oil

a large bowl and place the dough in it, turning once to oil the top. Cover with a towel and let rise in a warm place until doubled in bulk, about 2 hours.

4. Butter and flour a large baking sheet.

5. On a lightly floured surface, knead the dough lightly to eliminate air bubbles. Knead in the figs, nuts, and raisins. Shape the dough into a 12- by 6-inch loaf. Place the loaf on the prepared baking sheet. Cover and let rise for 1 hour, or until slightly puffy.

6. Preheat the oven to 400°F.

7. Bake for 25 to 30 minutes, or until lightly browned. Transfer to a wire rack to cool.

Torta di Grano Saraceno

BUCKWHEAT CAKE

Serves 8

Andreas Hellrigl is the chef and owner of New York's Palio Restaurant. This is an adaptation of his recipe for a traditional cake from Merano, his hometown. The cake is traditionally made with *mirtilli rossi*, red blueberries. Andreas suggests substituting cranberries or blueberries. The fruit is made into a kind of jam that is used both as a filling for and an accompaniment to the cake. Fior di Latte is served alongside.

Buckwheat flour, called Saracen grain, can be purchased at most health food shops.

JAM

½ to 1 cup sugar

¼ cup water

1 cinnamon stick

4 cups fresh or frozen cranberries or blueberries

CAKE

⅔ *cup buckwheat flour*

⅓ *cup potato starch*

½ *teaspoon baking powder*

12 *tablespoons (1½ sticks) unsalted butter, softened*

¾ *cup sugar*

4 *large eggs, separated*

1 *cup almonds, toasted and coarsely chopped*

1 *teaspoon vanilla extract*

Fior di Latte (page 225) or whipped cream

1. To make the jam: In a large saucepan, combine the sugar, water, and cinnamon stick; if using cranberries use the larger amount of sugar. Bring to a simmer over medium heat and cook, stirring occasionally, for 3 minutes, or until the sugar is dissolved.

2. Add the berries and cook, stirring occasionally, until the berries begin to burst. With a slotted spoon, transfer the berries to a bowl. Let the juices that remain in the pan simmer until thickened and reduced to a thick syrup. Discard the cinnamon stick. Pour the thickened juices over the berries and let cool.

3. To make the cake: Preheat the oven to 325°F. Butter and flour a 9-inch springform pan.

4. Combine the flour, potato starch, and baking powder.

5. In a large bowl, beat the butter and ½ cup of the sugar until light and fluffy. Add the egg yolks one at a time, beating well after each addition. Beat in the almonds and vanilla. Fold in the dry ingredients.

6. In a large bowl, beat the egg whites until foamy. Gradually beat in the remaining ¼ cup sugar and beat until soft peaks form. Fold one third of the whites into the butter mixture to lighten it. Then gradually fold in the remaining whites.

7. Pour the batter into the prepared pan. Bake for 35 to 40 minutes, or until a cake tester inserted in the center comes out clean. Let cool in the pan for 10 minutes, then remove from the pan and let cool completely on a wire rack.

8. With a long serrated knife, cut the cake in half horizontally. Spread the bottom half with a thin layer of the jam, and cover with the top half. Serve the remaining jam and the Fior di Latte or whipped cream alongside the cake.

Bocca di Dama

PARMA ALMOND CAKE

Serves 8

The name of this rich cake means "mouth of a lady" and probably comes from the fact that it is so delicious, it is fit for the mouth of a fine lady. It is very easy to make and can be served plain or dressed up. Try splitting it and filling with raspberry or apricot jam.

1½ cups blanched almonds

1 cup sugar

½ cup all-purpose flour

¼ teaspoon baking powder

4 tablespoons unsalted butter, at room temperature

4 large eggs, at room temperature

1 teaspoon vanilla extract

½ teaspoon almond extract

3 tablespoons sliced almonds

1. Preheat the oven to 325°F. Butter an 8-inch round cake pan. Line the bottom of the pan with a circle of wax paper. Butter the paper and sprinkle the pan with flour. Tap out the excess.

2. In a food processor or blender, combine the blanched almonds and ¼ cup of the sugar. Process until very finely ground. Add the flour and baking powder and pulse to blend.

3. In the large bowl of an electric mixer, beat the butter and the remaining ¾ cup sugar until light and fluffy. Beat in the eggs one at a time beating well after each addition. Beat in the extracts. Gently fold in the ground almond mixture.

4. Scrape the batter into the prepared pan. Sprinkle with the sliced almonds.

5. Bake for 45 to 50 minutes, or until the top of the cake is golden brown and a cake tester inserted in the center comes out clean. Let cool for 10 minutes on a wire rack.

6. Run a thin spatula around the side of the pan and invert the cake onto a rack. Turn the cake right side up onto another rack and cool completely. Serve plain or with Raspberry Sauce (page 217) and whipped cream.

$\mathcal{T}$orta di Nocciole

HAZELNUT CAKE

Serves 8

❧ Hazelnut cake is a specialty of Piedmont. It is delicious served plain or with chocolate sauce and ice cream.

1½ cups hazelnuts, toasted and skinned (page 3)

½ cup all-purpose flour

½ teaspoon baking powder

½ teaspoon salt

8 tablespoons (1 stick) unsalted butter, softened

⅔ cup sugar

3 large eggs, at room temperature

1. Preheat the oven to 350°F. Butter a 9-inch springform pan.

2. In a food processor, finely chop the hazelnuts. Add the flour, baking powder, and salt and pulse just to blend.

3. In the large bowl of an electric mixer, beat the butter until light and creamy. Gradually add the sugar and beat until fluffy. Scrape the sides of the bowl. Beat in the eggs one at a time, beating well after each addition. Stir in the dry ingredients just until blended.

4. Spread the butter evenly in the prepared pan. Bake for 30 minutes, or until a cake tester inserted in the center comes out clean.

5. Cool in the pan for 5 minutes. Then unmold the cake onto a wire rack and cool completely.

Torta di Semolina

SEMOLINA CAKE

Serves 8

Semolina is a kind of meal made from coarsely ground hard wheat. It usually is used for making pasta and bread, but sometimes it is cooked like cereal and baked into a pudding. This is another recipe from my friend Carla, who comes from the mountainous Piedmont region. A warm slice of this cake would be comforting on a cold winter night.

> 1 quart milk
>
> 2/3 cup sugar
>
> 1/2 teaspoon salt
>
> 1 teaspoon grated lemon zest
>
> 1 1/4 cups fine semolina
>
> 2 large eggs, beaten
>
> 1 teaspoon vanilla extract
>
> 1/2 cup raisins
>
> 1/4 cup pine nuts

1. Preheat the oven to 400°F. Butter a 9-inch springform pan.

2. In a medium saucepan bring the milk to a simmer over medium-low heat. Add the sugar, salt, and lemon zest. Stir in the semolina and cook over low heat, stirring constantly, for 5 minutes. Remove from the heat and let cool slightly, stirring occasionally.

3. In a medium bowl, beat the eggs and vanilla until blended. Stir the beaten eggs, raisins, and pine nuts into the cooled semolina. Pour the mixture into the prepared pan.

4. Bake the cake for 45 minutes, or until golden brown on top. Cool in the pan on a wire rack. Serve warm or chilled.

Torta Croccante

CRUNCHY CAKE

Serves 8

✺ Only five ingredients are needed to make this crunchy cookielike torte. The sugar and almonds form a crackling topping for the buttery shortbread layers. This is great with tea. Cutting it into even slices is impossible, so I just break it into irregular chunks.

¾ *cup sugar*

1 *cup slivered almonds*

½ *pound (2 sticks) unsalted butter, softened*

1 *teaspoon salt*

2 *cups all-purpose flour*

1. Preheat the oven to 350°F. Line the bottom and sides of a 9-inch round cake pan with aluminum foil. Butter the foil.

2. Sprinkle ¼ cup of the sugar and ½ cup of the almonds over the bottom of the prepared pan.

3. In the large bowl of an electric mixer, beat the butter, the remaining ½ cup sugar, and the salt until light and fluffy. On low speed, beat in the flour until a crumbly dough forms.

4. Scatter half of the dough over the bottom of the prepared pan and press it with your fingertips into an even layer. Sprinkle with the remaining ½ cup almonds. Scatter the remaining dough over the almonds and press it into an even layer.

5. Bake for 45 minutes, or until the top is lightly browned. Let cool for 10 minutes on a wire rack. Then invert the cake onto a rack, carefully lift off the foil, and let cool completely. Serve upside down.

Torta Sbricciolona

CRUMBLY CAKE

Serves 12

✿ This cake looks more like a giant cookie than a traditional cake. Instead of cutting it into wedges, I like to let everyone break off chunks they can eat with their hands. It is a fine informal dessert to dunk and nibble with a glass of dessert wine. Nobody will leave the table until the last crumb is gone.

½ pound (2 sticks) unsalted butter, softened

1 cup sugar

½ teaspoon salt

1 large egg

½ cup fine yellow cornmeal

2 teaspoons grated lemon zest

1 teaspoon vanilla extract

2 cups all-purpose flour

1½ cups blanched almonds, toasted and finely chopped

½ cup slivered almonds

Confectioners' sugar

1. Preheat the oven to 350°F. Butter a 12- by 1-inch round pizza pan or a large baking sheet.

2. In a large bowl, beat the butter with an electric mixer on medium speed until light and fluffy. Beat in the sugar and salt. Beat in the egg. Beat in the cornmeal, lemon zest and vanilla just until blended. On low speed, beat in the flour just until combined. Stir in the chopped nuts.

3. Turn the dough out into the prepared pan, and pat the dough out into a 12-inch circle. Sprinkle with the slivered almonds and lightly press them into the dough. Bake for 30 minutes, or until the cake is lightly browned and feels firm when touched lightly in the center.

4. Transfer the pan to a rack to cool for 5 minutes. If using a pizza pan, invert the cake onto a rack, then invert it again onto another rack to cool completely. If using a baking sheet, just slide the cake onto a rack to cool. Sprinkle with confectioners' sugar before serving.

Ciambella di Polenta
CORNMEAL CAKE
Serves 12

A frosty mist had settled over Bologna one winter day and we felt chilled to the bone. We stopped at a pasticceria, where we warmed up with hot chocolate and slices of freshly made *ciambella di polenta*. It is something like a pound cake but with a rich golden color and slight crunchiness that comes from cornmeal.

Use a fine stone-ground cornmeal or the texture may be too coarse. Dried Fruit Compote (page 125) goes well with this cake.

1¼ cups all-purpose flour

½ cup fine yellow cornmeal

2 teaspoons baking powder

12 tablespoons (1½ sticks) unsalted butter, softened

1 cup sugar

5 large eggs, separated

1½ teaspoons grated lemon zest

1 teaspoon vanilla extract

¼ teaspoon salt

Confectioners' sugar

1. Preheat the oven to 350°F. Butter and flour an 8-cup ring mold.
2. Sift together the flour, cornmeal, and baking powder.
3. In a large bowl, beat the butter with an electric mixer at medium speed until light and fluffy. Gradually beat in the sugar. Beat in the egg yolks one at a time, beating well after each addition. Beat in the lemon zest and vanilla.
4. In another large bowl, using clean beaters, beat the egg whites with the salt at medium speed until foamy. Increase the speed to high and beat until soft peaks form. Gently fold the whites into the egg yolk mixture. Fold in the dry ingredients.
5. Pour the batter into the prepared pan and smooth the top. Bake for 35 to 40 minutes, or until a cake tester inserted in the center comes out clean.
6. Let cool in the pan for 10 minutes. Then invert onto a rack and let cool completely. Sprinkle with confectioners' sugar before serving.

Torta di Mascarpone

MASCARPONE CHEESECAKE

Serves 10

🌀 I love the atmosphere at Manhattan's Remi restaurant. Its unique painted murals and Venetian glass lamps make dining there like taking a gondola ride along Venice's Grand Canal.

The restaurant serves marvelous individual-size creamy cheesecakes made with a mascarpone topping on a bed of fresh pears. This version, modeled on theirs, is made with apples.

CRUST

1 cup all-purpose flour

2 tablespoons sugar

¼ teaspoon salt

5 tablespoons unsalted butter, softened

1 large egg yolk

1 teaspoon vanilla extract

APPLE FILLING

2 tablespoons unsalted butter

2 large Golden Delicious apples, peeled, cored, and thinly sliced

2 tablespoons sugar

¼ teaspoon ground cinnamon

TOPPING

1 pound (2 cups) mascarpone, softened

2 3-ounce packages cream cheese, softened

½ cup sugar

2 large eggs, at room temperature

2 tablespoons fresh lemon juice

1. Preheat the oven to 350°F. Butter a 9-inch springform pan. Place the pan on a 12-inch square of heavy-duty aluminum foil, and mold the foil tightly around the outside of the pan so that water cannot enter.

2. To make the crust: In a large bowl, combine the flour, sugar, and salt. With a pastry blender, cut in the butter until the mixture resembles coarse meal. Beat together the egg yolk and vanilla, and stir into the dry ingredients just until a dough forms.

3. Pat the dough into the bottom of the prepared pan, and prick it all over with a fork. Bake for 20 minutes or until lightly browned. Cool on a wire rack.

4. To make the filling: In a large skillet, melt the butter over medium heat. Add the apples, sugar, and cinnamon and cook, stirring occasionally, until the apples are tender, about 10 minutes. Remove from the heat and let cool.

5. To make the topping: In a large bowl, beat both cheeses, the sugar, eggs, and lemon juice until well blended.

6. Spread the apples evenly over the cooled crust. Scrape the cheese mixture over the apples and level the top. Place the springform pan in a large roasting pan and set it on the middle rack of the oven. Pour hot water to a depth of 1 inch into the roasting pan. Bake for 1 hour or until just set.

7. Turn off the oven and prop the door open with the handle of a wooden spoon. Let the cake cool for 1 hour in the turned-off oven, then remove the foil and refrigerate for several hours or overnight.

8. When ready to serve, run a knife around the inside of the pan. Remove the rim and slide the cake, on its base, onto a serving dish.

Torta di Ricotta al Dante

DANTE'S CHEESECAKE

Serves 12 to 16

Caffè Dante in Greenwich Village is my favorite café, outside of Italy, for cappuccino. The walls are covered with murals depicting Florence through the ages and the place is always lively and packed with throngs of students and local characters. In the warmer months, the tables spill out onto the sidewalk.

The glass-enclosed showcases up front are full of sophisticated cakes and pastries, but I always order my favorite Italian cheesecake. Dante's version is sublime, smooth and creamy with a light, almost custardlike consistency. The cake itself is immense, and the portions it's cut into are thick slabs, each easily enough to serve two.

This is my scaled-down version of Caffè Dante's cheesecake, though it still makes a big cake. To achieve a smooth, creamy consistency, the ricotta is first puréed in a blender or processor and the eggs are beaten only enough to blend them without incorporating air. Baking the cake in a water bath insulates it and helps it to bake evenly. As a result, the cake rises very little as it bakes, and so does not sink in the center or crack as many cheesecakes do.

> 8 large eggs
>
> 2 teaspoons vanilla extract
>
> 1 teaspoon grated orange zest
>
> 1½ cups sugar
>
> ½ cup all-purpose flour
>
> 3 pounds (6 cups) whole-milk ricotta cheese

1. Preheat the oven to 350°F. Butter and flour a 9-inch springform pan. Place the pan on a 12-inch square of heavy-duty aluminum foil, and mold the foil tightly around the pan so that water cannot enter.

2. In a large bowl, beat the eggs, vanilla, and orange zest just until blended. Beat in the sugar and flour.

3. In a food processor or blender, purée the ricotta until very smooth. Add the cheese to the egg mixture and stir well with a wooden spoon.

4. Pour the batter into the prepared pan. Place the pan inside a large roasting pan and set it on the middle rack of the oven. Pour hot water to a depth of 1 inch into the roasting pan. Bake for 1 hour 30 minutes, or until the top is golden and a knife inserted 2 inches from the center of the cake comes out clean.

5. Turn off the oven and prop the door open with a wooden spoon. Let the cake cool for 30 minutes in the turned-off oven. Remove from the oven and remove the foil wrapping. (Do not worry if there is some liquid in the foil that has seeped out from the cake.) Cool completely on a wire rack.

6. The cake is best at room temperature or slightly chilled. Store in the refrigerator.

Cassola

SKILLET CHEESECAKE

Serves 4

𝄢 This small, simple cake is adapted from a Roman-Jewish recipe. The technique for making it is somewhat unusual as the cake is partially baked in a skillet on top of the stove and is finished in the oven. It is best when freshly made and served with fresh berries or a fruit sauce.

1 15-ounce container whole-milk ricotta cheese

2 teaspoons extra-virgin olive oil

¼ cup sugar

1 tablespoon cornstarch

1 large egg

2 large egg yolks

Confectioners' sugar

Fresh raspberries or strawberries

1. To drain the excess liquid from the ricotta, line a large strainer with cheesecloth and place the strainer over a bowl. Spoon the ricotta into the strainer and fold the cloth over the cheese. Place a plate on top and weight it down with several heavy cans. Refrigerate for 24 hours.

2. Preheat the oven to 350°F. Brush an 8-inch ovenproof nonstick skillet with the olive oil.

3. Unwrap the drained ricotta and place it in a large bowl. With a wooden spoon, beat in the sugar and cornstarch. With a whisk, beat in the egg and yolks until well blended.

4. Spoon the ricotta mixture into the oiled skillet, and set the skillet over very low heat. Cook for 20 minutes, or until the cheesecake mixture is set 1 inch in from the sides of the skillet. Watch carefully so that the bottom does not burn.

5. Transfer the skillet to the oven and bake for 10 to 15 minutes, or until the cheesecake is puffed and lightly browned on top.

6. Invert the cake onto a serving plate. Let cool to lukewarm. Sprinkle with confectioners' sugar and cut into wedges. Garnish with fresh raspberries or strawberries.

Migliaccio

AUNT LORETTA'S CHEESECAKE

Serves 12

Migliaccio is a name applied to any number of puddinglike desserts made throughout Italy. This particular version was given to me by my aunt, Loretta Balsamo, who got it from an Italian friend. This cake is traditionally made at Easter time.

The farina gives the cake a light, moist, creamy texture that is absolutely delicious.

6 large eggs, at room temperature

3 cups (about 1½ pounds) whole-milk ricotta cheese

1 cup sugar

1 teaspoon grated orange zest

1 teaspoon grated lemon zest

1 tablespoon orange liqueur

2 cups milk

1 cup water

¾ cup uncooked farina

1 teaspoon salt

¼ cup finely chopped candied citron

1. Preheat the oven to 350°F. Butter a 9- by 3-inch springform pan.
2. In a large bowl, beat the eggs until foamy. Beat in the ricotta, sugar, orange and lemon zests, and the liqueur.
3. In a medium saucepan, combine the milk and water, and bring to a simmer over medium heat. Add the farina in a fine stream, stirring constantly. Stir in the salt and cook, stirring, for 3 minutes, or until thick and creamy.
4. Stir the cooked farina into the ricotta mixture, then stir in the citron. Pour into the prepared pan.
5. Bake for 1 hour and 10 minutes, or until the top of the cake is golden and a knife inserted in the center comes out clean. Cool on a wire rack. Serve at room temperature or slightly chilled. Store in the refrigerator.

Torta Gianduja

CHOCOLATE HAZELNUT CAKE

Serves 8 to 10

In Piedmont, the combination of hazelnuts and chocolate is called *gianduja*. The combination of flavors is very popular and it appears in candies, ice cream, puddings, and cakes.

This version of gianduja cake is a favorite. As it bakes, the cake forms a firm, crusty surface while the inside remains moist and fudgy. The glaze is not essential since the cake is so rich, but it does make it look quite elegant.

> 8 tablespoons (1 stick) unsalted butter, softened
>
> 1 cup sugar
>
> 5 large eggs, separated
>
> 6 ounces semisweet chocolate, melted and cooled
>
> 1½ cups hazelnuts, toasted, skinned (page 3), and finely chopped
>
> ¼ teaspoon salt

GLAZE

> 6 ounces semisweet chocolate
>
> 2 tablespoons unsalted butter

> 2 tablespoons toasted, skinned, and finely chopped hazelnuts

1. Preheat the oven to 350°F. Butter a 9- by 2-inch round cake pan.

2. In a large bowl, beat the butter with an electric mixer at medium speed until light and fluffy. Gradually beat in the sugar. Add the egg yolks and beat until smooth. Stir in the melted chocolate and hazelnuts.

3. In another large bowl, with clean beaters, beat the egg whites and salt on medium speed until foamy. Increase the speed to high and beat until soft peaks form. Gently fold a large spoonful of the whites into the chocolate mixture to lighten it. Then gradually fold in the remainder.

4. Scrape the batter into the prepared pan. Shake the pan gently to level the surface. Bake for 55 to 60 minutes, or until the cake is firm around the edge but slightly moist in the center. Let cool for 15 minutes on a wire rack. Then unmold the cake onto a rack, invert onto another rack, and let cool right side up.

5. To make the glaze: Break the chocolate into pieces and place it in a small heatproof bowl. Add the butter and place the bowl over a saucepan of simmering water. Heat over low heat until the chocolate is softened. Remove from the heat and stir until smooth.

6. Cut four narrow strips of wax paper and place them around the edges of a cake plate. Center the cake on the plate. Pour the glaze on top of the cake, and, with a long metal spatula, spread the chocolate over the top of the cake, allowing a small amount to drip over the sides. Smooth the sides with the spatula. Sprinkle the chopped nuts around the edge of the cake. Carefully remove the wax paper. Let stand in a cool place until the glaze is set.

7. Serve at room temperature. Store in the refrigerator.

Torta di Cioccolata alla Grappa

CHOCOLATE GRAPPA CAKE

Serves 8

My husband likes grappa and frequently brings home new brands to try. As a result, I found myself with a cabinet full of grappa bottles. I began to use it in cooking and discovered that its raisin-y flavor goes very well with chocolate, among other things. You don't have to use an expensive brand of grappa for cooking.

½ cup dark raisins

9 ounces semisweet or bittersweet chocolate, coarsely chopped

8 tablespoons (1 stick) unsalted butter

¾ cup plus 1 tablespoon all-purpose flour

6 large eggs, separated

½ cup sugar

⅓ cup grappa

1 teaspoon vanilla extract

⅓ cup pine nuts

Pinch of salt

Confectioners' sugar

Whipped cream

1. Place the raisins in a small bowl and add warm water to cover. Let stand for 20 minutes.

2. Preheat the oven to 350°F. Butter and flour a 9-inch springform pan.

3. In a heatproof bowl or the top of a double boiler set over simmering water, melt the chocolate with the butter. Remove from the heat and stir until completely smooth. Let cool slightly.

4. Drain the raisins and pat dry with paper towels. In a small bowl, toss the raisins with 1 tablespoon of the flour.

5. In a large bowl, whisk the egg yolks, sugar, grappa, and vanilla until well blended. Stir in the chocolate mixture a spoonful at a time. Stir in the remaining ¾ cup flour just until blended. Fold in the raisins and pine nuts.

6. In a large bowl, beat the egg whites with the salt until soft peaks form. Fold one third of the whites into the chocolate mixture to lighten it. Then gently fold in the remaining whites.

7. Scrape the mixture into the prepared pan and level the top. Bake for 45 to 50 minutes, or until the cake is puffed and slight cracks appear on the surface. The center should be slightly moist. Let the cake cool in the pan for 10 minutes. Remove the rim of the pan and place the cake on a wire rack to cool completely.

8. Sprinkle the cake with confectioners' sugar. Serve with whipped cream.

Torta della Nonna

GRANDMOTHER'S CAKE

Serves 8

Florence's Piazza Michelangelo is surely among the most beautiful spots in the world. Not only is it the best place to take in the sight of the magical city on the River Arno, but it is a great location for people-watching. On warm summer evenings, all of Florence—natives, students, tourists—seems to gather there to look at the view, catch the breeze, watch the setting sun, stroll, meet friends and family, flirt, eat gelati, take pictures, have a drink, and just about anything else one can think of to have a good time.

There are several caffès to sit in and one grand restaurant, called La Loggia, where I first tasted this lovely cream-filled torte, a favorite in many parts of Tuscany.

FILLING

1 cup milk

3 large egg yolks

⅓ cup sugar

1½ teaspoons vanilla extract

2 tablespoons all-purpose flour

2 tablespoons orange liqueur

CAKE

1⅔ cups all-purpose flour

½ cup sugar

1 teaspoon baking powder

¼ teaspoon salt

8 tablespoons (1 stick) unsalted butter, cut into bits and softened

1 large egg, lightly beaten

1 teaspoon vanilla extract

1 *egg yolk beaten with 1 teaspoon water, for egg wash*

2 *tablespoons pine nuts*

Confectioners' sugar

1. To make the filling: In a medium saucepan, heat the milk until bubbles form around the edges. Remove from the heat.

2. In a medium bowl, whisk the egg yolks, sugar, and vanilla until pale yellow. Whisk in the flour. Gradually add the hot milk, whisking constantly. Transfer the mixture to the saucepan and cook over low heat, stirring constantly, until it comes to a boil. Reduce the heat and simmer for 1 minute. Scrape the custard into a bowl. Stir in the orange liqueur. Place a piece of plastic wrap directly on the surface of the custard to prevent a skin from forming, and refrigerate until chilled, 1 hour or overnight.

3. Preheat the oven to 350°F. Butter a 9-inch round cake pan.

4. To make the cake: In a large bowl, combine the flour, sugar, baking powder, and salt. With a pastry blender, cut in the butter until the mixture resembles coarse crumbs. Add the egg and vanilla and stir until a dough forms. Divide the dough in half.

5. Press one half of the dough evenly into the bottom of the prepared pan and ½ inch up the sides. Spread the chilled custard cream over the center of the dough, leaving a 1-inch border around the edges.

6. On a lightly floured surface, roll out the remaining dough to a 9½-inch circle. Drape the dough over the rolling pin and place it over the filling. Pinch the edges of the dough together to seal. Brush the egg wash over the top of the cake. With a small knife, make several slits in the top to allow steam to escape. Sprinkle the top with the pine nuts.

7. Bake for 30 to 35 minutes, or until golden brown on top. Let cool on a wire rack for 10 minutes. Invert the cake onto a wire rack, then invert onto another rack to cool completely. Sprinkle with confectioners' sugar before serving. Store in the refrigerator.

$\mathcal{L}$a Pastiera di Grano

NEAPOLITAN EASTER CAKE

Serves 12

No matter what else was served on Easter Sunday, one dessert we all looked forward to was *la pastiera*, or "pizza gran," as we called this delicious cake made with wheat grain and ricotta. I still have the pan my grandmother used to make hers. It is twelve inches wide by five inches deep—needless to say, there was always plenty. Grandma would also make miniature versions, to be given as gifts or exchanged with other family members and friends for their holiday desserts, though everyone preferred Grandma's.

Some historians trace la pastiera to the cloistered nuns who devised such a cake as a symbol of the Resurrection, with the grain representing rebirth and the spices and flavorings representing spring. But others trace it back even further, dating it to a time when sweet cakes made with grain were prepared to honor Demeter, the pagan goddess of fertility.

This is my mother's version of the cake as she learned it from my father's mother. The pastry, called *pasta frolla*, is quite unusual. Made with confectioners' sugar, it has a tender, melt-in-your-mouth texture. When I was a child, I used to love rolling out scraps of the dough in sugar and shaping it into cookies.

For the filling, you will need to buy hulled soft wheat, which has a creamy white color. Do not buy hard red wheat. The hull has not been removed and it will remain tough no matter how long it is cooked. Soft wheat is available in Italian markets and many health food stores. It must be soaked overnight before cooking. Some Italian markets sell the grain already cooked in cans and jars at holiday time.

The characteristic flavoring in pastiera is orange flower water. This delightful essence is available in many Italian, Greek, and Middle Eastern markets.

8 ounces hulled wheat

CRUST

2 cups all-purpose flour

½ teaspoon ground cinnamon

¼ teaspoon salt

8 tablespoons (1 stick) unsalted butter, softened

¾ cup confectioners' sugar

1 large egg

1 large egg yolk

1 teaspoon orange flower water

FILLING

½ teaspoon salt

8 tablespoons (1 stick) unsalted butter, softened

1 cup hot milk

1 teaspoon grated orange zest

1 pound (2 cups) whole-milk ricotta cheese

4 large eggs

⅔ cup sugar

3 tablespoons orange flower water

½ teaspoon ground cinnamon

½ cup chopped candied citron

½ cup chopped candied orange peel

Confectioners' sugar

1. Place the wheat in a large bowl, add water to cover, and let soak overnight in a cool place.

2. To make the dough: Combine the flour, cinnamon, and salt.

3. In a large bowl, beat the butter and confectioners' sugar until light and fluffy. Add the egg and egg yolk and beat until smooth. Beat in the orange flower water. Add the dry ingredients and stir just until blended. Shape the dough into two disks, one slightly larger than the other. Wrap in plastic wrap and chill for at least 1 hour, or overnight.

4. To make the filling: Drain the soaked wheat and place it in a medium saucepan with fresh water to cover. Add the salt and bring to a simmer over medium heat. Cook, stirring occasionally, until the wheat is tender, 20 to 30 minutes. Drain, and place in a large bowl. Stir in the butter, milk, and orange zest. Let cool.

5. Preheat the oven to 350°F.

6. In a large bowl, combine the ricotta, eggs, sugar, orange flour water, and cinnamon. Beat until blended. Stir in the wheat mixture, citron, and candied orange peel.

continued

7. Roll out the larger piece of dough to a 15-inch circle. Fit the dough into a 9- by 3-inch springform pan. Pour in the filling and smooth the top.

8. Roll out the remaining piece of dough to a 10-inch circle. With a fluted pastry cutter, cut the dough into ½-inch-wide strips. Place the strips over the filling in a lattice pattern. Press the ends against the bottom pastry to seal. Bake for 1½ hours, or until well browned on top. Let cool in the pan for 15 minutes. Remove the rim of the pan and let cool completely on a wire rack.

9. Sprinkle the cake with confectioners' sugar before serving. Store in the refrigerator.

Torta di Noci e Canditi

CHOCOLATE, WALNUT, AND ORANGE TORTE

Serves 8 to 10

This rich cake comes from Liguria, where walnuts are used in many recipes both sweet and savory. It is delicious served with Raspberry and Red Wine Sorbet (page 203).

6 ounces semisweet chocolate, chopped

1⅔ cups walnuts

6 large eggs, separated

⅔ cup sugar

2 tablespoons orange liqueur

⅓ cup finely chopped candied orange peel

Confectioners' sugar

1. Preheat the oven to 350°F. Butter a 9-inch springform pan and dust it lightly with flour. Tap out the excess.

2. Place the chocolate in a food processor fitted with a steel blade, and process until coarsely chopped. Add the walnuts and process until finely ground.

3. In a large bowl, beat the egg yolks until well blended. Gradually add ⅓ cup of the sugar and beat until very light and fluffy. Beat in the orange liqueur. Beat in the chocolate mixture and orange peel.

4. In a large bowl, beat the egg whites until foamy. Gradually beat in the remaining ⅓ cup sugar, and beat until soft peaks form.

5. Fold one third of the egg whites into the chocolate mixture to lighten it. Gradually fold in the remainder.

6. Scrape the batter into the prepared pan. Bake in the center of the oven for 45 minutes, or until the cake is puffed but the center is still moist. Cool completely on a wire rack. Run a spatula around the inside of the rim of the pan to release it. Remove the rim and place the cake on a serving plate. Just before serving, sprinkle with confectioners' sugar.

Panettone

Serves 10 to 12

Christmas in Italy would not seem like Christmas without panettone. The tall, cylindrical, fruit-studded yeast cakes have become an essential part of the holiday celebration. During the Christmas season, Italians eat panettone throughout the day—at breakfast with coffee, for between-meal snacks with Marsala or another dessert wine, and after a meal with spumante.

A romantic legend with many variations is told about the origins of panettone. Supposedly, there was a Milanese baker named Toni di Borgo alle Grazie who had a beautiful daughter called Adalgisa. A young baker wanted to marry Adalgisa. In order to win her father's approval, the young man developed a special sweet bread, filled with fruits and other rich ingredients, that made Toni's bakery famous. People began to call the bread "pan ad Toni," or Toni's bread. Toni became wealthy and, of course, allowed the young man to marry his daughter.

Leftover panettone has many uses. Serve it toasted and spread with butter or mascarpone for breakfast or use it to make French toast. It is also wonderful in bread pudding (page 158). Traditionally, a small piece of panettone is reserved at Christmas to eat on February 3, in honor of the feast of Saint Blaise.

½ cup milk

½ cup sugar

6 tablespoons unsalted butter

2 packages active dry yeast

½ cup warm water

2 large eggs

2 large egg yolks

¾ cup finely chopped candied citron

½ cup dark raisins

½ cup finely chopped candied orange peel

1 teaspoon grated lemon zest

5½ cups all-purpose flour

1. In a small saucepan, heat the milk until small bubbles form around the edges of the pan. Remove from the heat. Add the sugar and butter and let stand, stirring occasionally, until the butter is melted and the mixture has cooled to lukewarm.

2. In a large bowl of an electric mixer, sprinkle the yeast over the warm water. Let stand for 5 minutes, then stir until the yeast is dissolved. Add the milk mixture, eggs, and yolks, and beat at low speed until blended. Stir in the citron, raisins, orange peel, and lemon zest, add the flour, and beat until a stiff dough forms.

3. Scrape the dough into a large buttered bowl and turn it once to grease the top. Cover with a towel and let rise in a warm place until doubled in bulk, about 1½ hours.

4. Butter a 9- by 4-inch springform pan. (If your pan is less than 4 inches deep, make a collar for the pan: Tear off a 3-foot length of aluminum foil, and fold it in half lengthwise. Butter one side of the foil, and wrap it around the outside of the pan, buttered side in. Tie with string to secure.)

5. Punch the dough down to eliminate air bubbles. Place the dough in the prepared pan, cover with a towel, and let rise until doubled in bulk, about 1 hour.

6. Preheat the oven to 350°F. Adjust an oven rack to the lowest level.

7. With a sharp knife, slash a cross in the top of the panettone. Bake for 1 hour, or until browned on top. Cool for 10 minutes. Remove the rim of the springform, and let the cake cool completely on a wire rack before removing it from the base.

Crostate

~~~~
TARTS

Crostate, the Italian version of dessert tarts, are popular all over Italy. There are all kinds of crostate—filled with fresh or dried fruit, pastry cream, nuts, rice custard, ricotta, or chocolate. The crust also varies, often flavored with ground nuts, cocoa, or spices. Some crostate are made free-form, without a tart pan, and those sold in bakeries may be small or large, baked in long sheet pans, and sold by the slice.

Though the crust is generally a bit thicker and the fillings have a distinctly Italian accent, crostate are similar to French dessert tarts. But many historians credit the Florentine Caterina dei Medici with teaching the French the art of pastry making, and presumably crostate, for she arrived in France before her marriage to the future King Henry II with an entourage of Italian chefs and all of their equipment.

Tips for Making Crostate

- The pastry for Italian-style tarts is called *pasta frolla*, meaning "tender pastry," and it is an apt description. It has a high proportion of butter, sugar, and eggs to flour and needs to be well chilled and handled gently, especially in warm or humid weather. Chilling the dough for at least one hour or even overnight after assembling it helps to make it easier to roll. After chilling, the butter will have hardened, and it will be necessary to let the dough warm up slightly at room temperature before rolling it out.

- Use a minimum amount of flour on the rolling surface and pin, or the pastry will toughen. Rolling the dough between two sheets of wax paper is much simpler than flouring and reflouring a work surface. Just remember to rotate and turn the dough over frequently. As you do so, lift the paper away from the dough with each turn so that it does not become embedded in the dough. If it should become too soft at any point, rechill it.

- Drape the rolled-out dough over the rolling pin and transfer it to the pan. Chill the dough again after fitting it into the pan. This second chilling will help to prevent the dough from shrinking as it bakes.

- If you are in a hurry, you can pat the dough into the pan rather than rolling it immediately after it is made. Chill it for at least thirty minutes before proceeding with the recipe.

- A lattice topping can be fashioned from bits of dough simply formed into long ropes, as opposed to one made by rolling out the dough with a rolling pin and cutting it into strips. A lattice topping is easy to make. The dough strips do not need to be woven together. Just lay four or five strips of dough one inch apart across the filling, pressing the ends against the rim of the pastry until they adhere. Trim off the excess. Lay four or five more strips crosswise over the first batch, and seal and trim as before.

- Pasta frolla can be made into delicious butter cookies. Just roll out the dough ¼ inch thick, cut into shapes, and sprinkle with sugar. Bake until lightly browned.

- Pastry dough can be frozen for up to one month. Thaw it overnight in the refrigerator before using.

Single-Crust Pasta Frolla

Makes 1 9-inch crust

1⅓ cups all-purpose flour

3 tablespoons sugar

½ teaspoon salt

Grated zest of 1 lemon or 1 orange

8 tablespoons (1 stick) cold unsalted butter, cut into bits

1 large egg, lightly beaten

1 teaspoon vanilla extract

1. In a large bowl, combine the flour, sugar, salt, and zest. With a pastry blender or fork, blend in the butter until the mixture resembles coarse meal. Add the egg and vanilla extract and toss the mixture with a fork until the egg is incorporated.

2. Gather the dough together and shape it into a disk. Wrap it in plastic wrap. Chill for at least 1 hour, or overnight.

Double-Crust Pasta Frolla

Makes 2 9-inch crusts

2⅓ cups all-purpose flour

⅓ cup sugar

½ teaspoon salt

Grated zest of 1 lemon or 1 orange

12 tablespoons (1½ sticks) cold unsalted butter, cut into bits

1 large egg plus 1 large egg yolk, lightly beaten

1 teaspoon vanilla extract

1. In a large bowl, combine the flour, sugar, salt, and zest. With a pastry blender or fork, blend in the butter until the mixture resembles coarse meal. Add the egg and egg yolk and the vanilla extract and toss with a fork until the liquid is incorporated.

2. Gather the dough together and shape it into two disks, one slightly larger than the other. Wrap each disk in plastic wrap. Chill for at least 1 hour, or overnight.

Crostata di Marmellata

JAM TART

Serves 6 to 8

🍥 This tart also works well with a high-quality store-bought jam used as the filling. Cherry, blueberry, or plum jams are particularly good. You will need about 1½ cups.

1 recipe Double-Crust Pasta Frolla, (page 82), made with lemon zest

FILLING
2 cups fresh or frozen blackberries
1 cup sugar

1 egg yolk beaten with 1 teaspoon water, for egg wash
Confectioners' sugar

1. On a lightly floured surface, roll out the larger piece of dough to an 11-inch circle about ⅛ inch thick. Fit the dough into a 9-inch fluted tart pan with a removable bottom. Trim off all but a ½-inch border of dough. Fold the excess dough in against the inside of the pan and press into place. Chill the tart shell for 30 minutes.

2. Place the berries in a medium saucepan and crush them with a spoon. Bring to a simmer over low heat and cook for 10 minutes. Stir in the sugar and bring to a boil. Cook, stirring occasionally, until the mixture is very thick, about 10 minutes. Let cool.

3. Preheat the oven to 350°F. Place an oven rack on the lowest level.

4. Spread the jam in the bottom of the prepared shell. Roll out the remaining dough to a 10-inch circle about ⅛ inch thick and, with a fluted pastry wheel, cut it into ½-inch-wide strips. Arrange the strips across the jam, forming a lattice pattern of strips about 1 inch apart. Press the ends of the strips against the sides of the tart shell to seal. Brush the dough with the egg wash.

5. Bake for 30 to 35 minutes, or until the pastry is golden brown. Let cool on a wire rack for 10 minutes. Then remove the pan rim and let the tart cool completely. Just before serving, sprinkle with confectioners' sugar.

Crostata di Fichi

FIG TART

Serves 6 to 8

✺ This crostata is reminiscent of Fig Newtons.

1 recipe Double-Crust Pasta Frolla (page 82), made with orange zest

FILLING

1 package (16 ounces) diced Calimyrna figs, coarsely chopped

¼ cup sugar

⅓ cup fresh orange juice

¾ cup water

1 egg yolk beaten with 1 teaspoon water, for egg wash
Confectioners' sugar

1. On a lightly floured surface, roll out the larger piece of dough to an 11-inch circle about ⅛ inch thick. Press the dough into a 9-inch fluted tart pan with a removable bottom. Trim off all but a ½-inch border of dough. Fold the excess dough in against the inside of the pan and press into place. Chill the tart shell for 30 minutes.

2. In a medium saucepan, combine the figs, sugar, orange juice, and water and bring to a simmer over medium heat. Cook, stirring occasionally, for 10 minutes or until thickened. Let cool.

3. Preheat the oven to 350°F. Place an oven rack on the lowest level.

4. Spread the fig mixture in the bottom of the prepared shell. Roll out the remaining dough to a 10-inch circle about ⅛ inch thick and, with a fluted pastry wheel, cut it into ½-inch-wide strips. Arrange the strips across the filling, forming a lattice pattern of strips about 1 inch apart. Press the ends of the strips against the sides of the tart shell to seal. Brush the dough with the egg wash.

5. Bake for 30 to 35 minutes, or until the pastry is golden brown. Let cool on a wire rack for 10 minutes. Then remove the pan rim and let the tart cool completely. Just before serving, sprinkle with confectioners' sugar.

Crostata di Pignoli

PINE NUT TART

Serves 8

Malvasia di Lipari, a delightful apricot-flavored dessert wine from the Lipari Islands, off the coast of Sicily, goes extremely well with this tart. Serve the wine slightly chilled.

1 recipe Single-Crust Pasta Frolla (page 81), made with orange zest

FILLING
⅓ cup apricot jam
2 large eggs, separated
½ cup sugar
½ teaspoon vanilla extract
1¼ cups toasted pine nuts

Confectioners' sugar

1. On a lightly floured surface, roll out the dough to an 11-inch circle about ⅛ inch thick. Press the dough into a 9-inch fluted tart pan with a removable bottom. Trim off all but a ½-inch border of dough. Fold the excess dough in against the inside of the pan and press into place. Chill the tart shell for 30 minutes.

2. Preheat the oven to 350°F. Place an oven rack on the lowest level.

3. Spread the jam over the bottom of the prepared shell.

4. In a large bowl, combine the egg yolks, sugar, and vanilla. Whisk until pale yellow.

5. In another large bowl, beat the egg whites until soft peaks form. Fold the whites into the yolk mixture. Gently fold in the pine nuts. Scrape the mixture into the tart shell.

6. Bake for 30 to 35 minutes, or until the tart is puffed and golden. Let cool on a wire rack for 10 minutes. Remove the pan rim and let the tart cool completely. Just before serving, sprinkle with confectioners' sugar.

Crostata di Limone e Cioccolata

LEMON AND CHOCOLATE CREAM TART

Serves 8

My mother's mother came from Afragola, near Naples. She was an expert baker and this lemon and chocolate bull's-eye tart was one of her specialties.

1 recipe Double-Crust Pasta Frolla (page 82), made with lemon zest

FILLING

1¾ cups milk

3 large egg yolks

½ cup sugar

⅓ cup all-purpose flour

1½ ounces semisweet chocolate, finely chopped

½ teaspoon grated lemon zest

Confectioners' sugar

1. On a lightly floured surface, roll out the larger piece of dough to an 11-inch circle about ⅛ inch thick. Press the dough into a 9-inch fluted tart pan with a removable bottom. Trim off all but a ½-inch border of dough. Fold the excess dough in against the side of the pan and press it into place. Chill the tart shell for 30 minutes.

2. In a small saucepan, heat the milk until small bubbles form around the edges of the pan. Remove from the heat.

3. In a large bowl, beat the egg yolks and sugar until well blended. Beat in the flour. Slowly beat in the hot milk. Transfer the mixture to the saucepan and cook over medium-low heat, stirring constantly, until the mixture is thick and coats the back of a spoon; do not allow to boil. Divide the mixture between two bowls. Stir the chocolate into one bowl of filling until melted and smooth. Stir the lemon zest into the second bowl. Let cool to room temperature.

4. Preheat the oven to 350°F. Adjust an oven rack to the lowest level. Spoon the chocolate filling evenly around the outer edge of the prepared shell. Spoon the lemon filling into the center. (The two fillings will run together).

5. Roll out the remaining piece of dough to a 10-inch circle about ⅛ inch thick. Lay the dough over the filling. Press the top and bottom edges together and crimp to seal. With a small sharp knife, cut several slits in the top crust to allow the steam to escape. Bake for 35 to 40 minutes, or until puffed and golden brown.

6. Let the tart cool on a wire rack for 10 minutes. Remove the pan rim and let the tart cool completely. Just before serving, sprinkle with confectioners' sugar. Store any leftover tart in the refrigerator.

Crostata di Prugne

PRUNE TART

Serves 8

An unusual walnut crust complements the prune filling in this tart.

CRUST

1⅔ cups all-purpose flour

½ cup finely ground toasted walnuts

⅓ cup sugar

½ teaspoon salt

Grated zest of 1 orange

12 tablespoons (1½ sticks) cold unsalted butter, cut into bits

1 large egg plus 1 large yolk, lightly beaten

1 teaspoon vanilla extract

FILLING

1 12-ounce box pitted prunes

1 cup dark raisins

1 cup water

Grated zest of 1 orange

¼ cup dark rum

2 tablespoons honey

½ teaspoon ground cinnamon

1 cup chopped toasted walnuts

1 egg yolk beaten with 1 teaspoon water, for egg wash

Confectioners' sugar

1. To make the crust: In a large bowl, combine the flour, walnuts, sugar, salt, and orange zest. With a pastry blender or fork, blend in the butter until the mixture resembles coarse meal. Add the egg and egg yolk and the vanilla and toss the mixture with a fork until the liquid is incorporated. Gather the dough together. Shape the dough into two disks, one slightly larger than the other. Wrap each disk in plastic wrap. Chill for at least 1 hour, or overnight.

2. In a medium saucepan, combine the prunes, raisins, and water. Cover and cook over low heat until the prunes are soft, about 10 minutes. Let cool.

3. On a lightly floured surface, roll out the dough to an 11-inch circle about ⅛ inch thick. Fit the dough into a 9-inch fluted tart pan with a removable bottom. Trim off all but a ½-inch border of dough. Fold the excess dough in against the inside of the pan and press into place. Chill the tart shell for 30 minutes.

4. Preheat the oven to 350°F. Place an oven rack on the lowest level.

5. To make the filling: In a food processor, combine the prunes and raisins with their liquid and the orange zest. Process until finely chopped. Add the rum, honey, and cinnamon and process to blend. Transfer to a bowl and stir in the walnuts.

6. Spread the prune mixture in the bottom of the prepared tart shell. Roll out the remaining dough to a 10-inch circle about ⅛ inch thick and, with a fluted pastry wheel, cut it into ½-inch-wide strips. Arrange the strips over the prune filling to form a lattice pattern of strips about 1 inch apart. Press the ends of the strips against the side of the tart shell to seal. Brush the dough with the egg wash.

7. Bake for 30 to 35 minutes, or until golden brown. Let cool on a wire rack for 10 minutes. Remove the pan rim and let the tart cool completely. Just before serving, sprinkle with confectioners' sugar.

Crostata di Riso

RICE TART

Serves 6 to 8

❧ A creamy rice custard fills this crostata. It is thicker than most crostate so it is baked in a springform pan rather than a tart pan.

You will need to use a short-grain rice, such as the kind used to make risotto, to get the right consistency.

1 recipe Single-Crust Pasta Frolla (page 81), made with orange zest

FILLING

3 cups milk

¼ cup Arborio, Vialone Nano, or other short-grain rice

½ cup sugar

2 tablespoons unsalted butter

2 large eggs

1 teaspoon grated orange zest

2 tablespoons finely chopped candied citron

2 tablespoons golden raisins

1. On a lightly floured surface, roll out the dough to a 10-inch circle about ⅛ inch thick. Fit the dough into an 8-inch springform pan, pressing it up against the sides. Chill the pastry shell for 30 minutes.

2. In a medium saucepan, bring the milk to a simmer. Add the rice, sugar, and butter and cook over low heat, stirring occasionally, for 30 minutes or until the rice is very tender. Transfer to a bowl and let cool, stirring occasionally.

3. Preheat the oven to 350°F. Place an oven rack on the lowest level.

4. In a medium bowl, beat the eggs and orange zest. Stir into the cooled rice mixture. Stir in the citron and raisins. Pour the mixture into the prepared shell.

5. Bake for 40 to 45 minutes, or until the filling is set and the top is very lightly browned. Let cool on a wire rack for 10 minutes. Remove the pan rim and let the tart cool to room temperature. Store any leftovers in the refrigerator.

Crostata di Mandorle

ALMOND TART

Serves 6 to 8

1 recipe Single-Crust Pasta Frolla (page 81), made with
  lemon zest

FILLING

3 large eggs, at room temperature

¼ cup sugar

1 8-ounce can almond paste

½ cup all-purpose flour

¾ cup cherry or raspberry jam

½ cup sliced almonds

Confectioners' sugar

1. On a lightly floured surface, roll out the dough to an 11-inch circle about ⅛ inch thick. Press the dough into a 9-inch fluted tart pan with a removable bottom. Trim off all but a ½-inch border of dough. Fold the excess dough in against the inside of the pan and press it into place. Chill the tart shell for 30 minutes.

2. Preheat the oven to 350°F. Place an oven rack on the lowest level.

3. In a medium bowl, beat the eggs until foamy. Gradually beat in the sugar. Crumble the almond paste into the egg mixture and beat until smooth. Fold in the flour.

4. Spread the jam over the bottom of the prepared shell. Spread the almond paste mixture over the jam. Sprinkle with the sliced almonds.

5. Bake for 30 to 35 minutes, or until puffed and golden. Let cool on a wire rack for 10 minutes. Remove the pan rim and let the tart cool completely. Just before serving, sprinkle with confectioners' sugar.

Crostata di Frutti di Bosco

BERRY TART

Serves 8

I love the look of this gorgeous tart with its berries piled high under a snowy dusting of sugar. You can make the pastry shell and the filling up to a day ahead of time, but the tart is best assembled no more than two hours before serving.

1 recipe Single-Crust Pasta Frolla (page 81), made with lemon zest

FILLING
1 cup milk
2 large egg yolks
1/3 cup sugar
3 tablespoons all-purpose flour
1/4 teaspoon salt
2 tablespoons orange liqueur
1 teaspoon vanilla extract
1 pint blackberries
1 pint raspberries

Confectioners' sugar

1. On a lightly floured surface, roll out the dough to an 11-inch circle. Fit the dough into a 9-inch fluted tart pan with a removable bottom. Trim off all but a ½-inch border of dough. Fold the excess dough in against the inside of the rim and press it into place. Chill the tart shell for at least 30 minutes.
2. Preheat the oven to 400°F.
3. With a fork, prick the bottom of the tart shell at 1-inch intervals. Butter a sheet of aluminum foil and place it buttered side down over the pastry. Fill the pan with beans or pie weights. Bake for 20 minutes, then remove the

foil and beans, prick the dough again, and bake for 5 to 10 minutes longer, or until lightly browned. Let cool completely on a wire rack.

3. In a medium saucepan, heat the milk until small bubbles form around the edges. Remove from the heat.

4. In a small bowl, whisk the egg yolks and sugar until blended. Beat in the flour and salt just until smooth. Gradually beat in the warm milk. Pour the mixture into the saucepan and cook over low heat, stirring constantly, until it comes to a boil. Cook, whisking constantly, for 3 minutes more. Remove from the heat. Stir in the orange liqueur and vanilla. Place a piece of plastic wrap over the surface to prevent a skin from forming. Refrigerate until chilled, or overnight.

5. Place the pastry shell on a serving platter. Spread the cream evenly over the bottom of the shell. Pile the berries on top. Sprinkle generously with confectioners' sugar. Serve chilled.

Crostata di Cioccolata

PARMA CHOCOLATE TART

Serves 8

At one time the city of Parma was a part of the Austrian Empire. The Austrians brought much to Parma. Among their legacies is the burnished yellow color that much of the city is painted. They also left behind a taste for chocolate.

This rich tart has a delicious chocolate cookie crust and a creamy center, something like a fallen soufflé. This dough tends to be sticky, so roll it out between sheets of wax paper.

CRUST

1¼ cups all-purpose flour

3 tablespoons Dutch-process cocoa powder

3 tablespoons sugar

½ teaspoon salt

8 tablespoons (1 stick) unsalted butter, cut into bits

1 large egg, lightly beaten

1 teaspoon vanilla extract

FILLING

4 tablespoons unsalted butter

4 ounces semisweet chocolate

3 large eggs

¼ teaspoon salt

½ cup sugar

1 teaspoon vanilla extract

½ cup all-purpose flour

1. To make the crust: In a large bowl, combine the flour, cocoa, sugar, and salt. With a pastry blender or fork, blend in the butter until the mixture resembles coarse meal. Add the egg and vanilla and toss with a fork until the

egg is incorporated. Gather the dough together and shape it into a disk. Wrap in plastic wrap and chill for several hours, or overnight.

2. Roll out the dough between two sheets of wax paper to an 11-inch circle. Fit the dough into a 9-inch fluted tart pan with a removable bottom. Trim off all but a ½-inch border of dough. Fold the excess dough in against the inside of the pan and press into place. Chill the tart shell for 30 minutes.

3. Preheat the oven to 350°F.

4. Prick the bottom of the pastry shell at ½-inch intervals with a fork. Bake for 10 minutes. Prick the dough again and bake for 5 minutes more. Let cool on a wire rack.

5. To make the filling: In a small heatproof bowl set over a pan of simmering water, melt the butter and chocolate. Stir until completely smooth, and let cool slightly.

6. In a large bowl, beat the eggs and salt until foamy. Gradually beat in the sugar and beat until thick and pale yellow. Beat in the vanilla. Stir in the melted chocolate. Sift the flour over the mixture and stir until just combined. Pour into the partially baked tart shell.

7. Bake for 25 minutes, or until the top is firm when touched lightly with a fingertip. Let cool for 10 minutes on a wire rack. Remove the pan rim and cool the tart completely. Store any leftover tart in the refrigerator.

Crostata di Fragole
STRAWBERRY TART
Serves 8

⟨⟩ This tart should be served within one hour after it is assembled.

1 recipe Single-Crust Pasta Frolla (page 81), made with orange or lemon zest

FILLING

8 ounces (1 cup) mascarpone

2 tablespoons sugar

¼ cup heavy cream

1 pint strawberries

GLAZE

½ cup seedless raspberry jam

2 tablespoons sugar

1. On a lightly floured surface, roll out the dough to an 11-inch circle. Fit it into a 9-inch fluted tart pan with a removable bottom. Trim off all but a ½-inch border of dough. Fold the excess dough in against the inside of the rim and press it into place. Chill the tart shell for at least 30 minutes.

2. Preheat the oven to 400°F.

3. With a fork, prick the bottom of the tart shell at 1-inch intervals. Butter a sheet of aluminum foil and place it buttered side down over the dough. Fill the pan with beans or pie weights. Bake for 20 minutes. Remove the foil and beans, prick the dough again, and bake for 5 to 10 minutes longer, or until lightly browned. Let cool on a wire rack.

4. To make the filling: In a medium bowl, combine the mascarpone, sugar, and the cream and beat until light and spreadable. Spread the mixture evenly over the bottom of the baked tart shell.

5. Slice the strawberries thinly and arrange them over the filling.

6. To make the glaze: In a small saucepan, combine the jam and the sugar and bring to a simmer over medium heat. Cook until lightly thickened, 3 to 5 minutes. Brush the glaze over the strawberries. Serve the tart within 1 hour.

Pizza di Ricotta alla Romana

ROMAN-STYLE RICOTTA TART

Serves 8

A popular bakery in Rome's Campo dei Fiore market makes little ricotta cheesecakes with a decidedly rummy taste. Some friends and I could never agree on which type of ricotta tart we liked best: the rum-flavored variety or the chocolate cherry cheesecakes from another Roman bakery.

One day we had tickets to attend a performance of the opera *Aïda* at the magnificent Baths of Caracalla. The performance started early, so we had no time for dinner beforehand. Instead, we bought some of each kind of cheesecake and as we sat under the stars and listened to Verdi's masterpiece, we ate cheesecake to our hearts' content. Now, whenever I hear *Celeste Aïda*, I get a craving for cheesecake.

I have decided that this version is my favorite. Like many Roman-style cheesecakes, this one is rather thin. In fact, the cheese topping is of equal thickness with the buttery crust, so the tart looks something like a white pizza, as the name implies.

CRUST

1½ cups all-purpose flour

⅓ cup sugar

½ teaspoon salt

½ teaspoon baking powder

8 tablespoons (1 stick) unsalted butter, softened

1 large egg, lightly beaten

FILLING

1 3-ounce package cream cheese, softened

¼ cup sugar

1 tablespoon dark rum

1 large egg yolk

1 cup (8 ounces) whole-milk ricotta cheese

continued

1. To make the crust: In a large bowl, combine the flour, sugar, salt, and baking powder. With a pastry blender or a fork, cut in the butter until the mixture resembles coarse meal. Stir in the egg until a soft dough forms. Pat into the bottom and up the sides of a 9-inch fluted tart pan with a removable bottom. Refrigerate for 30 minutes.

2. Preheat the oven to 350°F.

3. To make the filling: In a large bowl, beat together the cream cheese, sugar, and rum. Beat in the egg yolk until well blended. Add the ricotta and beat until smooth.

4. Pour the cheese mixture into the prepared tart shell. Bake for 45 minutes, or until puffed and golden brown. Cool for 10 minutes on a wire rack. Remove the pan rim and let the tart cool completely. Serve at room temperature or lightly chilled. Store in the refrigerator.

Crostata di Ricotta

RICOTTA TART

Serves 8

1 recipe Double-Crust Pasta Frolla (page 82), made with orange zest

FILLING

⅓ cup dark raisins

2 tablespoons grappa or brandy

1 15-ounce container whole-milk ricotta cheese

2 large eggs

½ cup sugar

1 teaspoon vanilla extract

1 teaspoon grated orange zest

2 ounces semisweet or bittersweet chocolate, chopped (about ⅓ cup)

1 egg yolk beaten with 1 teaspoon water, for egg wash

Confectioners' sugar

1. On a lightly floured surface, roll out the larger piece of dough to an 11-inch circle about ⅛ inch thick. Fit the dough into a 9-inch fluted tart pan with a removable bottom. Trim off all but a ½-inch border of dough. Fold the excess dough in against the inside of the pan and press it into place. Chill the tart shell for 30 minutes.

2. In a small bowl, combine the raisins and grappa. Let stand for 30 minutes.

3. Preheat the oven to 350°F.

4. In a large bowl, combine the ricotta, eggs, sugar, vanilla, and orange zest and beat until blended. Stir in the raisins and grappa and then the chocolate. Spoon the filling into the prepared shell.

5. Roll out the remaining dough to a 10-inch circle about ⅛ inch thick and, with a fluted pastry wheel, cut it into ½-inch-wide strips. Arrange the strips about 1 inch apart over the filling, forming a lattice pattern. Press the ends of the strips against the sides of the tart shell to seal. Brush the dough with the egg wash. Bake for 50 minutes, or until the filling is puffed and the pastry is golden brown.

6. Let cool on a wire rack for 10 minutes. Remove the rim of the pan and cool the tart completely. Just before serving, sprinkle with confectioners' sugar.

Crostata di Mirtillo

BLUEBERRY TART

Serves 8

✿ The cornmeal in the crust of this crostata gives it a pleasantly crunchy texture. During the summer months when flavorful blueberries are plentiful, I make up big batches of the fresh-tasting blueberry jam used as the tart filling. I freeze the mixture in pint containers so that I have it available all winter long for tarts or as a delicious spread for toast.

FILLING

 3 *cups blueberries, picked over and rinsed*

 1 *cup sugar*

 ⅛ *teaspoon ground cinnamon*

CRUST

 2 *cups all-purpose flour*

 ⅓ *cup yellow cornmeal*

 ½ *cup sugar*

 1 *teaspoon baking powder*

 ½ *teaspoon salt*

 12 *tablespoons (1½ sticks) cold unsalted butter, cut into bits*

Grated zest of 1 lemon

 1 *large egg*

 1 *large egg yolk*

Confectioners' sugar

1. To make the filling: In a heavy medium saucepan, combine the blueberries, sugar, and cinnamon. Cover and bring to a simmer over medium heat. Uncover and cook, stirring occasionally, until the blueberries have burst and the mixture has thickened, about 20 minutes. Transfer to a bowl and let cool, then cover and chill. The mixture will thicken further as it cools. (There should be about 1¾ cups.)

2. To make the crust: In a large bowl, combine the flour, cornmeal, sugar, baking powder, and salt. With a pastry blender or a fork, cut in the butter until the mixture resembles coarse crumbs. Stir in the lemon zest. Beat the egg and yolk together and stir lightly into the flour mixture just until mixed. The dough should remain crumbly.

3. Preheat the oven to 350°F.

4. Scatter about two-thirds of the crust mixture over the bottom of a 9-inch fluted tart pan with a removable bottom. Press the crumbs evenly over the bottom and up the sides of the pan to form a pastry shell. Spoon the chilled blueberry mixture into the shell and smooth the top.

5. On a lightly floured surface, roll the remaining crust mixture into ½-inch-thick ropes. Place the ropes 1 inch apart across the filling to form a lattice pattern. Press the ends against the inside rim of the tart shell to seal.

6. Bake the tart for 45 to 50 minutes, or until golden brown. Let cool on a wire rack for 10 minutes. Remove the rim of the pan and let cool completely. Just before serving, sprinkle with confectioners' sugar.

Torta di Verdura

SWEET VEGETABLE TART

Serves 8

Dessert tarts made with vegetables are not uncommon in Italy, where everyone who can keeps a small garden. There are many versions of pumpkin or winter squash pies, and in Parma I came across a delicious tart made with green tomato preserves. A tart from Southern Italy that I have read about but never tried is made with eggplant and chocolate.

This particular sweet vegetable pie is from Tuscany. I first tasted it at Vipore, a lovely restaurant perched on a hilltop outside of Lucca. The restaurant has its own superb herb and vegetable garden, which supplies the chef with many of his ingredients.

continued

1 recipe *Double-Crust Pasta Frolla (page 82), made with orange zest*

FILLING

1 pound *Swiss chard*

½ teaspoon *salt*

1 *15-ounce container whole-milk ricotta cheese*

2 tablespoons *butter, melted*

1 cup *sugar*

1 large *egg*

½ teaspoon *grated orange zest*

½ teaspoon *ground cinnamon*

¼ teaspoon *grated nutmeg*

¼ cup *golden raisins*

¼ cup *pine nuts*

1. On a lightly floured surface, roll out the larger piece of dough to an 11-inch circle about ⅛ inch thick. Press the dough into a 9-inch fluted tart pan with a removable bottom. Trim off all but a ½-inch border of dough. Fold the excess dough in against the inside of the pan and press it into place. Chill the dough for 30 minutes.

2. Wash the Swiss chard well in several changes of cool water. Trim off the stem ends. Place the chard and salt in a large pot, add ½ cup water, cover, and bring to a simmer. Cook for 10 minutes, or until tender. Drain and let cool. Wrap the chard in a kitchen towel and squeeze out the excess liquid. Finely chop the chard.

3. Preheat the oven to 350°F. Place an oven rack on the lowest level.

4. In a large bowl, combine the ricotta, melted butter, sugar, egg, orange zest, cinnamon, and nutmeg and beat well. Stir in the chard, raisins, and pine nuts. Pour the mixture into the prepared tart shell.

5. Roll out the remaining dough to a 10-inch circle about ⅛ inch thick and, with a fluted pastry wheel, cut it into ½-inch-wide strips. Arrange the strips about 1 inch apart across the filling, forming a lattice pattern. Press the ends of the strips against the sides of the tart shell to seal.

6. Bake for 45 minutes, or until the filling is puffed and the pastry is golden brown. Let cool on a wire rack for 10 minutes. Remove the rim of the pan and let cool completely.

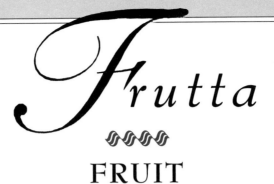

Frutta

FRUIT

After touring the United States, Alfredo and Luciana Currado, owners of the Vietti winery in Piedmont, came to visit us at our home. Though they enjoyed dinner, they were particularly delighted with the bowl of fresh fruit I offered them for dessert. Since they had been eating mostly in restaurants, they had been unable to find the good ripe fruit they were accustomed to having daily in Italy.

Fruit is, without a doubt, the most popular Italian dessert. Whether at home or in a restaurant, Italians are likely to choose fruit in one form or another as part of every lunch and dinner. It is light and healthful and essential to the Italian diet. Besides, one can always go for a stroll afterwards and stop at a caffè for gelati or a pastry.

During the summer months, Italians serve whole fruits along with a bowl of ice water. The idea is to dip the fruits in the water to rinse and refresh them before eating. Most fruits taste best at room temperature or just slightly chilled. Too cold, and their flavor and texture are lost. Ice water cools them just enough.

After their cold water bath, fruits like peaches and apples are peeled and eaten with a knife and fork. Having chased many a slippery peach around my plate, all I can say is that this is an art that requires some practice, though most Italians seem to accomplish it with ease and elegance.

Desserts made with fruits are also very popular. Macedonia, or fruit salad, is usually available, made from a combination of fruits chosen according to the season. (The word macedonia comes from the country of the same name, formed from a conglomeration of small states after they were conquered by Alexander the Great.) And any kind of fruits may be poached or marinated in wine, fruit juice, or liqueurs.

Agrumi ❧ Citrus Fruits

Many kinds of citrus fruits are grown in Italy, especially in Sicily, so Italians eat them all year round. With the exception of blood oranges, which have only recently begun to be available here, most varieties are familiar to us. Blood oranges are tart with bright red flesh and juice. Their orange skin usually has patches of red blush.

When buying any kind of citrus fruits, weigh them in your hand first. If they feel heavy for their size, they are full of juice.

Citrus fruits keep well in the refrigerator in the vegetable crisper. Remove them from their plastic bags to prevent them from becoming moldy.

Citrus fruits are easier to squeeze when they are at room temperature.

The zest, or colored part of the rind, contains oils that add flavor to many desserts. To grate the zest, first wash and dry the fruit. Rub the fruit over the fine holes of a grater, turning the fruit often to avoid digging into the bitter white pith. Remove the zest that collects on the grater with a pastry brush.

Fichi ❧ Figs

Fresh figs have a short season, from late summer to early fall. There are three kinds of fresh figs that are generally available, the dark purple or black mission variety and the green Calimyrna and Kadota varieties. When ripe, a fresh fig is very soft and tender. The best have a drop of nectar in the opening at the blossom end. Ripe figs should be eaten as soon as possible after purchasing. Though the Italians frequently serve them peeled, the skin is thin and can be eaten as well.

Since the fresh fig season is brief, I tend to use dried figs quite a bit. Look for dried figs that are moist and tender. Avoid fruits that are too dry and leathery. Dried figs from California are superior in flavor and texture to the imported variety.

Frutti di Bosco ❧ Berries

Soft, tender berries must be handled with care. Look them over carefully before purchase to be sure there are no traces of white or greenish mold, crushed berries, or other signs of spoilage. Use fresh berries as soon as possible after purchase. In warm weather, you may need to keep them in the refrigerator, but they should be served at room temperature for best flavor.

Do not wash berries until you are ready to use them as they become moldy if they are damp. Always dry berries well before serving since water droplets will dilute their delicate flavor.

In Italy, all types of berries are often served, singly or in combination, with a sprinkling of lemon juice and sugar to enhance their flavor.

Blueberries (*mirtilli*) should have a dark blue color with a white or silvery "bloom." The bloom disappears if the berries become overripe. Reddish berries are underripe. Avoid moist or wrinkled berries.

Raspberries (*lampone*) and blackberries (*more*) should be firm and dry with no traces of mold. The sweetest raspberries can be bright red or golden yellow according to their variety. Blackberries are larger and plumper, with heavy seeds. Their color should be evenly black.

Strawberries (*fragole*) should be a bright shiny red with no traces of green or white. Their aroma should be sweet and appetizing. Fresh strawberries should be eaten as soon as possible after purchase. Their flavor and aroma are best when they are at room temperature.

Wash strawberries in cool water just before you are ready to use them. Dry them well before removing the green hulls so that water does not get inside the berries.

In Italy, early spring brings *fragoline del bosco*, small wild strawberries with a delicious aroma. They are sometimes available in specialty markets here.

In Italy, a favorite way to prepare strawberries is to slice them, sprinkle with sugar and a few drops of balsamic vinegar or lemon juice, and allow them to stand briefly before serving.

Mele ⚘ *Apples*

Of the many kinds of apples available for eating out of hand and cooking, Golden Delicious are my favorite all-purpose variety, especially for Italian desserts. Their flavor is mild and sweet when raw but becomes more intense and concentrated when they are cooked. They also hold their shape well when baked or sautéed. What is more, Golden Delicious apples are always available.

When buying them, look for apples with a pale yellow or slightly greenish cast. Occasionally, they have a pink blush. Dark yellow apples may be overripe.

When I want a tarter apple for cooking, I generally choose Granny Smith apples. Granny Smiths should have an even bright green color with hard, crisp flesh.

All apples should be firm and free of wrinkles and bruises. Apples should be stored in a plastic bag or the vegetable crisper of the refrigerator, away from foods like onions and garlic so that they do not pick up off flavors.

Meloni ✺ *Melons*

When choosing a cantaloupe, look for a golden netting covering a creamy yellow background. The melon should feel heavy for its size and have a sweet, musky aroma. The blossom end (opposite the stem end) should yield slightly when pressed. At room temperature, cantaloupes will continue to ripen and soften.

Honeydew melons are a creamy yellow or white color and the shell should give slightly when pressed. Keep honeydew melons at room temperature until they reach the desired softness and ripeness.

Roadside stands all along the Italian highways sell watermelon, called *anguria* or *cocomero* depending on the region. The best way to judge a watermelon is by its weight; the heavier it is, the more full of juice it will be. The skin should be green with only one small yellow patch where the melon rested as it was maturing in the field. In Sicily, watermelon is used to make ices and pudding.

Pere ✺ *Pears*

Pears are one of the few fruits that ripen well off the tree. Let pears ripen at room temperature until they are soft and aromatic. The skin of some pear varieties changes color as they ripen, while that of others does not.

Yellow-green Bartlett and golden-brown Bosc pears are good for cooking as well as eating out of hand, though Anjou pears are also good. For poaching or baking whole, "slim" pears such as Bosc are the best choice since they cook through evenly.

Ripe fresh pears are especially good with cheese.

Pesche ✺ *Peaches*

A ripe peach has a creamy white or yellow background color. The amount of red blush depends on the variety and so does not always indicate ripeness.

Avoid peaches that are green or that have brown spots or wrinkles. Peaches are picked when mature but not quite ripe. Let them stand at room temperature for a few days to soften. Once they are ripe, serve them immediately or store them in the refrigerator.

To peel peaches and other soft fruits for salads or ice cream, bring a saucepan of water to a boil. Add the peaches (or other fruit) and keep them submerged for thirty seconds. Remove with a slotted spoon and drop them into a bowl of ice water. The skins should slip off easily, though I have occasionally bought peaches that will not release their peel after blanching them this way. In that case, peel them with a knife, or use them with the skins on.

Uve & Grapes

Green grapes are the sweetest and most flavorful once their color has turned from green to yellow or golden.

One of the most interesting green grape varieties is the Muscat. These big round golden grapes, which appear on the market in the fall, have a sweet, honeylike flavor.

Red and black grapes should be firm with vibrant color and no bruises.

All grapes should be crisp with the fruit securely attached to the stems. There should be a fine white bloom on the skins. Store grapes in the refrigerator.

Pesche Noce con More

GLAZED NECTARINES WITH BLACKBERRIES

Serves 8

A simple and refreshing combination of fruits. Substitute raspberries or blueberries if blackberries are not available.

¼ cup sugar

½ cup orange juice

2 tablespoons fresh lemon juice

2 tablespoons honey

8 medium ripe nectarines, peeled, pitted, and cut into thin wedges

3 tablespoons amaretto

1 teaspoon shredded orange zest

½ pint blackberries

1. In a medium saucepan, combine the sugar, orange and lemon juices, and honey. Bring to a simmer over medium heat. Gently stir in the nectarines, and simmer for 5 minutes.

2. Remove from the heat and stir in the amaretto and orange zest. Cover and chill.

3. Just before serving, stir in the blackberries.

Macedonia in Gelatina

INDIVIDUAL FRUIT TIMBALES

Serves 6

1 envelope unflavored gelatin

1 cup cold water

¾ cup sugar

½ cup dry white wine

2 tablespoons fresh lemon juice

1 cup small strawberries, halved or quartered

1 cup raspberries

1 cup blueberries

1 cup seedless green grapes

1 navel orange, peeled and cut into bite-size pieces

Strawberry Sauce (page 207)

1. In a small saucepan, sprinkle the gelatin over the water. Let stand for 5 minutes, until softened. Stir in the sugar and cook over low heat, stirring constantly, until the gelatin is dissolved. Stir in the wine and lemon juice. Transfer to a large bowl and let cool.

2. Add all the fruit to the cooled liquid, and stir gently to mix.

3. Spoon the fruit and liquid into six 6-ounce custard cups, pressing down with the back of the spoon so that all of the fruits are submerged. Chill for several hours, or until set.

4. Unmold the timbales onto serving plates. Spoon the strawberry sauce around the timbales.

Sottoboschi con Crema di Ricotta

BERRIES WITH CANNOLI CREAM

Serves 8

This luscious cream is usually used as the filling for cannoli, crisp-fried pastry tubes. But it is also delicious served over fresh berries. You can vary the cream by adding finely chopped bittersweet chocolate or pistachio nuts.

1 *15-ounce container whole-milk ricotta cheese*

2 *to 4 tablespoons sugar*

1 *teaspoon grated orange zest*

1 *teaspoon vanilla extract*

1 *pint blueberries*

1 *pint raspberries*

2 *tablespoons orange, cherry, or other fruit-flavored liqueur*

Mint leaves

1. In a food processor or blender, combine the ricotta, 2 tablespoons sugar, the orange zest, and vanilla. Process until smooth and creamy. Transfer to a bowl, cover, and chill until ready to serve.

2. Wash the berries and gently pat them dry. Set aside a few small berries for garnish. Place the remainder in a serving bowl and toss with the liqueur and with 2 tablespoons sugar if desired. Top with the ricotta cream. Garnish with mint leaves and the reserved whole berries.

Sottoboschi Caldi con Gelato

WARM BERRIES WITH CINNAMON ICE CREAM

Serves 4

Italians love all kinds of berries. In the early spring, there are tiny *fragoline del bosco*, the wild strawberries the French call *fraises des bois*, firm little berries that seem to have more aroma than flavor. In the summer, blackberries as fat as your thumb appear. And blueberries, currants, raspberries, and gooseberries all have their seasons.

When there is a profusion of berries available, a favorite technique is to serve them warmed so that they "melt" into a sauce. Cinnamon gelato is a perfect complement but vanilla, lemon, or honey would also be delicious.

1 *cup blueberries*

1 *cup raspberries*

1 *cup strawberries*

1 *cup blackberries*

¼ *cup water*

¼ *cup sugar, or more to taste*

1 *quart Cinnamon Ice Cream (page 173)*

1. Rinse the berries and remove the hulls or stems. Cut the strawberries into halves or quarters if they are large.

2. In a medium saucepan, combine the berries, water, and ¼ cup sugar. Bring to a simmer over medium heat. Cook, stirring occasionally, until the berries are soft and the juices are slightly thickened, about 5 minutes. Taste and add additional sugar if necessary. Remove from the heat and let cool to warm.

3. Spoon the berries into four goblets and top each serving with a scoop of the ice cream. Serve immediately.

$\mathcal{P}$esche al Prosecco
PEACHES IN PROSECCO
Serves 6

🌀 Prosecco is a dry sparkling wine from the Veneto region. It is best known as an ingredient in Bellinis, the delicious cocktails made with puréed white peaches, invented at Harry's Bar in Venice. Another dry sparkling wine can be substituted if Prosecco is not available.

> **6 medium peaches, thinly sliced**
>
> **¼ cup sugar**
>
> **¼ cup Grand Marnier or other orange liqueur**
>
> **1½ cups chilled Prosecco**

1. In a serving bowl, combine the peaches, sugar, and Grand Marnier and toss well. Chill for 1 hour.

2. Just before serving, pour on the wine. Serve immediately.

$\mathscr{P}$esche al Vino Rosso

PEACHES IN RED WINE

Serves 6

When I was a child, my grandfather had a white peach tree in his garden on Staten Island. The peaches it produced were ivory colored with a rosy blush and they had an intense peach aroma. One whiff and my mouth would start to water. We picked the ripe, sweet peaches and sliced them right into the wine glasses so that every last drop of the precious juice was saved.

White peaches are sometimes available at farmer's markets during the summer months but good yellow peaches will do very well. Amaretti cookies are a nice accompaniment.

6 firm white or yellow peaches

½ cup sugar

1 bottle (750 milliliters) fruity red wine

Juice of 1 lemon

1. Peeling the peaches is optional: To peel them, bring a large saucepan of water to a boil. Drop the peaches into the water and leave for 30 seconds. Remove with a slotted spoon. Starting at the stem end, pull off the skin, using a sharp knife and your fingers.

2. Cut the peaches into bite-size pieces.

3. In a large bowl, combine the sugar, wine, and lemon juice. Add the peaches and toss well. Cover and refrigerate for 2 to 3 hours.

4. Spoon the peaches and the liquid into wine goblets, and serve.

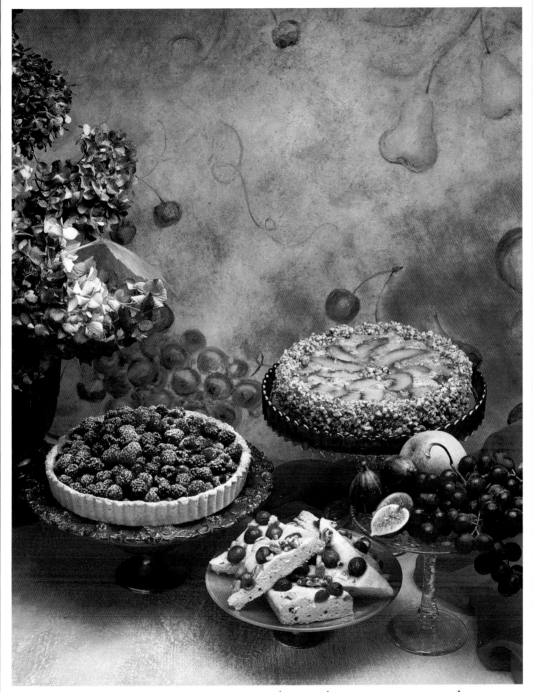

Left to right: Berry Crostata (*Crostata di Frutti di Bosco*), page 92; Upside-Down Peach Poppyseed Cake (*Torta Rovesciata alle Pesche*), page 42; and Grape Focaccia (*Focaccia all'Uva*), page 49

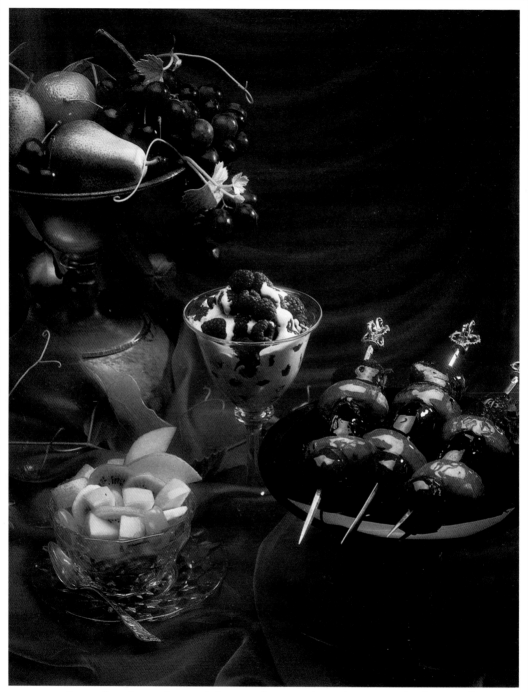

Left to right: Green Fruit Salad (*Macedonia Verde*), page 117; Zabaglione with Balsamic Vinegar and Raspberries (*Zabaglione al Balsamico con Lampone*), page 44; and Venetian Caramelized Fruit Skewers (*Golosezzi Veneziani*), page 132

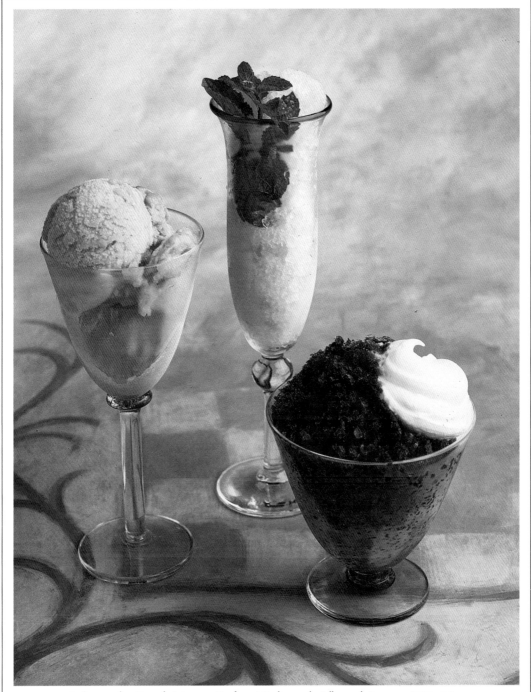

Left to right: Dried Apricot Sorbet (*Sorbetto di Albicocche*), page 202; Mint Granita (*Granita di Menta*), page 191; and Coffee Granita (*Granita di Caffè*), page 187

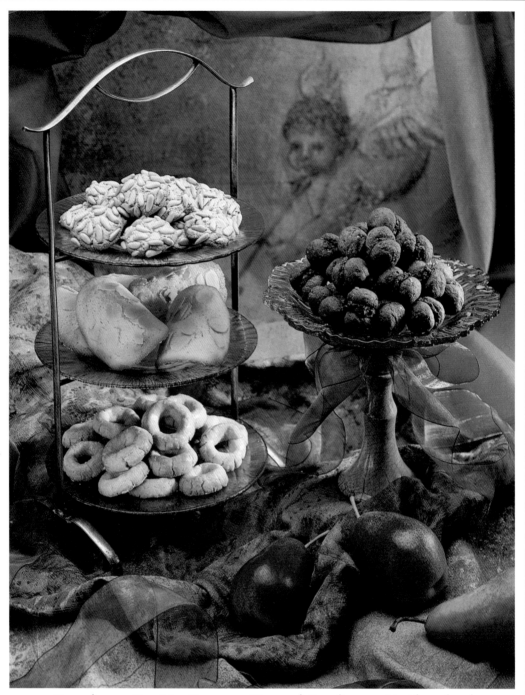

Top to bottom: Pine Nut Macaroons (*Biscotti di Pignoli*), page 26; Almond and Orange Tiles (*Tegoline*), page 34; Venetian Butter Rings (*Bussolai*), page 23; and *right*, Juliet's Kisses (*Baci di Giulietta*), page 38

Composta di Frutta alla Grappa

HONEYED GRAPPA COMPOTE

Serves 6

🌀 Grappa makes an interesting marinade for citrus fruits.

⅓ **cup honey**

⅓ **cup grappa**

1 **tablespoon fresh lemon juice**

2 **pink grapefruits**

2 **navel oranges**

1 **pint strawberries, hulled and sliced**

1 **cup halved seedless green grapes**

1. In a large serving bowl, whisk together the honey, grappa, and lemon juice.

2. With a serrated knife, cut away the peel and pith from the grapefruits and oranges. Cut the fruits crosswise into thin slices.

3. Add the grapefruit, oranges, strawberries, and grapes to the serving bowl and toss gently. Chill, covered, for at least 1 hour or up to 4 hours before serving.

Fragole e Arancie Marinate
STRAWBERRIES AND ORANGES
Serves 6

2 cups dry red wine

½ cup sugar

2 tablespoons raspberry jam

1 3-inch cinnamon stick

2 cloves

4 navel oranges, peeled and cut into wedges

1 teaspoon grated lemon zest

1 pint strawberries, hulled and sliced

1. In a large saucepan, combine the wine, sugar, jam, and spices. Bring to a simmer over medium heat for 10 minutes, or until the liquid is reduced by half. Let cool.

2. Place the oranges in a serving bowl. Strain the syrup over them. Stir in the lemon zest. Cover and chill.

3. Just before serving, stir in the strawberries.

Macedonia Verde

GREEN FRUIT SALAD

Serves 6

Fruit salad is the perennial Italian dessert, appropriate after every meal and always welcome. All kinds of fruit can be combined with wine, liqueur, or fruit juice, but I was particularly impressed by this lovely combination of green, yellow, and white fruits served by an Italian friend.

2 *cups seedless green grapes, halved lengthwise*

3 *kiwis, peeled and thinly sliced*

1 *green or yellow apple, cored and diced*

1 *ripe pear, cored and diced*

1 *banana, sliced*

3 *tablespoons honey*

3 *tablespoons fresh lemon juice*

1. In a large bowl, combine all the fruits.
2. Stir together the honey and lemon juice, and pour over the fruit. Stir well. Serve slightly chilled.

Fragole con Crema di Mascarpone

STRAWBERRIES IN MARSALA WITH HONEY MASCARPONE CREAM

Serves 4

This delicious *crema* is good on all kinds of fruits, cakes, and tarts. If you cannot find mascarpone, ricotta or sour cream can be substituted.

2 pints strawberries

¼ cup sweet Marsala

3 tablespoons sugar, or to taste

2 ounces (¼ cup) mascarpone

2 tablespoons honey

½ cup heavy cream

1. Rinse the strawberries in cold water and gently pat them dry. Set aside 4 perfect berries for garnish. Hull the remaining berries and slice them. In a bowl, combine the strawberries, Marsala, and sugar. Let stand at room temperature for 30 minutes.

2. In a large bowl, whisk the mascarpone and honey until smooth. In a medium bowl, whip the cream until soft peaks form. Fold the cream into the mascarpone.

3. Divide the strawberries and juices among four dessert bowls. Spoon on the mascarpone cream. Garnish with the reserved whole strawberries.

Arancie e Mandorle

ORANGES AND ALMONDS

Serves 6

🍊 Whenever I have been doing a lot of baking, I wind up with a collection of "bald" oranges in my refrigerator—that is, oranges with the zest, as the colored part of the peel is called, grated away. That's when I make this very refreshing fruit and nut combination inspired by some of Sicily's best products: Marsala wine, oranges, and almonds.

4 large navel oranges

¼ cup sugar, or to taste

½ cup golden raisins

1 cup sweet or dry Marsala

½ cup sliced almonds, lightly toasted

1. Peel the oranges, removing all of the white pith. Cut crosswise into thin slices.

2. In a large bowl, combine the oranges, sugar, raisins, and wine. Cover and refrigerate for 2 hours.

3. Just before serving, sprinkle the almonds over the oranges.

Ciliege al Vino Rosso

CHERRIES IN RED WINE

Serves 4

There is no need to look at a menu at Restaurant Arnaldo in Reggio Emilia. Each course, except for the pasta, arrives at the table on its own specially designed wheeled cart. First there is the antipasto cart, filled with locally made prosciutto and salami sliced to your order. After the pasta course, the next cart appears laden with *arrosto* and *bollito misto*, perfectly roasted or boiled meats and poultry, also sliced and served to order. Finally, the dessert cart arrives with tarts and cakes and beautiful cut-crystal bowls full of fruits poached in a variety of wine and spice-scented syrups.

I could not resist the bright red cherries that sparkled like rubies in a rich red wine sauce. They were topped with a cloud of softly whipped cream touched with almond flavor. Three young ladies at the next table, who were obviously regulars, liked the cream so much that that was all they ordered for dessert—big bowls of whipped cream!

Pitting the cherries is a lot less tedious if you invest in an inexpensive cherry pitter, available in most cooking supply stores. Otherwise you will have to cut the cherries in half to remove the pits.

¾ *cup sugar*

1 *3-inch cinnamon stick*

2 *cups dry red wine, such as Barbera*

1 *pound ripe cherries, pitted*

1 *cup heavy cream*

2 *tablespoons amaretto*

3 *tablespoons sliced almonds, toasted*

1. In a large saucepan, combine the sugar, cinnamon stick, and wine. Bring to a simmer over medium heat and cook, stirring occasionally, for 5 minutes.

2. Stir in the cherries and simmer until tender, about 15 minutes. Let cool to tepid, then refrigerate until completely chilled, at least 1 hour.

3. In a large bowl, using an electric mixer with chilled beaters, whip the cream with the amaretto until soft peaks form.

4. Spoon the cherries and their syrup into goblets, and top with the whipped cream and toasted almonds.

Mele al Forno con Salsa di Caramella

CARAMEL BAKED APPLES

Serves 8

8 *Golden Delicious apples*

1½ *cups dry white wine or vermouth*

1 *cup sugar*

1 *3-inch strip orange zest*

1 *cup heavy cream*

1. Preheat the oven to 350°F.

2. Remove the peel from the top third of each apple. In a baking pan just large enough to hold the apples, combine the wine, ½ cup of the sugar, and the orange zest. Add the apples. Bake for 30 to 40 minutes, or until tender.

3. Transfer the apples to a serving dish. Pour the juices from the pan into a small heavy saucepan, and discard the orange zest. There should be about ½ cup juice. Add the remaining ½ cup sugar and bring to a boil over medium heat. Cook, swirling the pan occasionally, until the sugar caramelizes and the liquid turns a light amber. Remove the pan from the heat and let cool slightly.

4. Stir the cream into the caramel carefully, as the caramel may sputter, and pour the sauce around the apples. Refrigerate until chilled.

Mele al Forno con Crostini di Polenta

WINE-BAKED APPLES WITH SWEET POLENTA CROSTINI

Serves 8

In the Val d'Aosta, baked apples are served on slices of golden polenta crusty with butter and sugar. This is a hearty dessert that I like to serve during the fall or winter after a rustic meal of soup, bread, and cheese.

POLENTA

3½ cups water

1 cup yellow cornmeal

1 teaspoon salt

WINE-BAKED APPLES

8 medium Golden Delicious apples (about 2½ pounds)

⅔ cup muscat raisins or dark raisins

¼ cup toasted pine nuts

⅓ cup sugar

1½ cups dry white wine

4 cloves

1 3-inch cinnamon stick

Zest of ½ lemon, cut into strips

3 tablespoons unsalted butter

1 tablespoon corn oil

2 tablespoons sugar

Whipped cream (optional)

1. To make the polenta: In a medium saucepan, bring 2 cups of the water to a boil. In a bowl, stir together the cornmeal and 1½ cups water.

2. Add the salt to the boiling water, then stir in the cornmeal mixture. Cook, stirring frequently, for 30 minutes, or until very thick. Pour the polenta into an 8- by 4-inch loaf pan and smooth the top. Cover with plastic wrap and chill for at least 4 hours. (The polenta can be prepared up to 3 days ahead.)

3. To make the apples: Preheat the oven to 375°F.

4. Core the apples and peel them two-thirds of the way down. Place the apples in a baking dish just large enough to hold them upright. Combine the raisins and pine nuts and stuff the mixture into the apples. Sprinkle the tops with the sugar. Pour the wine into the pan and scatter the cloves, cinnamon stick, and lemon zest around the apples. Bake for 40 minutes, basting occasionally with the pan juices, until the apples are tender when pierced with a knife. Let cool to lukewarm.

5. Meanwhile, run a knife around the sides of the pan and unmold the polenta onto a cutting board. Cut the polenta into 16 slices. Arrange the slices on a wire rack and let dry for 1 hour.

6. To serve: In a large nonstick skillet, melt 2 tablespoons of the butter with the oil over medium heat. Add half the polenta slices, and sauté for 5 to 6 minutes on each side, or until lightly browned. Sprinkle 1 tablespoon of the sugar over the polenta. Transfer to a heated plate and keep warm. Melt the remaining 1 tablespoon butter, cook the remaining polenta, and sprinkle with the remaining 1 tablespoon sugar.

7. Place two polenta croutons on each plate and top with a baked apple. Drizzle with some of the wine syrup. Serve with whipped cream if desired.

Melone al Balsamico

MELON WITH BALSAMIC VINEGAR

Serves 4

❦ Ripe melon with a wedge of lemon or lime is a classic combination. The same principle works here with the acid in balsamic vinegar substituting for the acid of the lemon, but the balsamico adds a special richness. Use a good-quality balsamico, one that is mellow and not harsh.

8 *thin slices peeled ripe cantaloupe*

8 *thin slices peeled ripe honeydew melon*

2 *teaspoons balsamic vinegar*

10 *to 12 fresh mint leaves*

Arrange alternate slices of the cantaloupe and honeydew on a large platter. Sprinkle with the vinegar. Tear the mint leaves into pieces and scatter over the melon. Serve immediately.

Composta di Frutta Secca

DRIED FRUIT COMPOTE

Makes 8 cups

🌀 This compote can be served plain or with a topping of Honey Mascarpone Cream (page 118). It would make a delicious dessert for a brunch, accompanied by the Cornmeal Cake (page 59).

1 cup dried apricots

1 cup dried peaches

1 cup dried figs, quartered if large

1 cup dried pitted prunes

1 cup Muscat raisins or other raisins

1 cup sugar

1 cup sweet Marsala

Zest and juice of 1 small orange

1. In a large bowl, combine all the fruits. Add cool water to cover by 1 inch. Cover and refrigerate for several hours, or overnight.

2. Drain the soaking liquid from the fruits into a large pot. Add the sugar and bring to a simmer over medium heat. Cook, stirring, until the sugar is dissolved. Add the fruits, Marsala, and orange zest and juice. Cover and cook for 15 minutes, or until the fruits are tender. Remove from the heat and let cool.

3. Serve warm or chilled.

Fichi Secchi al Cioccolato

STUFFED FIGS WITH CHOCOLATE

Makes about 18

✜ Instead of chocolate or candies, these easy-to-make sweets from the Naples area are delightful after a meal. Packed in an attractive tin lined with cellophane, they make a sensational Christmas gift.

4 ounces semisweet chocolate

2 tablespoons unsalted butter

1 pound soft dried Calimyrna figs

About 1 cup toasted walnut halves

About ½ cup candied orange or lemon peel

1. In the top half of a double boiler set over warm water, melt the chocolate and butter. Remove from the heat and stir until smooth.

2. Make a slit in the base of each fig. Stuff each fig with a walnut half and a piece of candied orange peel. Pinch the figs to close the slits.

3. Dip each fig in the melted chocolate and place on a wire rack until the chocolate is set.

4. To store: When the chocolate is set, pack the figs in an airtight box, separating each layer with wax paper. Refrigerated, these keep for up to 1 month.

Fichi alla Contadina
COUNTRY-STYLE FIGS
Serves 6 to 8

A charming Italian fable tells of a wealthy man who instructs his servants to pick his figs when they are at their best, "with tears in their eyes"—that is, when a tiny drop of nectar appears in the opening at the flower end of the fruit.

In Tuscany, fig trees grow just about everywhere, and the fruit is abundant in late summer and early fall. Since fresh figs may be hard to come by here, I have adapted this recipe for dried figs so that I can enjoy them all year round. These keep very well. They are great with nutty biscotti.

1 *pound dried dark (Mission) figs*

4 *cups water*

1 *3-inch strip lemon zest*

2 *tablespoons honey*

1 *tablespoon sugar*

1 *cup vin santo, Marsala, or dry red wine*

1. In a large bowl, combine the figs and water. Cover and chill overnight.

2. Pour the figs and water into a large saucepan. Add the remaining ingredients and bring to a simmer over medium heat. Cover and cook, 15 minutes, or until the figs are very tender.

3. With a slotted spoon, transfer the figs to a bowl. Simmer the cooking liquid until thickened and slightly reduced, about 10 minutes. Pour over the figs and let cool. Chill before serving. (These keep for up to 1 week in the refrigerator.)

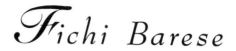

Fichi Barese

BARI-STYLE FIGS

Makes about 1 quart

Nicola Marzovilla and his mother, Dora, are the owners of Tempo Restaurant in New York. Dora makes wonderful pasta and desserts, including these simple baked figs. She keeps them in big glass jars and they are always good with a glass of dessert wine.

1½ pounds dried figs

About 1 cup toasted unblanched almonds

¼ cup bay leaves

1 tablespoon fennel seeds

1. Preheat the oven to 350°F.

2. Cut a small slit in the thickest part of each fig. Place an almond inside and pinch the slit closed. Place on a baking sheet and bake for 15 to 20 minutes, or until lightly browned. Let cool completely.

3. In a wide-mouth 1-quart jar or crock with a tight-fitting lid, layer the figs and bay leaves, sprinkling each layer with fennel seeds. Cover and store in a cool place for at least 1 week before serving.

$\mathcal{P}$ere al Forno

SPICED BAKED PEARS

Serves 6

Poached pears are delicious, but peeling and coring them can be a pain. This version is my all-time favorite since they are so easy, yet taste so great. Baked with red wine, spices, and sugar, the pears take on a beautiful red glaze, and they are delicious warm or cold. Chunks of Parmigiano-Reggiano are a nice accompaniment, or you can opt for whipped cream if you like.

They are practically infallible, too, as I learned when I demonstrated this recipe to a cooking class in Los Angeles. A tremendous rainstorm was raging outside and not long after I placed the pears in the preheated oven, the electricity went out and so did the oven. I did the best I could to cook the remaining recipes on the gas stovetop, but the pears remained in the darkened oven unattended for well over an hour. At last the lights came back on. When I checked the pears, I was amazed to find them ready to eat and perfectly delicious.

Use medium-size pears for this recipe. Very large or wide pears tend to remain hard in the center even after the outsides are well cooked. Slim brown Anjou pears are perfect.

6 firm ripe pears, such as Anjou or Bartlett

1 cup fruity red wine

½ cup sugar

1 3-inch cinnamon stick

1. Preheat the oven to 450°F.
2. In a baking dish just large enough to hold the pears upright, combine the wine, sugar, and cinnamon stick. Stir to dissolve the sugar.
3. Stand the pears in the dish, and spoon the wine over them. Bake the pears, basting frequently with the pan juices, for 45 to 60 minutes, or until the pears are tender when pierced with a knife and the juices are syrupy. Add a tablespoon or so of warm water if the liquid threatens to evaporate too quickly.
4. Let the pears cool to room temperature in the baking dish, basting them occasionally with the wine syrup. Serve plain or with whipped cream.

Pere al Vino con Gorgonzola

POACHED PEARS WITH GORGONZOLA

Serves 8

A sophisticated sweet and tangy dessert. Serve with a chilled dessert wine such as Recioto di Soave.

1 bottle (750 milliliters) dry white wine

2 cups water

¼ cup fresh lemon juice

2 cups sugar

1 ½-inch strip lemon zest

8 firm ripe pears, such as Anjou, peeled, cored, and halved lengthwise

4 ounces Gorgonzola

2 ounces (¼ cup) mascarpone

Mint leaves

1. In a large saucepan, combine the wine, water, lemon juice, sugar, and lemon zest. Bring to a simmer over medium heat and cook for 10 minutes. Add the pear halves and simmer until tender, about 10 minutes. With a slotted spoon, remove the pears to a shallow dish.

2. Simmer the syrup over medium high heat until reduced and thickened. Pour the liquid over the pears and let cool to room temperature.

3. In a bowl, mash the Gorgonzola and mascarpone until smooth and well blended. Place a spoonful of the mixture in the hollow of each pear half.

4. Refrigerate until slightly chilled. Garnish with mint, and serve with some of the cooking juices.

Pere al Balsamico

SAUTÉED PEARS WITH BALSAMIC VINEGAR

Serves 4

We tend to think of vinegar mostly in terms of salad dressing, but balsamic vinegar has many more uses. In fact, the Italians prefer to use a few drops of *aceto balsamico* as a condiment on meat or eggs or to brighten the flavor of fruits or sauces rather than in salads.

Balsamico is even believed to have mild medicinal properties. A small amount taken after meals is said to aid digestion and act as a restorative. Lucrezia Borgia, an early fan of balsamico, recommended it to alleviate the pain of childbirth.

Obviously, balsamico is not ordinary vinegar. To make it, Trebbiano grape juice is cooked until concentrated, then aged in a series of wood barrels of decreasing size made from oak, cherry, mulberry, ash, and chestnut. Authentic balsamico must be aged for a minimum of twelve years, and some families in the Emilia-Romagna region where it is made treasure balsamico that is over a hundred years old. As the vinegar ages, the sweet and sour flavor becomes more concentrated but mellower.

2 medium firm ripe pears, such as Anjou or Bartlett

2 tablespoons unsalted butter

1 tablespoon sugar

About 1 teaspoon balsamic vinegar

1. Cut each pear into 8 wedges and remove the cores and stems.
2. In a large skillet, melt the butter over medium heat. Add the pears and sugar. Cook, stirring gently, until lightly browned, about 5 minutes.
3. Divide the pears among four plates. Drizzle each serving with a few drops of vinegar. Serve warm.

$\mathcal{G}$olosezzi Veneziani

VENETIAN CARAMELIZED
FRUIT SKEWERS

Serves 8

*If you liked candy apples as a child, you will love these delicious fruits encased in a crackling caramel coating. Many kinds of fresh or dried fruits can be used. Though they are simple to make, there are a few things to keep in mind: Do not attempt to make these on a humid day—the caramel will not harden properly. Use tongs to handle the skewers to avoid burns from the molten sugar. Serve within two hours of making or the caramel will begin to soften.

In Venice, caramelized fruit skewers are traditionally served with the ring-shaped butter cookies called Bussolai (page 23).*

8 *strawberries*

8 *seedless green grapes*

1 *tangerine, divided into sections*

8 *pitted dates, preferably fresh*

1 *cup sugar*

½ *cup light corn syrup*

¼ *cup water*

1. Wash the strawberries and grapes and pat thoroughly dry. Thread 1 tangerine section and one each of the other fruits on each of eight 6-inch bamboo skewers, leaving about ¾ inch free on the blunt ends.

2. In a 10-inch skillet, combine the sugar, corn syrup, and water. Cook over low heat, stirring occasionally, until the sugar is dissolved. Raise the heat to medium high and boil without stirring until the syrup begins to turn golden around the edges. Swirl the pan gently over the heat so that the syrup colors evenly. Do not allow the syrup to turn brown, or it will be bitter.

3. Remove the pan from the heat. Using tongs, quickly dip each skewer in the syrup, turning to coat the fruit lightly but thoroughly. Let the excess syrup drain back into the pan. Place the skewers on a wire rack to cool and harden. If the syrup in the pan hardens before all of the skewers have been dipped, reheat it gently. Serve at room temperature. (These can be prepared up to 2 hours ahead of serving if the weather is not humid.)

Frutta allo Zabaglione

FRUITS GRATINÉED WITH ZABAGLIONE

Serves 4

2 oranges

2 ripe kiwis, peeled and thinly sliced

1 pint strawberries, hulled and thinly sliced

⅓ cup sugar

1 large egg

2 large egg yolks

⅓ cup dry Marsala

1. Grate ½ teaspoon zest from one of the oranges, and reserve. Peel both oranges, removing all of the white pith.

2. Thinly slice the oranges crosswise. Layer the oranges, kiwis, and strawberries in a 10- by 8- by 2-inch flameproof baking dish.

3. Preheat the broiler.

4. In a heatproof bowl, or the top of a double boiler, combine all the remaining ingredients. With a whisk or portable mixer, beat until foamy. Place the bowl or pot over simmering water, and beat until the mixture is very light and fluffy and holds a soft shape when dropped from the whisk or beaters.

5. Remove from the heat and pour the zabaglione over the fruits. Run the baking dish under the broiler for 1 to 2 minutes, or until the zabaglione is lightly browned. Serve immediately.

Ananas all'Arancia

PINEAPPLE IN ORANGE SAUCE

Serves 4

✿ Almonds, hazelnuts, walnuts, pine nuts, and chestnuts are produced in abundance in Italy, but not pecans. Even peanuts, called *noccioline Americani*, or "little American nuts," are popular but pecans do not seem to be available there. Too bad, because I am sure Italians would love them. I tried pecans on this pineapple dessert that is usually made with almonds and the results were terrific.

2 tablespoons butter

2 tablespoons sugar

½ cup orange juice

4 slices ripe pineapple, about ½ inch thick

¼ cup orange liqueur

1 pint vanilla ice cream

1 cup chopped toasted pecans or almonds

1. In a large nonstick skillet, melt the butter over medium heat. Stir in the sugar and orange juice and bring to a simmer.

2. Add the pineapple and cook, turning the slices in the liquid, for 5 minutes, or until the sauce is reduced and thickened. Stir in the orange liqueur and cook for 1 minute longer.

3. Spoon the pineapple and sauce onto four dessert plates. Top each serving with a scoop of the ice cream. Sprinkle with the nuts.

Spiedini alla Frutta

GRILLED FRUIT SKEWERS

Serves 4

🌀 An unusual dessert to serve at a barbecue.

1 banana, cut into 1-inch chunks

2 Golden Delicious apples, cored and cut into 1-inch chunks

Juice of 1 lemon

1 cup fresh pineapple cubes

2 peaches, cut into 1-inch chunks

1 bunch of mint, stemmed

2 tablespoons sugar

1. Prepare a barbecue grill.

2. Toss the banana and apple chunks with the lemon juice to prevent darkening.

3. Thread all the pieces of fruit onto 4 short skewers, placing a mint leaf between each piece. Sprinkle with the sugar.

4. Grill the skewers, turning frequently, until the fruits are lightly browned, about 5 minutes. Serve immediately.

Marroni alla Grappa
CHESTNUTS IN GRAPPA
Serves 6

No Christmas dinner would be complete without a basket of fresh roasted chestnuts. This is the way they serve them in the Val d'Aosta.

1 pound whole chestnuts

2 to 4 tablespoons grappa, to taste

2 to 4 tablespoons sugar, to taste

1. Preheat the oven to 425°F.

2. Wash the chestnuts in cold water. Place the chestnuts flat side down on a cutting board. With a small sharp knife, cut a "T" in each chestnut. Place the chestnuts in a metal baking pan just large enough to hold them in one layer. Bake until tender, about 45 minutes.

3. Peel the chestnuts while still hot. In a small bowl, toss them with the grappa and sugar. Serve immediately.

$\mathcal{G}$ratinata di Pesche
e Pere

PEACH AND PEAR GRATIN

Serves 6

§ Those amaretti cookies that are individually wrapped in paper and come in big red tins have many uses. They are great crushed over ice cream or sliced fruit, dunked whole in wine, or as a topping for gratinéed fruits, such as in this recipe.

4 medium peaches, peeled and cut into thin wedges

2 large pears, peeled, cored, and cut into thin wedges

¼ cup white wine or vermouth

2 tablespoons apricot jam

2 tablespoons sugar

½ cup crushed amaretti cookies

1 tablespoon unsalted butter, softened

1. Preheat the oven to 350°F. Butter an 11- by 8- by 2-inch oval baking dish.

2. Arrange the peach and pear slices in the dish. Stir together the wine and jam and pour over the fruit. Sprinkle with the sugar and cookie crumbs. Dot with the butter.

3. Bake for 45 minutes to 1 hour, until the fruit is tender. Serve warm.

Marmellata di Pere

PEAR JAM

Makes about 2½ cups

The Giardino di Felicin is a family-run inn and restaurant in Monforte d'Alba in Piedmont. It was founded by the father of the current proprietor, Giorgio Rocca. Giorgio and his lovely wife, Rosina, work in the kitchen while their son acts as sommelier. The kitchen turns out the most delicate *tajarin* (the Piemontese version of fettuccine), rich game dishes, and sublime desserts.

In addition to being a wonderful cook, Giorgio is also a most gracious host. He speaks five languages and delights in introducing the many foreigners who visit his inn to each other and instigating lively conversations.

One morning, he served us a beautiful golden jam with an intense honeyed pear flavor. Giorgio told us that the pears from trees just outside the door were not so good for eating, but they sure did make great jam.

I have tried this with several varieties of pears and it always turns out well.

> 2½ *pounds ripe pears*
> 2 *tablespoons fresh lemon juice*
> 2 *cups sugar*

1. Peel and quarter the pears. Remove the cores and cut the pears into ½-inch chunks. Sprinkle with the lemon juice.

2. In a heavy medium saucepan, combine the pears and sugar. Cook over medium-low heat, stirring frequently, until most of the liquid has evaporated and the mixture has thickened. Let cool.

3. Spoon into sterilized containers. Refrigerate for up to 1 month or freeze for up to 6 months.

Dolci da Cucchiaio

§§§§

SPOON DESSERTS

The Italians call puddings, gelatins, mousses, and all kinds of soft desserts dolci da cucchiaio, or spoon desserts. In this chapter you will find a collection of desserts that have that one thing in common—they can be eaten with a spoon. Some are made with gelatin, some are puddings, and some are mousses. Some are very easy and can be put together in minutes, while others are more elaborate, suitable for the most important occasions.

Zabaglione

Serves 4 to 6

§ The name *zabaglione* is derived from that of San Giovanni Baylon, venerated in Turin as the patron saint of pastry makers. Though it is usually eaten for dessert, the Italians also think of zabaglione as a soothing, healthful food. Invalids are sometimes given zabaglione to build up their strength. The Romans consider zabaglione invigorating, the type of dessert the amorous Casanova might have chosen.

Zabaglione can take many forms. It usually appears as a warm pudding or sauce for cake, gelati, puddings, or fruit, though it also can be the base for ice cream or semifreddo. Cooled zabaglione, lightened with whipped cream, is served as a kind of mousse or used as a filling for layer cakes and pastries.

Typically, zabaglione is made with egg yolks, sugar, and a fortified wine, usually Marsala, beaten over simmering water until pale, light, and fluffy.

In her excellent book *La Cucina di Lidia* Lidia Bastianich—the owner, with her husband, Felix, of Felidia Restaurant in New York—explains the chemistry of zabaglione and the importance of using the proper proportion of ingredients and a careful technique. Lidia says the right ratio is "1 egg yolk to 1 tablespoon sugar to 1 tablespoon Marsala." She emphasizes that "these ingredients must be thoroughly blended before being subjected to heat, and once the heating has begun, temperature must remain constant and moderate." For a light fluffy zabaglione, these proportions can vary only slightly. If the heat is too high, the evaporating alcohol will escape too quickly, leaving the zabaglione flat or, worse yet, curdled.

There are any number of ways to vary zabaglione by substituting other liquids for the Marsala, and you should feel free to experiment. Using cordials such as amaretto or orange liqueur in place of Marsala is tricky, however, because their higher alcohol content will make them evaporate too rapidly. I have found that the best way to incorporate liqueurs is to substitute them for just a portion of the Marsala.

Zabaglione is best when it is freshly made, so plan to serve it immediately. It is good on its own, over cake, with berries or fruit salad, as a dip for biscotti, or as a sauce over ice cream or pudding.

4 large egg yolks

¼ cup sugar

¼ cup dry Marsala

1. In the bottom of a double boiler or in a medium saucepan, bring about 2 inches of water to a simmer.

2. In the top half of the double boiler or in a heatproof bowl that will fit comfortably over the saucepan, beat the egg yolks, Marsala, and sugar with a hand-held electric mixer or a whisk until well blended. Place the top of the double boiler or the bowl over the simmering water; the bottom should not be in contact with the water. Do not allow the water to boil. Beat or whisk the mixture until it is pale, light, and fluffy and holds a soft shape when dropped from the beaters or whisk, 3 to 5 minutes. Serve immediately.

Vin Santo Zabaglione. Substitute vin santo for the Marsala.

Zabaglione Freddo
COLD ZABAGLIONE
Serves 6

ZABAGLIONE
4 large egg yolks
¼ cup granulated sugar
¼ cup dry Marsala

1 cup heavy cream
2 tablespoons confectioners' sugar
2 tablespoons orange liqueur

1. Make the zabaglione according to the instructions on pages 140 to 141. Immediately place the bowl of zabaglione into a large bowl filled with ice water, and whisk the zabaglione until cold.

2. In a large chilled bowl, using an electric mixer with chilled beaters, beat the cream and confectioners' sugar until stiff. Beat in the orange liqueur.

3. Fold the cold zabaglione into the whipped cream. Spoon into large goblets. Cover and chill until serving time. (The recipe can be prepared up to 1 day ahead.)

Zabaglione al Cioccolata
CHOCOLATE ZABAGLIONE
Serves 4

✿ This tastes like a rich chocolate mousse, yet it is very quick and easy to make. Serve it warm or cold.

3 ounces semisweet chocolate, coarsely chopped

¼ cup heavy cream

4 large egg yolks

¼ cup sugar

2 tablespoons dry Marsala

2 tablespoons orange liqueur or rum

1. In a small saucepan, combine the chocolate and cream. Heat gently over low heat, stirring until the chocolate has melted and the mixture is smooth. Remove from the heat.

2. In the bottom of a double boiler or in a medium saucepan, bring about 2 inches of water to a simmer.

3. In the top of the double boiler or in a medium heatproof bowl, beat the egg yolks and sugar until light. Beat in the Marsala and rum or liqueur. Place over the simmering water; the bottom should not be in contact with the water. Do not allow the water to boil. Beat or whisk the mixture until it is pale, light, and fluffy and holds a soft shape when dropped from the beaters or whisk, 3 to 5 minutes.

4. Remove from the heat. Gently fold in the chocolate mixture. Serve immediately.

To serve cold: After folding in the chocolate, set the top of the double boiler or the bowl into a large bowl filled with ice water. Beat until the zabaglione feels cold to the touch. Divide among four goblets. Cover and chill until serving time.

Espresso Zabaglione

Serves 4 as a dessert, 8 as a sauce

4 large egg yolks

¼ cup sugar

¼ teaspoon ground cinnamon

⅓ cup cooled brewed espresso or 1½ teaspoons instant espresso powder dissolved in ⅓ cup hot water and cooled

2 tablespoons Cognac, rum, or coffee liqueur

1. In the bottom of a double boiler or in a medium saucepan, bring about 2 inches of water to a simmer.

2. In the top half of the double boiler or in a heatproof bowl that will fit comfortably over the saucepan, beat all of the ingredients with a hand-held electric mixer or a wire whisk until well blended. Place the top of the double boiler or the bowl over the simmering water; the bottom should not be in contact with the water. Beat on high speed or whisk until the mixture has quadrupled in volume and is pale, light, and fluffy, 3 to 5 minutes. Serve immediately.

Zabaglione al Balsamico con Lampone

ZABAGLIONE WITH BALSAMIC VINEGAR AND RASPBERRIES

Serves 6

The sweet and sour taste of balsamic vinegar complements many kinds of fruit and adds piquancy to zabaglione. At Restaurant Picci in Cavriano near Parma, it is used to make zabaglione and served as a sauce over raspberries in a cookie cup. Use as much balsamico as is needed for a balanced flavor.

3 *large egg yolks*

3 *tablespoons sugar*

2 *tablespoons Marsala*

2 *to 3 teaspoons balsamic vinegar, to taste*

6 *Cookie Cups (page 35)*

1 *pint raspberries*

1. In the bottom of a double boiler or in a medium saucepan, bring about 2 inches of water to a simmer.

2. In the top half of the double boiler or in a heatproof bowl that will fit comfortably over the saucepan, beat the egg yolks, sugar, Marsala, and vinegar with a hand-held electric mixer or a wire whisk until well blended. Place the top of the double boiler or the bowl over the simmering water; the bottom should not be in contact with the water. Beat on high speed or whisk until the mixture has quadrupled in volume and is pale, light, and fluffy, 3 to 5 minutes. Remove from the heat.

3. Place the Cookie Cups on individual serving plates. Divide the raspberries among the cups, and spoon on the zabaglione. Serve immediately.

Spuma di Cioccolato e Lampone

CHOCOLATE RASPBERRY CREAM

Serves 6

This rich dessert takes only minutes to prepare.

2 cups raspberries

1 tablespoon sugar

2 tablespoons raspberry or orange liqueur

3 ounces semisweet chocolate, melted and cooled

½ cup (4 ounces) mascarpone

1 cup heavy cream

Chocolate shavings

1. Set aside a few berries for garnish. In a bowl, toss the remaining raspberries with the sugar and raspberry or orange liqueur.

2. In a large bowl, whisk the melted chocolate into the mascarpone until smooth.

3. In a large chilled bowl, using an electric mixer with chilled beaters, whip the cream until stiff. Gradually fold in the whipped cream into the chocolate mixture.

4. Spoon half the chocolate cream into six goblets. Spoon the raspberries with the liqueur over the cream. Top with remaining chocolate cream. Garnish with the reserved raspberries and chocolate shavings. Serve immediately.

Budino di Riso con Salsa di Cioccolata

VANILLA RICE PUDDING WITH LIGHT CHOCOLATE SAUCE

Serves 8

Sometimes I find rice pudding cloying because it is can be so heavy and rich, but this version is different. It has a light, fluffy consistency and is chunky with chopped chocolate. The chocolate sauce is light too, since it is made with cocoa and milk instead of chocolate and cream. The pudding tastes just fine on its own though, so you can serve it plain if you prefer.

6 cups milk

1 cup Arborio rice

½ vanilla bean, split lengthwise

½ teaspoon salt

1 cup sugar

2 tablespoons dark rum or Cognac

1 cup heavy cream

3 ounces semisweet chocolate, finely chopped

LIGHT CHOCOLATE SAUCE

2 tablespoons Dutch-process cocoa powder

3 tablespoons sugar

1 teaspoon cornstarch

2 cups cold milk

1. In a large saucepan, bring the milk to a simmer. Stir in the rice, vanilla bean, and salt. Simmer, stirring occasionally, until the rice is tender, about 30 minutes. Remove the vanilla bean, and stir in the sugar. Let cool to room temperature, then stir in the rum or Cognac.

2. In a large chilled bowl using an electric mixer with chilled beaters, whip the cream until stiff. Fold the cream into the cooled rice, then fold in the

chocolate. Spoon into a large serving bowl or individual goblets. Cover and chill.

3. To make the sauce: In a small saucepan, combine the cocoa, sugar, and cornstarch. Stir in a tablespoon or two of the milk, just enough to form a smooth paste. Gradually stir in the remaining milk. Place over medium heat and cook, stirring constantly, until the mixture thickens and comes to a boil. Reduce the heat and simmer for 1 minute more. Let cool. Cover and chill until ready to serve.

4. To serve, spoon the sauce over the pudding.

Gelo di Tarocchi

BLOOD ORANGE JELLY

Serves 4

🌀 Any fresh orange juice can be used for this very refreshing jelly, though blood orange juice is particularly attractive. This dessert is a far cry from packaged gelatin desserts, a revelation of how good a fruit gel can be. Serve it plain or with whipped cream or sugared strawberries.

2 envelopes unflavored gelatin

½ cup cold water

¾ cup sugar

3 cups fresh blood orange or other orange juice

¼ cup light rum

1. In a small saucepan, sprinkle the gelatin over the water. Let stand for 5 minutes to soften.

2. Add the sugar and heat oven medium-low heat, stirring constantly, until the gelatin is completely dissolved. Stir in the orange juice and rum. Pour into a 1-quart mold or bowl. Cover and chill several hours or until set.

3. To unmold, dip the mold in warm water for 30 seconds. Run a small knife around the edge of the mold and invert the jelly onto a serving plate. Serve immediately or refrigerate until ready to serve.

$\mathscr{P}$an di Caffè

ESPRESSO CREAM

Serves 6

At La Chiusa, a magnificent Tuscan country inn in Montefollonico, this rich coffee custard is served with an assortment of chocolate desserts.

The owner told us that it is a very old recipe from his grandmother. Though similar to crème caramel, it contains no milk or cream, so the texture is rather dense, but it is not too rich.

1½ *cups sugar*

2 *tablespoons water*

5 *large eggs*

2 *cups very strong espresso*

1 *tablespoon light rum*

Whipped cream

1. Preheat the oven to 350°F.

2. In a small saucepan, combine ¾ cup of the sugar and the water. Wash down any sugar crystals on the sides of the pan with a pastry brush dipped in water, and bring to a boil. Cook over medium heat without stirring until the mixture begins to darken and caramelize. Then swirl the pan over the heat until the syrup is an even golden brown. Immediately pour the caramel into six 6-ounce custard cups. Let cool.

3. In a large bowl, whisk the eggs and the remaining ¾ cup sugar until light. Beat in the espresso and rum. Strain the mixture into the custard cups.

4. Place the cups in a large roasting pan and set it in the oven. Carefully pour hot water around the custard cups to a depth of 1 inch. Bake for 30 minutes, or until a knife inserted ¼ inch from the center of the custards comes out clean. Remove the custard cups from the roasting pan and let cool. Chill completely.

5. Run a thin knife around the inside of each cup. Invert onto individual serving plates. Serve with whipped cream.

Panna Cotta

Serves 6

🌀 *Panna cotta* means "cooked cream," but I like to think of it as the essence of cream. It is just a simple gelatin creation made with milk, cream, vanilla, and a bit of sugar but it is delicious. If you can find fresh cream—that is, not the ultrapasteurized kind that seems to be everywhere lately—it will taste even better.

At one time this simple homemade dessert was served only in Piemonte, where it seems to have originated. Now, however, panna cotta can be found in trendy restaurants all over Italy. The basic cream remains the same but the sauce changes according to the season and the cook. As an alternative, you can caramelize the molds as for the Chocolate Crème Caramel (page 151).

1 package unflavored gelatin

2 cups cold milk

1 cup heavy cream

1 vanilla bean, split

¼ cup sugar

Hot Chocolate Sauce (page 208), cooled to room
temperature

Raspberry Sauce (page 217)

Fresh raspberries

1. In a small saucepan, sprinkle the gelatin over ⅓ cup of the milk. Let stand for 5 minutes to soften.

2. Place over low heat and cook, stirring, until the gelatin is completely dissolved, about 5 minutes. Stir in the remaining 1⅔ cups milk, the cream, and vanilla bean and cook, stirring frequently, until small bubbles appear around the edges. Remove from the heat and let cool slightly.

3. Remove the vanilla bean, and scrape the seeds into the liquid. Pour the mixture into six 4-ounce ramekins or custard cups. Cover and chill until set.

4. Dip the cups in warm water for 30 seconds. Run a small spatula around the edges to release the creams. Invert onto serving plates. Spoon a pool of Raspberry Sauce to one side and a pool of Chocolate Sauce to the other of each panna cotta. Garnish with fresh raspberries.

Crema di Melone con Salsa di Fragola

CANTALOUPE CREAM WITH STRAWBERRY SAUCE

Serves 6

ᡀ Any kind of cups or glasses can be used to mold this unusual dessert. Disposable clear plastic drinking cups are the perfect size and shape.

2 packages unflavored gelatin

½ cup cold water

1 large ripe cantaloupe (about 2½ pounds), seeded and cut into chunks, at room temperature

¾ cup sugar

1 to 2 tablespoons fresh lemon juice, to taste

1 cup heavy cream

Strawberry Sauce (page 207)

Fresh strawberries

1. In a small heatproof cup, sprinkle the gelatin over the cold water. Let stand for 5 minutes to soften.

2. Place the cup in a small saucepan partially filled with simmering water. Heat the gelatin, stirring constantly, until completely dissolved, about 5 minutes. Remove from the heat.

3. In a food processor or blender, purée the cantaloupe. There should be about 3½ cups purée. Add the sugar and lemon juice to taste. Process until the sugar is completely dissolved. Add the gelatin and the cream and process until blended.

4. Pour the mixture into six 8- to 9-ounce cups or glasses. Chill until set, 2 to 3 hours.

5. Dip the cups in warm water for 15 seconds and unmold the cantaloupe creams onto dessert plates. Serve with the fresh Strawberry Sauce and garnish with strawberries.

Crema Rovesciato di Cioccolata

CHOCOLATE CRÈME CARAMEL

Serves 6

In an otherwise nondescript Roman trattoria, we were served a gorgeous chocolate version of crème caramel. The combination of chocolate and caramel is sublime.

1¼ *cups sugar*

2 *tablespoons water*

2 *cups milk*

4 *ounces semisweet chocolate, coarsely chopped*

4 *large eggs*

2 *large egg yolks*

1. Preheat the oven to 350°F.

2. In a small saucepan, combine ¾ cup of the sugar and the water. Wash down any sugar crystals on the sides of the pan with a pastry brush dipped in water and bring to a boil. Cook over medium heat without stirring until the mixture begins to darken and caramelize. Then swirl the pan over the heat until the syrup is an even golden brown. Immediately pour the caramel into six 6-ounce custard cups. Let cool.

3. In a medium saucepan, heat the milk until small bubbles form around the edges. Remove from the heat. Stir in the chocolate. Let stand until the chocolate is softened, then stir until smooth.

4. In a large bowl, whisk the eggs, yolks, and the remaining ½ cup sugar until light. Add the chocolate mixture and stir until blended. Strain the mixture into the prepared cups.

5. Place the cups in a large baking pan and set it in the oven. Carefully pour hot water to a depth of ½ inch around the cups. Bake for 20 to 25 minutes, or until a knife inserted about ¼ inch from the center comes out clean but the center is still slightly soft.

6. Remove the cups from the baking pan and let cool. Chill completely.

7. Just before serving, run a small knife around the edge of the custards. Invert them onto serving plates.

Crema di Yogurt con Salse di Frutta

YOGURT CREAM WITH FRESH FRUIT SAUCES

Serves 6

𝄢 I served this dessert to a visitor who was amazed to learn that Italians eat yogurt! They certainly do—for breakfast, as a snack, or in desserts.

This light and lovely yogurt cream was served to us at Da Delfina Restaurant in Artimino. Delfina was once the cook at a nearby royal hunting lodge. Now she presides over the restaurant kitchen, while her son Carlo runs the dining room.

You can make this as elaborate or as simple as you like. Though two or three sauces are very pretty, one is fine. Vary the sauces according to the season. For a special occasion, I like to center the creams on large dinner plates and spoon the sauces around them. A few slices of a fresh peach, banana, orange, or kiwi or some fresh berries make a beautiful finishing touch.

1 envelope unflavored gelatin

¼ cup cold water

½ cup sugar

1 pint plain yogurt

1 cup heavy cream

1 teaspoon vanilla extract

One or more Fresh Fruit Sauces (page 231)

Mint sprigs

1. In a small heatproof cup, sprinkle the gelatin over the water. Let stand for 5 minutes to soften.

2. Place the cup in a small saucepan partially filled with simmering water. Heat, stirring, until the gelatin is dissolved. Remove from the heat.

3. In a large bowl, beat the sugar, yogurt, ½ cup of the cream, and the vanilla until smooth. In a chilled medium bowl, using an electric mixer with

chilled beaters, whip the remaining ½ cup cream until stiff. Fold the whipped cream into the yogurt mixture. Pour into six 6-ounce custard cups. Chill until set.

4. Dip the cups into warm water and turn the creams out onto individual serving plates. Serve with one or more Fresh Fruit Sauces, spooning the sauce(s) around the creams. Garnish with mint sprigs.

Coppa di Mascarpone con Amaretti

MASCARPONE AND AMARETTI CREAM

Serves 6

½ *cup crushed amaretti cookies (about 8)*

½ *cup golden raisins*

⅓ *cup Cognac, rum, or amaretto*

8 *ounces (1 cup) mascarpone*

¼ *cup sugar*

1 *tablespoon fresh lemon juice*

1 *cup heavy cream*

2 *tablespoons toasted almonds*

1. In a small bowl, combine the cookies, raisins, and Cognac, and toss well.

2. In a large bowl, whisk the mascarpone with the sugar and lemon juice until smooth. In a chilled medium bowl, using an electric mixer with chilled beaters, whip the cream until it forms soft peaks. Gently fold the whipped cream into the mascarpone mixture.

3. Spoon half of the mascarpone mixture into six large wine goblets. Spoon the amaretti crumb mixture over the cream. Top with the remaining mascarpone cream. Chill completely.

4. Just before serving, sprinkle with the almonds.

Tiramisù

Serves 10 to 12

✿ *Tiramisù* means "pick-me-up," and as one story goes, this was a favorite dessert of Venetian courtesans who needed lots of energy for their amorous adventures. A less romantic but probably more likely story is that it was the creation of a thrifty cook with leftover biscuits and coffee.

There are as many versions of this luscious dessert as there are cooks in Italy. This is my favorite, though I like to experiment with it at times, substituting Marsala or amaretto for the orange liqueur or Cognac for the dark rum. Savoiardi are Italian-style ladyfingers that are available in packages at many shops selling imported foods. Ordinary ladyfingers or thin slices of plain cake can be substituted for the cookies.

1 pound (2 cups) mascarpone

3 tablespoons sugar

2 tablespoons orange liqueur

2 tablespoons dark rum

1 cup heavy cream

24 savoiardi or ladyfingers

1½ cups cold brewed espresso

8 ounces semisweet chocolate, finely chopped

1. In a large bowl, combine the mascarpone, sugar, liqueur, and rum and beat until smooth.

2. In a chilled bowl, using an electric mixer with chilled beaters, whip the cream until soft peaks form. Gently fold the whipped cream into the mascarpone mixture.

3. Pour the espresso into a cup. Lightly moisten 12 of the savoiardi in the espresso and arrange them in a single layer in the bottom of an 8-inch square cake pan.

4. Spread half the mascarpone mixture over the savoiardi and sprinkle with half the chocolate. Repeat with remaining ingredients.

5. Cover and refrigerate for at least 1 hour, or overnight. To serve, spoon onto individual serving plates.

Zuppa di Ricotta

RICOTTA TRIFLE

Serves 6

🌀 Sometimes the process of slicing biscotti yields a lot of crumbs. Gather them up and store them until you have enough to make this easy trifle. Of course, you can use crushed store-bought cookies. Chocolate wafers are especially good.

2 cups crumbled biscotti or other dry cookie crumbs (about 6 ounces)

⅓ cup blanched almonds, toasted and finely chopped

¼ cup amaretto, rum, or orange liqueur

1 15-ounce container whole-milk ricotta cheese

¼ cup sugar

1 teaspoon grated lemon zest

½ cup sour cream

Shaved chocolate

1. In a bowl, combine the crumbs and almonds. Add the amaretto and toss well.

2. In a food processor or blender, combine the ricotta, sugar, and lemon zest. Process until the mixture is smooth and creamy. Add the sour cream and pulse just until blended. Do not overmix.

3. Spread half of the cookie mixture in the bottom of a 1-quart serving bowl. Spoon on half of the ricotta mixture. Sprinkle with the remaining crumbs. Top with the remaining ricotta, and smooth the top. Garnish with chocolate shavings. Cover and refrigerate for several hours, or overnight.

Torta di Pane Raffermo

CHOCOLATE-RUM RAISIN BREAD PUDDING

Serves 8

An old adage says that good cooks waste nothing. Why should they, when some leftover bread and a few dry cookies can be turned into something so delicious as this delightful torta? The recipe is from the family of my friend Carla Simons, who comes from Novara in Piemonte.

1½ cups dark raisins

⅓ cup dark rum

2 cups cubed white Italian or French bread

2 cups cubed whole-wheat bread, preferably Italian or French

⅓ cup sugar

1 quart milk

½ cup Dutch-process cocoa powder

3 large eggs, lightly beaten

6 amaretti cookies, crumbled

½ cup chopped semisweet chocolate

1. In a small bowl, combine the raisins and rum. Let stand until the raisins are plumped, about 1 hour.

2. In a large bowl, combine the bread, sugar, and milk. Stir well. Let stand for 1 hour.

3. Preheat the oven to 400°F. Butter a shallow 2½- to 3-quart baking dish.

4. Mash the soaked bread with a fork. Add the cocoa, eggs, and amaretti and stir well to mix. Pour into the baking pan and smooth the top. Sprinkle with the chocolate. Bake for 40 minutes, or until a knife inserted 1 inch from the edge of the pudding comes out clean. Serve warm or chilled.

Budino di Mele

APPLE BREAD PUDDING

Serves 10 to 12

There are more apples than bread in this delicate bread pudding from the Val d'Aosta, so the texture is very light. I like to serve it at room temperature with a dollop of whipped cream.

4 *cups cubed Italian or French bread*

1 *quart milk*

8 *Golden Delicious apples (about 3 pounds)*

6 *tablespoons unsalted butter*

1¼ *cups sugar*

1 *cup golden raisins*

4 *large eggs*

1 *teaspoon grated lemon zest*

Confectioners' sugar

1. In a large bowl, combine the bread and milk. Set aside for 1 hour.
2. Preheat the oven to 325°F. Butter a shallow 2½- to 3-quart baking dish.
3. Peel and core the apples and cut them into ¼-inch slices.
4. In a large skillet, melt the butter over medium heat. Add the apples and ¼ cup of the sugar. Cook, stirring frequently, until the apples are tender. Stir in the raisins. Stir the mixture into the bread and milk.
5. In a large bowl, beat the eggs with the remaining 1 cup sugar and the lemon zest. Stir into the apple mixture, until well mixed.
6. Pour into the prepared dish. Bake for 50 to 60 minutes or until a knife inserted 2 inches from the center of the pudding comes out clean.
7. Slide the pudding under a preheated broiler and broil until the top is lightly browned, about 1 to 2 minutes. Serve warm or at room temperature. Sprinkle with confectioners' sugar just before serving.

Miascia all'Arancia
ORANGE BREAD PUDDING
Serves 8

🎵 This rich bread pudding is a good way to use up leftover holiday breads such as panettone or stöllen. If you use white bread, be sure it is a good-quality firm bread. Soft, airy white bread is unsuitable. If the bread contains raisins or candied fruits, you may not want to add more raisins.

⅔ cup golden raisins

6 ounces panettone, brioche, challah, or good-quality white bread, thinly sliced (about 8 slices)

2 cups milk

¾ cup sugar

1 cup heavy cream

¼ cup rum

¼ cup dry Marsala

3 large eggs

2 teaspoons grated orange zest

½ teaspoon ground cinnamon

Confectioners' sugar

1. Preheat the oven to 375°F. Butter a shallow 2½- to 3-quart rectangular baking dish.

2. Sprinkle half the raisins over the bottom of the dish. Layer half the bread slices over the raisins. Sprinkle with the remaining raisins and top with the remaining bread.

3. In a medium saucepan, combine the milk and sugar. Bring to a simmer and simmer just until the sugar is dissolved. Remove from the heat, and stir in the cream, rum, and Marsala.

4. In a large bowl, beat the eggs, orange zest, and cinnamon. Stir in the milk mixture. Slowly pour over the bread slices, pressing the bread down to keep it submerged. Let stand for 10 minutes.

5. Place the baking dish in a larger roasting pan. Pour hot water around

the baking dish to a depth of 1 inch. Bake for 30 minutes, or until a knife inserted 2 inches from the edge of the pudding comes out clean and the top is golden.

6. Serve warm or chilled, cut into squares. Just before serving, sprinkle with confectioners' sugar.

$\mathcal{B}$udino di Biscotti
BISCOTTI PUDDING
Serves 8 to 10

🍲 Don't discard leftover cookies, cake, or bread. They can be used in so many delicious ways such as this pudding. It goes well with Mascarpone Custard Sauce (page 226) or whipped cream.

6 cups cubed firm bread

3 cups coarsely chopped or crumbled biscotti or other dry cookies

6 cups milk

4 large eggs

1 cup sugar

¾ cup dark raisins

¾ cup chopped semisweet chocolate (about 3 ounces)

2 tablespoons slivered almonds

Confectioners' sugar

1. In a large bowl, combine the bread and cookies. Add the milk, cover, and let stand for 1 hour.

2. Preheat the oven to 375°F. Butter a shallow 3-quart baking dish.

3. In a large bowl, beat together the eggs and sugar. Stir the eggs, raisins, and chocolate into the bread mixture. Pour the mixture into the prepared pan and smooth the surface. Sprinkle with the almonds.

4. Bake for 1 hour, or until the top is browned and puffed. Serve warm, chilled, or at room temperature. Sprinkle with confectioners' sugar just before serving.

$\mathcal{B}$udino di Pere

PEAR AND GRAPPA PUDDING

Serves 6

¾ cup golden raisins

½ cup grappa, rum, or brandy

2½ pounds firm ripe pears (about 8)

2 tablespoons unsalted butter

⅓ cup sugar

1 teaspoon grated lemon zest

TOPPING

6 tablespoons unsalted butter, melted and cooled

⅓ cup sugar

3 large eggs, separated

½ cup all-purpose flour

⅔ cup milk

2 tablespoons grappa, rum, or brandy

1½ teaspoons vanilla extract

Pinch of salt

Confectioners' sugar

Whipped cream

1. In a small bowl, combine the raisins and grappa. Let stand for 30 minutes.

2. Peel and core the pears and cut them into ½-inch slices.

3. In a large nonstick skillet, melt the butter over medium heat. Add the pears and sugar. Cook, stirring occasionally, until the pears are almost tender, about 7 minutes. Add the raisins and grappa and simmer for 2 minutes. Stir in the lemon zest and remove from the heat.

4. Preheat the oven to 350°F. Butter a shallow 2½-quart baking dish. Spread the pear mixture evenly in the dish.

5. To make the topping: In a large bowl whisk together the butter, sugar, and egg yolks. Stir in the flour. Add the milk, grappa, and vanilla. Whisk until the batter is well combined.

6. In a large bowl, with an electric mixer, beat the egg whites with the salt until they just hold soft peaks. Fold the whites into the batter. (The batter will be very thin.) Pour the batter over the pears and bake for 20 to 30 minutes, or until the top of the pudding is golden and firm to the touch. Let cool to warm or room temperature.

7. Just before serving sprinkle with confectioners' sugar. Serve with whipped cream.

Mousse di Cioccolato Bianco

WHITE CHOCOLATE MOUSSE

Serves 6

Ⓢ I came across this easy mousse in an Italian food magazine called *Tutto Cucina*. Their version was scooped into egg shapes and surrounded with two berry sauces and big fat curls of white chocolate—it looked absolutely gorgeous. My version uses one sauce with assorted berries.

1 cup (8 ounces) whole-milk ricotta cheese

2 tablespoons amaretto, brandy, or rum

1 cup heavy cream

¼ cup sugar

4 ounces white chocolate, finely chopped

2 10-ounce packages frozen raspberries in syrup, thawed

Fresh blueberries or strawberries

White chocolate curls

1. In a large bowl, whip the ricotta and amaretto until smooth and creamy.

2. In a large chilled bowl, using an electric mixer with chilled beaters, whip the cream with the sugar until stiff peaks form. Beat in the ricotta mixture. Fold in the white chocolate. Chill completely.

3. In a food processor or blender, purée the raspberries with their juices until smooth. Strain the sauce through a fine sieve to remove the seeds.

4. To serve, spoon a pool of sauce onto each serving plate. Using a small ice cream scoop or two large tablespoons, place two scoops of the mousse on each plate. Garnish with berries and white chocolate curls.

Sformato Bianco alla Castagna

MOLDED CHESTNUT CREAM

Serves 8

🌀 A sophisticated dessert for a special autumn or winter dinner. Instead of the Mocha Sauce, the chestnut cream can be served with whipped cream and candied chestnuts.

8 ounces whole chestnuts

½ cup sugar

1 cup milk

2 tablespoons orange liqueur or rum

1 package unflavored gelatin

½ cup cold water

1 cup heavy cream

Mocha Sauce (page 227)

1. To peel the chestnuts: Bring a medium saucepan of water to a boil. With a small sharp knife, cut a T-shaped slit in the rounded side of each chestnut.

2. Drop the chestnuts into the boiling water and cook for 10 minutes. With a slotted spoon, remove the chestnuts one at a time from the water and peel off the outer shell and the inner skin. If they are difficult to peel, return the chestnuts to the boiling water for another minute.

3. In a large heavy saucepan, combine the chestnuts, sugar, and milk. Bring to a simmer over medium-low heat and cook for 30 to 40 minutes, or until the chestnuts are very tender. Drain the chestnuts, reserving the milk.

4. In a food processor or blender, purée the chestnuts. With the machine running, gradually blend in the liqueur and reserved milk until smooth. Transfer to a large bowl and let cool.

5. In a small heatproof cup, sprinkle the gelatin over the cold water. Let stand for 5 minutes to soften. Place the cup in a small saucepan partially filled with water and bring the water to a simmer. Stir the gelatin until completely dissolved. Remove from the heat.

continued

6. In a large chilled bowl, using an electric mixer with chilled beaters, whip the cream until stiff.

7. Stir the gelatin into the chestnut mixture. Gently fold in half the whipped cream just until blended, then fold in the remaining cream. Spoon into a 1-quart bowl or mold. Cover and refrigerate until set, at least several hours, or overnight.

8. Dip the bowl or mold in warm water for 30 seconds. Unmold the chestnut cream onto a serving plate. Serve with the Mocha Sauce.

Coppa di Mascarpone al Caffè

MASCARPONE AND COFFEE CUPS

Serves 6

〽 Serve this easy but sophisticated dessert with plain cookies.

⅓ cup hot strong espresso

¼ cup sugar

¼ cup dark rum

4 ounces (½ cup) mascarpone, at room temperature

1 cup heavy cream

½ cup chopped semisweet chocolate (about 2 ounces)

1. Combine the espresso and sugar. Stir until the sugar is dissolved. Stir in the rum. Let cool to room temperature.

2. In a large bowl, whisk the mascarpone and coffee together until smooth. In a chilled medium bowl, using an electric mixer with chilled beaters, whip the cream until soft peaks form. Gently fold the cream into the mascarpone mixture. Set aside 2 tablespoons of the chocolate for garnish, and fold the remaining chocolate into the mascarpone.

3. Spoon the mixture into six goblets. Sprinkle with the reserved chocolate. Chill for at least 1 hour, or overnight.

Gelati

§§§§

ICE CREAMS

Eating ice cream is a favorite indulgence of Italians, both young and old. Especially in the warmer months, the after-dinner passagiata, or stroll, generally ends at the local caffè for an ice cream cone. Sunday afternoons, whole families gather around tiny sidewalk tables, downing elaborate ice cream concoctions.

Many caffès advertise produzione proprio, meaning that their gelati are made in-house. Most offer an astonishing variety, and there is constant competition to come up with new and unusual flavors. One Roman bar is known for its special vegetable flavors such as zucchini, tomato, and potato. Another makes an assortment of flavors based on rice. But these exotic offerings are just novelties.

If you want to sample a new flavor, you can ask for an assaggio, and you will receive a tiny taste on a small plastic spoon. Popular flavors include the intense bacio (chocolate kiss), gianduja (chocolate hazelnut), and every fruit and nut flavor imaginable.

Since the Italians have been making ice cream since Roman times, it should come as no surprise that they are masters of the art—Italian ice cream is very special. Because it is generally lower in butterfat, the flavors are fresh and pure with none of the heavy, mouth-coating feeling you sometimes experience with other ice creams. What is more, genuine Italian gelati are not frozen as deeply as other ice creams, so they have a lighter, creamier texture.

Making gelati at home is not difficult, but you do need an ice cream maker. There are all kinds of ice cream makers available, and even the inexpensive ones work quite well. The important thing to remember is to follow the manufacturer's directions. Keep in mind that since homemade gelati contain no stabilizers or preservatives, they should be eaten soon after they are made.

The recipes in this chapter are for flavors that I feel work particularly well in a home ice cream maker. I have also included a few recipes for some typically Italian presentations for gelati.

About Custards

Many of the sauces and gelati in this book are based on a stirred custard, a simple mixture of cooked eggs and milk. When making this type of custard, cook the ingredients just until smooth and slightly thickened. The cooked custard will leave a coating that will be either thin or thick, depending on the number of egg yolks used, on the back of a wooden spoon.

Custards need to be cooked carefully, otherwise they may curdle. Always use a saucepan with a heavy bottom and cook over low heat. Stir constantly with a wooden spoon. As the custard mixture comes to the right temperature, watch the surface carefully. Any foam will disappear and wisps of steam will start to rise. The correct temperature for custard is 140°F., which can be measured with an instant-reading thermometer. As soon as the custard is ready, remove it from the heat and strain it through a sieve into a bowl to eliminate any cooked egg fibers and to stop the cooking.

If the custard should overcook and curdle, you may still be able to save it. Pour the curdled mixture into a blender and blend on high speed until smooth.

Place a piece of plastic wrap directly on the surface of a cooked custard to prevent a skin from forming. For gelati, let the custard cool slightly at room temperature, then chill it thoroughly before proceeding.

$\mathcal{G}$elato di Caffè

COFFEE ICE CREAM

Makes 1 quart

🍥 I always associate the aroma of good coffee with Italy. In fact, as I walk off the airplane on arrival in Milan or Rome, it is invariably the first smell to reach me. I have to stop for coffee even before I pick up my luggage. Then I really feel like I have arrived.

Good Italian coffee is not limited to a single role as a beverage. It appears frequently in desserts of all sorts from cakes to ice cream. The success of this ice cream depends on the quality of the coffee used, so buy a good-quality espresso roast coffee and brew it fresh.

2 cups milk

⅔ cup sugar

3 large egg yolks

1 cup (8 ounces) double-strength brewed espresso

¼ teaspoon ground espresso

1. In a small saucepan, stir the milk and sugar over low heat just until the sugar is dissolved. Remove from the heat.

2. In a large bowl, beat the egg yolks until pale yellow. Gradually add the warm milk mixture in a thin stream, beating constantly. Pour the mixture into the saucepan. Cook over low heat, stirring constantly with a wooden spoon, until slightly thickened; do not boil. Strain the mixture into a bowl. Stir in the brewed and ground espresso. Cover and let cool. Chill thoroughly.

3. Freeze the mixture in an ice cream freezer according to the manufacturer's instructions. Transfer to a covered container and place in the freezer until ready to serve. If frozen hard let soften in the refrigerator for 30 minutes before serving.

Gelato di Cappuccino. Top each portion with whipped cream and a sprinkling of cinnamon or unsweetened cocoa powder.

Gelato di Fichi

FIG ICE CREAM

Makes 1 quart

A winemaker in Sava in Apulia took us to visit his cousin who owned a pastry shop. The shop featured the most unusual flavors of gelati I have ever encountered. There were rose, mulberry, and jasmine, among others, but my husband's favorite was this *gelato di fichi* with a rich flavor that came from dried figs. We ate the gelato with fresh, moist almond macaroon cookies.

1 cup dried figs (about 4 ounces), very finely chopped

1 cup water

1 cup sugar

2½ cups milk

1. In a medium saucepan combine the figs and water. Simmer for 5 minutes over low heat. Stir in the sugar and cook, stirring occasionally, until dissolved. Pour into a bowl. Let cool.

2. Stir in the milk. Cover and chill thoroughly.

3. Freeze the mixture in an ice cream freezer according to the manufacturer's directions. Transfer to a covered container and place in the freezer until ready to serve. If frozen hard, let soften in the refrigerator for 30 minutes before serving.

Gelato di Gianduja

CHOCOLATE HAZELNUT ICE CREAM

Makes 1 quart

✹ Torino is a gracious old city with a nineteenth-century look to it. The streets are wide and many of the sidewalks are covered by porticos, making strolling and window shopping a pleasure.

Two dessert flavors I always associate with Torino are chestnuts, in the fall and winter, and, year round, the chocolate and hazelnut combination called *gianduja*. A flavor marriage made in heaven, gianduja is a specialty of Turin that appears in cakes, candies, and gelati.

> 3 cups milk
>
> 2 cups hazelnuts, toasted and skinned (page 3)
>
> 3 ounces semisweet chocolate
>
> 1½ ounces unsweetened chocolate, coarsely chopped
>
> 3 large egg yolks
>
> 6 tablespoons sugar

1. In a medium saucepan, heat the milk until small bubbles form around the edges. Remove from the heat.

2. In a food processor or a blender, finely chop the nuts. With the machine running, slowly add about 1 cup of the hot milk. Blend until smooth, scraping down the sides of the container as needed. Pour the mixture into the saucepan of hot milk. Let stand for 30 minutes.

3. Place a large sieve over a bowl and line the sieve with dampened cheesecloth. Strain the hazelnut milk, pressing on the solids in the sieve with a wooden spoon. Pour the liquid into a medium saucepan. Discard the solids. Add both chocolates and heat gently over low heat until the chocolate is softened. Remove from the heat and stir until completely melted.

4. In a large bowl, beat the egg yolks and sugar until thick and light colored. Gradually beat in the milk mixture. Transfer to a large saucepan and cook over low heat, stirring constantly, until the mixture is thickened and lightly coats the back of a spoon.

5. Pour into a bowl and let cool slightly. Cover and refrigerate for several hours or overnight.

6. Freeze the mixture in an ice cream freezer according to the manufacturer's instructions. Transfer to a covered container and place in the freezer until ready to serve. If frozen hard, let soften for 30 minutes in the refrigerator before serving.

Gelato di Datteri

DATE ICE CREAM

Makes 1 quart

1 cup pitted dates (about 4 ounces)

3 cups milk

½ cup sugar

2 large egg yolks

1½ tablespoons dark rum

1. In a medium saucepan, combine the dates and milk. Bring to a simmer over medium heat and cook for 10 minutes. With a slotted spoon, transfer the dates to a food processor or blender. Reserve the milk. Process the dates until smooth.

2. In a large bowl, whisk together the sugar, egg yolks, and rum. Gradually whisk in the reserved milk. Beat in the date purée.

3. Pour into a medium saucepan and cook over medium-low heat, stirring constantly, until the mixture has thickened slightly and coats the back of a spoon. Strain into a bowl. Stir in the rum. Let cool, then cover and chill.

4. Freeze the mixture in an ice cream freezer according to the manufacturer's directions. Transfer to a covered container and place in the freezer until ready to serve. If frozen hard, let soften in the refrigerator for 30 minutes before serving.

Gelato di Mandorle

TOASTED ALMOND ICE CREAM

Makes about 1½ quarts

2 cups milk

1 cup heavy cream

4 large egg yolks

1 cup sugar

2 teaspoons vanilla extract

½ teaspoon almond extract

1 cup toasted almonds, coarsely chopped

1. In a medium saucepan, heat the milk and cream until small bubbles form around the edges. Remove from the heat.

2. In a large bowl, whisk the egg yolks and sugar until blended. Gradually pour the milk into the egg yolks, whisking constantly. Return the mixture to the saucepan and cook over medium heat, stirring constantly with a wooden spoon, until the mixture thickens slightly and lightly coats the back of the spoon.

3. Strain the mixture through a fine sieve. Let cool. Stir in the vanilla and almond extracts. Cover and chill for several hours, or overnight.

4. Freeze the mixture in an ice cream freezer according to the manufacturer's instructions. When the ice cream is frozen, add the chopped almonds. Transfer to a covered container and place in the freezer until serving time. If the ice cream becomes too firm, place it in the refrigerator for 30 minutes before serving.

Gelato di Cannèlla

CINNAMON ICE CREAM

Makes about 5 cups

§ A subtle hint of cinnamon flavors this gelato. It is ideal with Warm Berry Sauce (page 112) or Hot Chocolate Sauce (page 208).

2 cups milk

1 cup heavy cream

1 2-inch strip of lemon zest

½ teaspoon ground cinnamon

4 large egg yolks

½ cup sugar

1. In a medium saucepan, combine the milk, cream, lemon zest and cinnamon. Heat until small bubbles form around the edges. Remove from the heat and let cool slightly.

2. In a large bowl, whisk the egg yolks and sugar until foamy. Gradually pour the warm milk into the egg yolks, whisking constantly. Return the mixture to the saucepan and cook over medium heat, stirring constantly with a wooden spoon, until the mixture thickens slightly and lightly coats the back of the spoon.

3. Strain the mixture through a fine sieve. Let cool. Cover and chill for several hours, or overnight.

4. Freeze the mixture in an ice cream freezer according to the manufacturer's instructions. Transfer to a covered container and place in the freezer until serving time. If the gelato becomes too firm, place it in the refrigerator for 30 minutes before serving.

Gelato di Crema. Omit the cinnamon and add 1 teaspoon vanilla extract to the strained cream.

Gelato di Arance

ORANGE ICE CREAM

Makes 5 cups

๑ This type of gelato, made with whipped cream and a sugar syrup, is sometimes called *spumone*. *Gelato di arance* is wonderful in Tartufi (page 178) instead of chocolate ice cream, or serve it with Hot Chocolate Sauce (page 208).

> 3 *navel oranges*
>
> 1 *cup water*
>
> ¾ *cup sugar*
>
> 6 *large egg yolks*
>
> 1 *cup heavy cream*

1. Finely grate the zest from the oranges and squeeze the juice. There should be about 3 tablespoons zest and ⅔ cup juice.

2. In a medium saucepan, combine the water and sugar. Cook over medium heat, stirring, until the sugar dissolves, about 3 minutes. Remove from the heat.

3. In a large bowl, whisk the egg yolks until very light. Slowly add the hot sugar syrup in a thin stream, whisking constantly. Pour into a large saucepan and cook over low heat, stirring with a wooden spoon, until slightly thickened.

4. Strain the mixture into a medium bowl, and set it in a larger bowl partially filled with ice water. Stir in the orange juice and zest. Let cool, stirring occasionally. (Or chill overnight in the refrigerator.)

5. In a large chilled bowl, using an electric mixer with chilled beaters, whip the cream until stiff peaks form. Fold the cream into the cooled orange custard mixture. Freeze in an ice cream freezer according to the manufacturer's instructions. Transfer to a covered container and place in the freezer until serving time. If the gelato becomes too firm, place it in the refrigerator for 30 minutes before serving.

Gelato di Caramello

CARAMEL ICE CREAM

Makes 1½ quarts

Caramel ice cream is luscious plain and maybe even better with a spoonful or two of aged dark rum.

1¼ cups sugar

¼ cup water

1 cup heavy cream

2 cups milk

5 large egg yolks

1 teaspoon vanilla extract

1. In a medium saucepan, combine 1 cup of the sugar and the water. Wash down any sugar crystals on the sides of the pan with a pastry brush dipped in water, and bring to a boil. Cook over medium heat without stirring until the syrup begins to darken and caramelize. Carefully swirl the pan over the heat until the syrup is an even golden brown.

2. Remove from the heat. When the syrup stops boiling, gradually stir in the cream. The caramel will harden. Return to the heat and reheat gently, stirring constantly, until smooth. Remove from the heat.

3. In a medium saucepan, heat the milk until small bubbles form around the edges. Remove from the heat.

4. In a large bowl, whisk the egg yolks and the remaining ¼ cup sugar until thick and light. Gradually whisk in the warm milk. Pour the mixture into the saucepan and cook over low heat, stirring constantly, until slightly thickened; do not boil.

5. Strain the custard into the caramel mixture, and stir until blended. Let cool. Stir in the vanilla extract. Cover and refrigerate for several hours, or overnight.

6. Freeze the mixture in an ice cream freezer according to the manufacturer's directions. Transfer to a covered container and place in the freezer until serving time. If the gelato becomes too firm, place it in the refrigerator for 30 minutes before serving.

Gelato di Castagna

CHESTNUT ICE CREAM

Makes about 1 quart

Down a narrow alley off the Via Coronari in Rome, there used to be a charming but extremely odd little restaurant. The owner, who spoke only Italian, insisted on reciting the long and elaborate menu at each table. Sometimes the wait seemed endless as he tried to explain the day's offerings to foreigners who did not understand a word of Italian. The result could be chaos. Though the owner was often as frustrated by the lack of communication as his customers, he refused to relent and supply a written menu—in any language.

While waiting, we would amuse ourselves watching his antics—something like an unrehearsed floor show. The food was usually good, but my favorite dessert was the creamy smooth chestnut gelato topped with chunks of candied chestnuts in syrup.

Canned sweetened chestnut purée can be substituted for the fresh chestnuts. Just stir in the milk, cream, and vanilla extract and freeze.

8 ounces whole chestnuts

½ cup sugar

2 cups milk

1 cup heavy cream

1 vanilla bean, split, or 1 teaspoon vanilla extract

1. With a small sharp knife, make a T-shaped slit in the rounded side of each chestnut. Bring a medium saucepan of water to a boil. Drop the chestnuts into the water and cook for 10 minutes. With a slotted spoon, remove the chestnuts one at a time and peel off the outer shell and inner skin. If they are difficult to peel, return the chestnuts to the water for another minute.

2. In a medium saucepan, combine the chestnuts, sugar, milk, and vanilla bean (do not add the vanilla extract at this point). Bring to a simmer and cook over low heat, stirring occasionally, until the chestnuts are very tender, about 40 minutes. Drain the chestnuts, reserving the liquid. Remove the vanilla bean.

3. In a food processor, purée the chestnuts until smooth. Add the reserved milk and cream and the vanilla extract if using, and process until blended. Cover and let cool. Refrigerate until thoroughly chilled.

4. Freeze the mixture in an ice cream freezer according to the manufacturer's directions. Transfer to a covered container and place in the freezer until ready to serve. If the gelato becomes too firm, let soften for 30 minutes in the refrigerator before serving.

Gelato di Miele

HONEY ICE CREAM

Makes 1½ quarts

2 cups milk
1 cup heavy cream
4 large egg yolks
½ cup honey

1. In a medium saucepan, heat the milk and cream until small bubbles appear around the edges. Remove from the heat.

2. In a large bowl, whisk the egg yolks and honey until blended. Gradually beat in the hot milk and cream. Pour the mixture into the saucepan and cook, stirring constantly, until slightly thickened; do not boil.

3. Immediately strain the mixture into a bowl. Let cool. Cover and chill thoroughly.

4. Freeze in an ice cream freezer according to the manufacturer's directions. Transfer to a covered container and place in the freezer until serving time. If the gelato becomes too firm, place it in the refrigerator for 30 minutes before serving.

Gelato al Torrone. Spoon Honey Ice Cream into serving bowls. Top each portion with chopped *torrone* (almond nougat) and a spoonful of rum or Cognac.

Tartufi

CHOCOLATE ICE CREAM TRUFFLES

Serves 6

꧂ Tre Scalini, a bar and restaurant in the Piazza Navona in Rome, is renowned for its decadently rich tartufo, a chocolate ice cream truffle. The truffle consists of a scoop of dark chocolate ice cream with a brandied cherry concealed in its center. The ice cream is rolled in a coating of crisp, thin semisweet chocolate flakes. Dieters can skip the whipped cream topping! One bite of this version will transport you to the Piazza Navona. All that's missing is Bernini's Fountain of the Four Rivers.

If you can find them, amarena, dark cherries in syrup, are the perfect filling for the tartufo. They are made by Fabbri and several other Italian manufacturers. Otherwise, homemade marinated cherries can be used—or substitute maraschino cherries, store-bought walnuts in syrup, tutti frutti, or candied chestnuts.

Work quickly and keep everything well chilled. The chocolate flakes used in this recipe make a nice topping for other desserts too.

6 fresh or frozen pitted cherries

1 tablespoon Cognac

1 teaspoon sugar

4 ounces semisweet or bittersweet chocolate, coarsely chopped

1 pint chocolate ice cream

Whipped cream (optional)

1. In a small bowl, combine the cherries, Cognac, and sugar. Stir well, and set aside to marinate for 1 hour.

2. Line a baking sheet with aluminum foil.

3. Place the chocolate in a bowl set over a saucepan of simmering water. Let stand until softened. Remove from the heat and stir until smooth. Pour the melted chocolate onto the prepared baking sheet. With a long metal spatula, spread the chocolate evenly and thinly over the foil. Chill in the refrigerator until firm.

4. Line a small metal pan with wax paper, and place it in the freezer.

5. Remove the baking sheet from the refrigerator. Lift the foil from the pan and peel off the chocolate sheet, breaking the chocolate into ½-inch flakes. Work quickly to prevent the chocolate from melting. Scatter the flakes over the baking sheet.

6. With a large ice cream scoop, gather up a ball of ice cream. Holding the ball of ice cream in the scoop, poke a hole in it with a teaspoon and insert a cherry. Smooth the ice cream over the cherry. Drop the ice cream ball onto the sheet of chocolate flakes and scatter more flakes over the ice cream, pressing them lightly so that they adhere. With a spatula, transfer the ice cream ball to the chilled metal pan. Return the pan to the freezer and make 5 more tartufi with the remaining ingredients, placing each one in the freezer. Freeze for 1 to 2 hours before serving.

7. Serve the tartufi with whipped cream if desired.

Gelato Affogato

DROWNED ICE CREAM

Serves 2

"Drowning" ice cream in coffee or liqueur is a nice way to dress it up. Other good combinations include Gelato di Caramello (page 175) with rum and chocolate gelato with amaretto.

4 scoops Gelato di Caffè (page 168)
½ cup hot brewed espresso

Divide the gelato between two serving dishes. Pour on the espresso. Serve immediately.

$\mathcal{G}$elato di Crema con Balsamico

VANILLA ICE CREAM WITH BALSAMIC VINEGAR

Serves 2

🍋 Gelato di Crema is similar to vanilla ice cream but it has a hint of lemon flavor. Vanilla ice cream can be substituted in this amazingly good combination presented at New York's Felidia Restaurant by the owner, Lidia Bastianich, to the members of Les Dames d'Escoffier, a professional wine and food society. Use only a well-aged balsamico, however.

2 scoops Gelato di Crema (page 173) or vanilla ice cream

1 teaspoon balsamic vinegar

Soften the ice cream slightly and stir in the balsamico. Serve immediately.

Mangia e Bevi
EAT AND DRINK
Serves 4

🌀 Great big goblets of fresh fruit salad and gelati are a favorite summertime dessert or afternoon snack in Italy. As the gelati melts, it mixes with the fruit and juices, hence the name.

1 *ripe banana, peeled and sliced*

1 *large ripe peach, peeled and sliced*

1 *cup sliced strawberries*

2 *kiwi, peeled and sliced*

¼ *cup orange juice*

1 *to 2 tablespoons orange liqueur (optional)*

2 *tablespoons sugar*

1 *pint (2 cups) Honey Ice Cream (page 177) or vanilla ice cream*

1. Combine the fruits, juice, liqueur, and sugar.
2. Divide the fruit mixture among four large goblets. Top with scoops of the gelato. Serve immediately.

Granite e Sorbetti

~~~~~

ICES AND SORBETS

F riends from Sicily often reminisce about their morning granita di caffè (coffee ice), into which they would dip their breakfast brioscia (sweet roll). What a refreshing way to start a hot summer day!

Granita comes from the word grana, meaning "grain" or "grainy." The technique for making granita results in a soft, almost slushy, granular ice. It is best to eat it slowly, allowing the ice crystals to melt in your mouth.

Granita is usually made with fruit juice and sugar syrup, though there are variations with coffee, tea, or other liquids. Freezing tends to dull flavors, so the base mixture must be very intense so that the flavor comes through after it is frozen.

One of the good things about granita, aside from its great taste, is that it is so easy to make at home. No special equipment is required—all you need is a pan and a spoon. If you should decide to make it in an ice cream freezer, it will be very good, though smooth and not granular—more like the Italian ices sold in this country, which are, in fact, closer to sorbetto than granita.

Though similar in their content, there are two important differences between granita and sorbetto. One is the technique: Granita is stirred as it freezes. Sorbetto is frozen solid first, then puréed until smooth. Second, a sorbetto often contains fruit solids while a granita is made with fruit juice or some other liquid. As a result, sorbetto has a soft, smooth, creamy texture in contrast to granita's granular and coarse texture.

Any of the granita recipes in this book can be prepared using the sorbetto technique, and they will turn out smoother and creamier. Most of the sorbetto mixtures do not work well as granita, however. The fruit pulp does not freeze into crystals and the result is unpleasantly gritty.

As with granita, no special equipment is needed to make sorbetto. After the ingredients are frozen solid, they can be broken into small chunks and puréed in a food processor or in a large bowl using an electric mixer. They are best served within a few hours of being made.

During the summer months when I make granita very often, I keep a large batch of sugar syrup in the refrigerator. It keeps well for a long time and I can make granita, or other ices, on a moment's notice.

Granita and Sorbetto Hints

- Keep a batch of sugar syrup chilled in a covered jar in the refrigerator to facilitate making granita and sorbetto. Equal parts sugar and water is the most useful mixture to have on hand. Then add it to taste to fruit juice or purée, diluting with water as needed. Remember that the fruit mixture should taste quite sweet for best results. Balance the flavor with fresh lemon or lime juice.

- Have all utensils and ingredients chilled, especially if the weather is warm. Chill the metal pan you are using in the freezer before adding the mixture to be frozen. Taking these steps makes a big difference in overall freezing time.

- When making granita, leave the cold spoon in the metal pan between stirrings so as not to raise the temperature unnecessarily.

Granita di Gelsomino

JASMINE TEA GRANITA

Makes 5 cups

Mary Taylor Simeti's incomparable book *Pomp and Sustenance: Twenty-five Centuries of Sicilian Food* (Knopf, 1989) traces the origins of modern-day gelati and granita to the Arabs, who used lumps of snow from the chilly summit of Mt. Etna to chill their *sarbat*, a forerunner of sherbet and other frozen desserts. Ms. Simeti, who lives in Sicily, describes one ice, flavored with jasmine flowers, that was a particular favorite of the Saracens.

Her recipe calls for freshly picked jasmine flowers, impossible to find in my neighborhood, so I tried it with jasmine tea. The result is deliciously light and fragrant, if a little unorthodox. Of course, other teas can be used, such as Earl Grey or even ordinary orange pekoe.

2½ **tablespoons jasmine tea leaves**

3 **cups water**

1 **cup sugar**

2 to 3 **tablespoons fresh lemon juice**

1. Place the tea leaves in a heatproof bowl. Bring the water to a boil and pour over the tea leaves. Let steep for 5 minutes. Strain.

2. Add the sugar and lemon juice and stir until the sugar is completely dissolved. Let cool.

3. Pour the mixture into a chilled 9-inch square metal pan. Freeze for 30 minutes, or until ice crystals form around the edges.

4. Stir the ice crystals into the center of the mixture. Return the pan to the freezer and continue freezing, and stirring every 30 minutes, until all of the liquid is frozen, about 2 to 2½ hours.

5. To serve, scoop the granita into serving dishes.

Granita di Caffè

COFFEE GRANITA

Makes 1½ quarts

One of the best ways to pass a hot summer afternoon in Rome is to find a shady table at an outdoor caffè and order a granita di caffè. If you make it yourself, you have the advantage of being able to use decaffeinated coffee if you prefer, and sweetening it or not, to your own taste. Even non–coffee lovers like this.

¾ cup finely ground Italian espresso

4 cups water

2 tablespoons sugar, or to taste

Whipped cream (optional)

1. In an espresso maker or drip coffeepot, make coffee according to the manufacturer's directions, using the espresso and water. Add the sugar if desired, and stir until dissolved. Let cool slightly, then cover and chill until cold.

2. Pour the coffee into a chilled 12- by 9- by 2-inch metal pan. Freeze for 30 minutes, or until ice crystals begin to form around the edges.

3. Stir the ice crystals into the center of the mixture. Return the pan to the freezer and continue freezing, stirring every 30 minutes, until all of the liquid is frozen, about 2 to 2½ hours.

4. Serve in large goblets, with whipped cream if desired.

Granita di Fragole

STRAWBERRY GRANITA

Makes 1½ quarts

This granita is a little different from most because whole fruit is used. Raspberries or blackberries can be substituted for strawberries. Adjust the amount of sugar to the sweetness of the fruit.

3 *cups water*

1 *cup sugar*

1 *pint strawberries, rinsed and hulled*

½ *cup fresh orange juice*

¼ *cup fresh lemon juice*

1. In a small saucepan, combine the water and sugar. Bring to a simmer over medium heat and cook until the sugar is dissolved, about 3 minutes. Let cool slightly, then refrigerate until cold.

2. In a food processor, purée the strawberries. Add the sugar syrup and orange and lemon juices, and pulse to blend.

3. Pour the mixture into a chilled 12- by 9- by 2-inch metal pan. Freeze for 30 minutes, or until ice crystals form around the edges.

4. Stir the ice crystals into the center of the mixture. Return the pan to the freezer and continue freezing, stirring every 30 minutes, until all of the liquid is frozen, about 2 to 2½ hours.

Granita di Limone

LEMON GRANITA

Makes 1½ quarts

Try adding a scoop of this lemon granita to a glass of ice tea.

4 cups water

1 cup sugar

1 teaspoon grated lemon zest

¾ cup fresh lemon juice

1. In a medium saucepan, combine the water and sugar. Bring to a simmer and cook over medium heat, stirring occasionally, until the sugar is dissolved, about 3 minutes. Let cool slightly, then refrigerate until cold.

2. Combine the sugar syrup, lemon zest, and lemon juice. Pour the mixture into a chilled 12- by 9- by 2-inch metal pan. Freeze for 30 minutes, or until ice crystals form around the edges.

3. Stir the ice crystals into the center of the mixture. Return the pan to the freezer and continue freezing, stirring every 30 minutes, until all of the liquid is frozen, about 2 to 2½ hours.

Misto di Bosco con Granita di Limone

BERRIES WITH LEMON GRANITA

Serves 4

1 cup blackberries

1 cup blueberries

1 cup sliced strawberries

1 cup raspberries

2 tablespoons sugar

1 pint (2 cups) Lemon Granita (page 189)

Grappa or vodka (optional)

1. Combine the berries and sugar and toss well.
2. Divide the berries among four serving dishes. Top with scoops of the granita. Drizzle with grappa or vodka if desired.

Granita di Menta

MINT GRANITA

Makes 1½ quarts

This granita is especially good served after a fish dinner. Either spearmint or peppermint can be used.

4 cups water

¾ cup sugar

2 bunches of fresh mint, stemmed and coarsely chopped (about 2 cups)

¼ cup fresh lemon juice

1. In a medium saucepan, combine the water and sugar. Bring to a simmer over medium heat and cook, stirring occasionally, until the sugar is dissolved, about 3 minutes. Add the mint and let cool. Refrigerate until chilled.

2. Strain the syrup, discarding the mint, and add the lemon juice. Pour the mixture into a chilled 12- by 9- by 2-inch metal pan. Freeze for 30 minutes, or until ice crystals form around the edges.

3. Stir the ice crystals into the center of the mixture. Return the pan to the freezer and continue freezing, stirring every 30 minutes, until all of the liquid is frozen, about 2 to 2½ hours.

Granita di Pompelmo e Campari

GRAPEFRUIT AND CAMPARI GRANITA

Makes 1½ quarts

🌀 I am not sure whether this is an American or an Italian creation. Whatever it is, I like its flavor and its rosy pink color.

½ cup sugar

1 cup water

4 to 5 medium grapefruits (pink or white)

¾ cup Campari

1. In a small saucepan, combine the sugar and water. Bring to a simmer and cook, stirring occasionally, until the sugar is dissolved, about 3 minutes. Remove from the heat and let cool. Cover and refrigerate until cold.

2. Grate ½ teaspoon zest from one of the grapefruit. Squeeze 3 cups juice from the grapefruits.

3. Combine the juice, sugar syrup, Campari, and zest. Pour into a chilled 12- by 9- by 2-inch metal pan. Freeze the mixture for 30 minutes, or until ice crystals form around the edges.

4. Stir the ice crystals into the center of the mixture. Return the pan to the freezer and continue freezing, stirring every 20 to 30 minutes, until all of the liquid is frozen, about 2 to 2½ hours.

Granita di Mandarino

TANGERINE GRANITA

Makes 1 quart

1 cup sugar

1 cup water

About 8 tangerines, mandarin oranges, or clementines

1 to 2 tablespoons fresh lemon juice to taste

1. In a medium saucepan, bring the water and sugar to a simmer over medium heat. Cook for 3 minutes, or until the sugar is dissolved. Let cool slightly, then refrigerate until cold.

2. Grate 1 teaspoon zest from 1 or 2 of the tangerines and set aside. Halve the tangerines and squeeze out the juice. Squeeze 1½ cups juice from the fruit.

3. Combine the juice, sugar syrup, and zest. Add lemon juice to taste. Pour the mixture into a 12- by 9- by 2-inch metal pan. Freeze for 30 minutes or until ice crystals begin to form around the edges.

4. Stir the ice crystals into the center of the mixture. Return to the freezer and continue freezing, stirring every 30 minutes, until all of the liquid is frozen, about 2 to 2½ hours.

Sorbetto di Mirtille

BLUEBERRY SORBET

Makes 1 quart

One of my favorite summer desserts. Try splashing on some grappa just before serving. This looks and tastes great in combination with Cantaloupe Sorbet (page 197).

1 cup water
1 cup sugar
1 pint blueberries, picked over
2 to 3 tablespoons fresh lemon juice, to taste

1. In a small saucepan, combine the water and sugar. Simmer over medium heat, stirring occasionally, until the sugar is dissolved, about 3 minutes. Let cool. Refrigerate until chilled.

2. Rinse the blueberries, and pat dry. In a blender or food processor, purée the berries. Add the sugar syrup and lemon juice to taste. Pour the mixture into a chilled 12- by 9- by 2-inch metal pan. Freeze until solid, several hours or overnight.

3. Break the sorbetto into small chunks. Place in a food processor and process until smooth and creamy. Serve immediately, or pack into a covered container and freeze for up to 2 hours.

Bellini Sorbetto

PEACH AND PROSECCO SORBET

Makes 5 cups

A Bellini is the white peach and sparkling white wine cocktail made famous by Harry's Bar in Venice. The same flavors make a fabulous iced dessert.

The typical wine used in a Bellini is Prosecco, a dry sparkling white wine from the Veneto area. An elegant way to serve this sorbetto is in large goblets, drizzled with additional Prosecco.

1¼ pounds ripe peaches (about 5)

½ cup sugar, or to taste

2 tablespoons fresh lemon juice

1 cup Prosecco or other dry sparkling white wine

1. Bring a medium saucepan of water to a boil. Add the peaches and simmer for 30 seconds. Remove the peaches with a slotted spoon and let cool. Remove the skins. Cut the peaches in half and remove the pits.

2. In a blender or food processor, combine the peaches, sugar, and lemon juice. Blend or process until the sugar is completely dissolved. Pour the mixture into a 12- by 9- by 2-inch square metal pan. Stir in the wine. Freeze until solid, several hours or overnight.

3. Break the sorbetto into small chunks. Place in a food processor and purée until smooth and creamy. Serve immediately, or pack into a covered container and freeze for up to 2 hours.

Sorbetto al Limone Verde con Aranciata

LIME SORBET WITH CANDIED ORANGE ZEST

Makes 5 cups

◊ This sorbetto is made with egg white, which gives it a smoother, creamy consistency. If you prefer, the egg white can be eliminated.

1 cup sugar

2 cups water

1 cup fresh lime juice

1 teaspoon grated lime zest

2 oranges

3 tablespoons honey

1 large egg white

1. In a small saucepan, combine the sugar and water. Bring to a simmer over medium heat. Cook until the sugar is dissolved, about 3 minutes. Let cool slightly, then refrigerate until cold.

2. Combine the sugar syrup, lime juice, and lime zest. Pour the mixture into a 9-inch square metal pan. Freeze until solid, several hours or overnight.

3. Meanwhile, with a vegetable peeler, remove zest from the oranges in long strips. Stack the strips and cut the zest into matchsticks.

4. Squeeze the juice from the oranges and set aside. Bring a small saucepan of water to a boil. Add the orange zest and simmer for 10 minutes. Drain and pat dry.

5. In a small saucepan, combine the orange juice, zest, and honey. Simmer until most of the liquid has evaporated and the peel is glazed; watch carefully so that the zest does not scorch. Let cool, then chill until ready to use.

6. In a food processor, process the egg white until foamy. Break the sorbetto into small chunks. Add to the food processor and purée until smooth and creamy. Serve immediately, or pack into a covered container and freeze for up to 2 hours.

7. Serve the sorbetto topped with the candied zest.

Sorbetto di Melone

CANTALOUPE SORBET

Makes 3 cups

🌀 Honeydew melon also makes an excellent sorbetto. The melons have a particular affinity for the lime flavor, though either fresh lime or lemon juice can be used.

1 cup sugar

1 cup water

1 ripe medium cantaloupe (about 1½ pounds), peeled, seeded, and cut into small chunks

2 to 3 tablespoons fresh lime or lemon juice, to taste

1. In a small saucepan, combine the sugar and water. Bring to a simmer over medium heat. Cook until the sugar is dissolved, about 3 minutes. Let cool slightly, then refrigerate until cold.

2. In a food processor, purée the melon until smooth. Add the sugar syrup and lime or lemon juice, and process until blended. Pour the mixture into a 9-inch square metal pan. Freeze until solid, several hours or overnight.

3. Break the sorbetto into small chunks. Place in a food processor and purée until smooth and creamy. Serve immediately, or pack into a covered container and freeze for up to 2 hours.

Sorbetto di Cioccolata

CHOCOLATE SORBET

Makes about 3 cups

This sorbetto is made with chocolate and milk instead of fruit juice. Kids love it.

2 cups milk

¼ cup sugar

3 ounces semisweet chocolate, coarsely chopped

1. In a medium saucepan, heat the sugar and milk until warm, stirring until the sugar is dissolved. Remove from the heat, add the chocolate, and let stand until softened. Whisk until smooth. Let cool, then refrigerate until chilled.

2. Pour the mixture into a chilled 9-inch square metal pan. Freeze until solid, several hours or overnight.

3. Break the sorbetto into small chunks. Place in a food processor and purée until smooth and creamy. Serve immediately, or pack into a covered container and freeze for up to 2 hours.

Sorbetto di Banana

BANANA SORBET

Makes 1 pint

This is so smooth and creamy, it is hard to believe it contains no cream or egg yolks.

½ **cup sugar**

½ **cup water**

2 **ripe medium bananas**

2 **tablespoons fresh lemon juice**

1. In a medium saucepan, combine the sugar and water and bring to a simmer over medium heat. Cook for 3 minutes, or until the sugar is dissolved. Let cool slightly, then refrigerate until cold.

2. In a food processor or blender, purée the bananas and lemon juice until smooth. Add the sugar syrup. Pour the mixture into a chilled 9-inch square metal pan. Freeze until solid, several hours or overnight.

3. Break the sorbetto into chunks. Place in a food processor and purée until smooth and creamy. Serve immediately, or pack into a covered container and freeze for up to 2 hours.

Sorbetto di Mele

APPLE SORBET

Makes 5 cups

1 cup dry white wine

1 cup water

¾ cup sugar

1 tablespoon fresh lemon juice

4 large Granny Smith apples, peeled, cored, and chopped

⅓ cup Calvados or apple brandy

1. In a large saucepan, combine the wine, water, sugar, lemon juice, and apples. Cover and bring to a simmer. Cook over low heat until the apples are very tender when pierced with a knife, about 20 minutes. Let cool.

2. Transfer the apple mixture to a food processor or blender, and purée until smooth. Add the Calvados and process to blend. Pour the mixture into a chilled 12- by 9- by 2-inch metal pan. Freeze until solid, several hours or overnight.

3. Break the sorbetto into chunks. Place in a food processor and purée until smooth and creamy. Serve immediately, or pack into a covered container and freeze for up to 2 hours.

Sorbetto di Ananas

PINEAPPLE SORBET

Makes 1 quart

A light and refreshing dessert. Sprinkle with dark rum or a dash of cinnamon for a tropical accent.

1 cup sugar

1 cup water

3 cups ripe pineapple chunks

2 to 3 tablespoons fresh lemon juice, to taste

1. In a medium saucepan, combine the sugar and water and bring to a simmer over medium heat. Cook for 3 minutes, or until the sugar is dissolved. Let cool slightly, then refrigerate until cold.

2. In a food processor or blender, purée the pineapple until smooth. Add the sugar syrup and lemon juice to taste. Pour the mixture into a chilled 12- by 9- by 2-inch metal pan. Freeze until solid, several hours or overnight.

3. Break the sorbetto into chunks. Place in a food processor and purée until smooth and creamy. Serve immediately, or pack into a covered container and freeze for up to 2 hours.

Sorbetto di Albicocche

DRIED APRICOT SORBET

Makes 1 quart

The season for fresh apricots is all too short, so this sorbetto is made with dried apricots, which are always available. It is inspired by one I tasted at a modern-looking Roman caffè known as Al Restoro della Salute, located across from the Coliseum. Healthy fruit- and vegetable-based drinks, ices, and gelati are the specialty of the house, and big boxes of fresh fruit and vegetables are piled up near the entrance, waiting to be used.

1 cup dried apricots

¾ cup sugar

3 cups water

1. In a small saucepan, combine all the ingredients. Bring to a simmer over medium heat. Cook until the apricots are tender, about 10 minutes. Remove from the heat and let stand until cool.

2. With a slotted spoon, transfer the apricots to a food processor. Purée until smooth. Add the cooking syrup and process to blend. Pour the mixture into a chilled 12- by 9- by 2-inch metal pan. Cover and freeze until firm.

3. Break the sorbetto into chunks and place in a food processor. Process until smooth and creamy. Serve immediately, or pack into a covered container and freeze for up to 2 hours.

Sorbetto di Lampone e Vino Rosso

RASPBERRY AND RED WINE SORBET

Makes 1 quart

꿁 The red wine in this sorbetto enhances and brings out the raspberry flavor. I like to serve it with chocolate cake or biscotti.

1 *pint raspberries*

1 *cup sugar*

1 *cup dry red wine*

2 *cups water*

1. In a small saucepan, combine all the ingredients. Bring to a simmer over medium heat and cook, stirring occasionally, for 15 minutes. Let cool. Refrigerate until chilled.

2. Strain the raspberry mixture through a sieve, pressing on the solids with the back of a spoon. Pour the mixture into a chilled 12- by 9- by 2-inch metal pan. Freeze until solid.

3. Break the sorbetto into small chunks. Place in a food processor and process until smooth. Serve immediately, or pack in a covered container and freeze for up to 2 hours.

Semifreddi

FROZEN MOUSSES

To me, a semifreddo is one of the most intriguing of Italian desserts. Whenever I order it, I am never sure what to expect.

Semifreddo means "half cold" and the name is derived from the fact that the concoction never freezes as hard as gelati. In Ada Boni's classic cookbook Il Talismano della Felicita (Casa Editrice Colombo, 1983), the author states that semifreddi are "those types of preparations that, having need of a more or less long stay in the freezer or refrigerator, must not give the palate the characteristic sensation of ice and for that reason they must not reach the temperature or consistency of frozen preparations." The author then lists within the category of semifreddo the following: Bavarians, biscuit glacés, charlottes, gelatin desserts, and mousselines.

Italians use the term semifreddo to describe many disparate types of desserts, cold or frozen, but to me the best ones are mousselike mixtures that are mixed or layered with fruit, chocolate, crumbled cookies or nuts and frozen either in individual servings or in loaf or dome shapes. The airy mousse and the chopped bits never freeze really hard and the result is creamy, yet chunky for an interesting texture. It is this type of semifreddo that you will find in this chapter. Gelatin desserts and puddings, though sometimes called semifreddi by Italians, can be found in the chapter on Spoon Desserts.

A semifreddo is very similar to ice cream in ingredients and preliminary preparation. Because air is incorporated in the form of whipped cream and/or eggs, churning is not needed to keep the mixture smooth and free of ice crystals. It is essential, though, to maintain the volume of air, so the ingredients should be folded in carefully and quickly and the utensils kept cold.

There really is nothing difficult about making semifreddi, but the recipes do entail several steps and a number of bowls and beaters. It helps if you have an extra set of attachments for your electric mixer. All of the semifreddi may be made up to three days before serving, as can most of the sauces in this chapter.

Semifreddo al Cioccolata Bianco

WHITE CHOCOLATE SEMIFREDDO WITH STRAWBERRY SAUCE

Serves 8

3 3½-ounce bars white chocolate, chopped

3 large eggs, separated, at room temperature

3 tablespoons sugar

2 tablespoons amaretto

1 cup heavy cream

STRAWBERRY SAUCE

1 pint strawberries, hulled and chopped

3 tablespoons sugar

¼ cup fresh orange juice

2 tablespoons amaretto

1. Line a 9- by 5- by 3-inch metal loaf pan with plastic wrap, leaving a 2-inch overhang on the ends. Chill in the freezer.

2. In a metal bowl set over hot but not simmering water, melt the white chocolate, stirring occasionally, until smooth. Let cool to lukewarm.

3. In a large bowl, beat together the egg yolks, sugar, and amaretto until thick and pale.

4. In the large bowl of an electric mixer, beat the egg whites just until they hold stiff peaks. In another bowl, whip the cream just until it holds stiff peaks. Gently but thoroughly fold the whites into the cream. Fold half the melted chocolate into the yolk mixture then fold in one quarter of the cream mixture. Gently but thoroughly fold in the remaining chocolate and the remaining cream mixture. Scrape into the chilled pan. Cover with plastic wrap and freeze for at least 8 hours, or overnight.

5. To make the sauce: In a food processor, purée the berries with the sugar, orange juice, and amaretto until smooth.

6. To serve, unmold the semifreddo onto a serving dish. Cut into slices and accompany with the Strawberry Sauce.

Semifreddo alle Mandorle con Salsa Calda al Cioccolata

ALMOND SEMIFREDDO WITH HOT CHOCOLATE SAUCE

Serves 8

⑨ Diana Restaurant in Bologna is a large, bustling trattoria. The food is straightforward—grilled fungi and scampi, great pasta, and bollito misto. It was there that I tasted the ultimate semifreddo. It was creamy with a subtle crunch of nuts and amaretti, and melted in the mouth.

The crowning touch was the velvety bittersweet chocolate sauce made with Majani chocolate, a local brand that does not seem to travel far from Bologna. At home, I make it with Tobler or Lindt extra-bittersweet chocolate, though a good semisweet works well too.

6 amaretti cookies, finely crushed

¼ cup toasted almonds, finely chopped

¾ cup sugar

¼ cup water

4 large eggs, at room temperature

¾ cup heavy cream

1 teaspoon vanilla extract

HOT CHOCOLATE SAUCE

6 ounces extra-bittersweet or semisweet chocolate

¾ cup heavy cream

1. Line a 9- by 5- by 3-inch metal loaf pan with plastic wrap, leaving a 2-inch overhang on the ends. Chill the pan in the freezer.

2. Combine the cookie crumbs and almonds and set aside.

3. In a small saucepan, combine the sugar and water. Bring to a simmer and cook without stirring until the sugar is completely dissolved, about 5 minutes. Meanwhile, in a large bowl, beat the eggs with an electric mixer on medium speed until pale yellow.

4. Slowly beat the hot sugar syrup into the eggs in a thin stream. Continue beating until the mixture is very light and fluffy and feels cool to the touch, 8 to 10 minutes.

5. In a large chilled bowl, beat the cream with the vanilla until it just holds stiff peaks. Gently but thoroughly fold the cream into the egg mixture. Set aside 2 tablespoons of the amaretti mixture for garnish, and stir the remainder into the egg mixture. Spoon into the prepared loaf pan. Cover with plastic wrap and freeze for at least 8 hours, or overnight.

6. When ready to serve, make the sauce: Combine the chocolate and cream in a large metal bowl set over barely simmering water, and stir until smooth. Keep warm over low heat.

7. Unmold the semifreddo onto a serving plate and sprinkle with the reserved amaretti mixture. Cut into slices and serve with the Hot Chocolate Sauce.

Semifreddo al Torrone
NOUGAT SEMIFREDDO
Serves 8

I can't imagine a more picturesque setting for a restaurant than that of the Antica Locanda Mincio in Valeggio sul Mincio near Verona. To reach it, you must cross over the Mincio River on an ancient stone bridge that was once part of a fortress. The river flows over a waterfall and under a small wooden footbridge just outside the restaurant's door. In the summer months, guests sit at tables along the riverbank in the shade of enormous linden trees while the waitresses and waiters dash back and forth carrying platters of homemade tortellini alla zucca, large ring-shaped pasta stuffed with a pumpkinlike squash, or fettuccine with wild mushroom sauce and grilled meats or fish from the river. For dessert, I can't resist their delicious individual-size semifreddi flavored with crunchy torrone.

Torrone is a honey and nut nougat candy. It is sold either as long bars or miniatures packed in tiny boxes decorated with women wearing Italian folk costumes. The little boxes were always tucked among the fruits and nuts in our holiday fruit bowl centerpieces. The kids loved to collect them to use for whatever purposes children use tiny boxes.

If torrone is not available, use a cup of crushed cookies instead.

continued

2 large eggs

¼ cup sugar

1 cup heavy cream

2 tablespoons rum or Cognac

4 ounces torrone (Italian nougat candy), finely chopped

2 ounces semisweet chocolate, finely chopped

Hot Chocolate Sauce (page 208)

1. Line a 9- by 5- by 3-inch metal loaf pan with plastic wrap, leaving a 2-inch overhang on the ends. Chill in the freezer.

2. In a metal bowl or the top half of a double boiler, beat the eggs and sugar until very light and fluffy. Place over simmering water, and with an electric mixer or wire whisk, beat until the mixture is very light and pale yellow and holds a soft shape.

3. Remove the bowl or top half of the double boiler from the heat and set it into a larger bowl filled with ice water. Let cool, whisking occasionally.

4. In a large bowl, whip the cream with the rum or Cognac until it just holds soft peaks. Fold the beaten eggs gently but thoroughly into the cream.

5. Fold in the torrone and chocolate. Scrape the mixture into the chilled pan. Cover with plastic wrap and freeze for at least 8 hours, or overnight.

6. Unmold the semifreddo onto a serving dish. Slice and serve with the Hot Chocolate Sauce.

Semifreddo al Cappuccino

CAPPUCCINO SEMIFREDDO

Serves 8

🌀 A coffee layer and a cinnamon cream layer make the flavors of this semifreddo reminiscent of cappuccino. Mocha Sauce (page 227) goes very well with it.

4 large eggs, separated, at room temperature

¾ cup sifted confectioners' sugar

⅛ teaspoon ground cinnamon

¾ cup chilled heavy cream

1 tablespoon instant espresso powder dissolved in 1 teaspoon warm water

Cocoa powder

1. Line a 9- by 5- by 3-inch metal loaf pan with plastic wrap, leaving a 2-inch overhang on the ends. Chill the pan in the freezer.

2. In the large bowl of an electric mixer, beat together the egg yolks, ¼ cup of the confectioners' sugar, and the cinnamon until thick and pale.

3. In a large bowl, beat the egg whites until they are foamy. Gradually add the remaining ½ cup confectioners' sugar, beating until the whites just hold stiff peaks.

4. In a large bowl, beat the cream until it just holds stiff peaks. Gently but thoroughly fold in the whites, and then fold the cream mixture into the yolk mixture. Pour half the mixture into the chilled pan and freeze it for 45 minutes. Stir the espresso into the remaining mixture, cover, and refrigerate.

5. Stir the espresso mixture and pour it over the frozen cinnamon layer, smoothing the top. Cover with plastic wrap and freeze for at least 8 hours, or overnight.

6. Unmold the semifreddo onto a serving dish. Sprinkle very lightly with cocoa powder.

Semifreddo alla Gianduja

CHOCOLATE HAZELNUT SEMIFREDDO

Serves 8

Don't try to make the zabaglione sauce ahead of time, as it will not hold. If you don't want to have to deal with it at the last minute, serve the semifreddo with Hot Chocolate Sauce (page 208) or whipped cream instead.

⅔ *cup hazelnuts, toasted and skinned (page 3)*

½ *cup hot milk*

6 *ounces semisweet chocolate, chopped*

3 *large egg whites, at room temperature*

3 *tablespoons sugar*

1 *cup heavy cream*

RUM ZABAGLIONE SAUCE

3 *large egg yolks*

¼ *cup sugar*

2 *tablespoons dark rum*

1. Line a 9- by 5- by 3-inch metal loaf pan with plastic wrap, leaving a 2-inch overhang on the ends. Chill the pan in the freezer.

2. In a food processor or blender, chop the hazelnuts fine. Add the hot milk and process until smooth.

3. In a large metal bowl set over barely simmering water, melt the chocolate, stirring occasionally until it is smooth. Stir in the hazelnut mixture. Remove the bowl from the heat and set it into a larger bowl filled with ice water. Let cool, whisking occasionally.

4. In the large bowl of an electric mixer, beat the egg whites until they are foamy. Gradually add the sugar and continue beating just until the whites hold stiff peaks.

5. In a chilled bowl, beat the cream until it just holds stiff peaks. Gently but thoroughly fold in the whites. Fold one quarter of the cream mixture into the chocolate mixture. Then fold in the remaining cream mixture. Pour into the chilled pan, cover with plastic wrap, and freeze for at least 8 hours, or overnight.

6. To make the zabaglione: In a metal bowl or the top half of a double boiler, beat the yolks, sugar, and rum until well blended. Place over barely simmering water, and beat until the mixture is thick and quadrupled in volume, about 5 minutes.

7. Immediately unmold the semifreddo onto a serving dish. Serve it sliced with the zabaglione.

Semifreddo al Cocco con Salsa di Arance

COCONUT SEMIFREDDO WITH BURNT ORANGE SAUCE

Serves 8

Coated with toasted coconut and served with a caramelized orange sauce, this semifreddo has a tropical flavor. To toast coconut, spread it in a baking pan and bake in a 350°F. oven, stirring occasionally, for five to ten minutes, until lightly browned.

BURNT ORANGE SAUCE

1 *cup sugar*

¼ *cup water*

1¼ *cups strained fresh orange juice*

2 *teaspoons orange zest cut into matchstick strips*

¾ *cup sugar*

¼ *cup fresh orange juice*

4 *large eggs, at room temperature*

1 *teaspoon grated orange zest*

¾ *cup heavy cream*

1⅓ *cups (3½ ounces) sweetened flaked coconut, lightly toasted*

continued

1. To make the sauce: In a medium saucepan, combine the sugar and water. Cook over medium heat, stirring and washing down the sugar crystals on the sides of the pan with a brush dipped in cold water, until the sugar is dissolved. Then bring to a boil and cook the mixture without stirring until it turns a golden amber. Carefully add 1 cup of the orange juice, pouring it near the side of the pan, and add the zest. Cook, stirring, until the caramel dissolves. Let the mixture cool, then stir in the remaining ¼ cup orange juice. Cover and chill.

2. Line a 9- by 5- by 3-inch metal loaf pan with plastic wrap, leaving a 2-inch overhang on the ends. Chill it in the freezer.

3. In a small saucepan, combine the sugar and orange juice and bring to a simmer. Cook, stirring, until the sugar is dissolved.

4. Meanwhile, in a large bowl, beat the eggs with an electric mixer on high speed until they are thick and pale.

5. Gradually beat in the hot orange syrup and continue beating until the mixture has doubled in volume and is cool to the touch, about 5 to 8 minutes. Beat in the grated zest.

6. In a large chilled bowl, beat the cream until it just holds stiff peaks. Fold the cream into the egg mixture. Pour into the chilled pan, cover with plastic wrap, and freeze for at least 8 hours, or overnight.

7. Unmold the semifreddo onto a serving dish. Coat it with the toasted coconut, pressing the coconut gently to make it adhere. Serve sliced, with the Burnt Orange Sauce.

Semifreddo alle Noce

WALNUT AND CARAMEL SEMIFREDDO

Serves 8

4 large eggs, at room temperature

1 cup sugar

2 tablespoons dark rum

1 teaspoon vanilla extract

1 cup heavy cream

¾ cup chopped walnuts, toasted

Toasted walnut halves

Whipped cream

1. Line a 9- by 5- by 3-inch metal loaf pan with plastic wrap, leaving a 2-inch overhang on the ends. Chill the pan in the freezer.

2. In the large bowl of an elecric mixer, beat the eggs on high speed until they are thick and pale.

3. Meanwhile, in a small saucepan, combine the sugar and ¼ cup water. Cook over medium heat, swirling the pan occasionally, until the syrup turns a deep golden amber.

4. Remove the pan from the heat and let the syrup stop bubbling. Gradually beat the syrup into the eggs, then beat the mixture for 5 to 8 minutes, or until it is cool to the touch. Beat in the rum and vanilla.

5. In a chilled bowl, beat the cream until it just holds stiff peaks. Fold the cream and chopped walnuts into the egg mixture. Scrape the mixture into the chilled pan. Cover with plastic wrap and freeze for at least 8 hours, or overnight.

6. Unmold the semifreddo onto a serving dish. Garnish with walnut halves and serve with whipped cream.

Semifreddo al Cioccolata con Salsa di Ciliegie

CHOCOLATE SEMIFREDDO
WITH CHERRY SAUCE

Serves 8

CHERRY SAUCE

1 12-ounce bag frozen pitted unsweetened dark cherries

½ cup Cognac

¼ cup sugar

1 teaspoon cornstarch dissolved in 1 tablespoon water

8 ounces semisweet chocolate, chopped

3 large eggs, separated, at room temperature

3 tablespoons sugar

1 teaspoon vanilla extract

1 cup heavy cream

Chocolate curls

1. To make the sauce: In a bowl, combine the cherries, Cognac, and sugar. Let stand for 1 hour.

2. Drain the cherries in a sieve set over a measuring cup, and reserve the liquid. Cut ½ cup of the cherries in half and reserve for making the semifreddo.

3. Add enough water to the measuring cup to equal 1 cup liquid. Pour into a small saucepan and bring to a simmer. Stir in the cornstarch mixture. Bring to a boil and cook for 1 minute. Stir in the whole cherries. Let cool, then cover and chill.

4. Line a 9- by 5- by 3-inch metal loaf pan with plastic wrap, leaving a 2-inch overhang on the ends. Chill it in the freezer.

5. In a metal bowl set over barely simmering water, melt the chocolate, stirring occasionally until smooth. Let cool slightly.

6. In the large bowl of an electric mixer, beat the egg yolks and sugar until the mixture is thick and pale. Beat in the vanilla.

7. In a large bowl, beat the egg whites until they just hold stiff peaks. In another large bowl, beat the cream until it just holds stiff peaks. Gently but thoroughly fold the whites into the cream. Fold half the chocolate into the yolk mixture, and then fold in one third of the cream mixture. Fold in the remaining chocolate and then the remaining cream mixture. Fold in the reserved halved cherries.

8. Scrape into the chilled pan, cover with plastic wrap, and freeze for at least 8 hours, or overnight.

9. Unmold the semifreddo onto a serving dish. Sprinkle with chocolate curls and serve sliced, with the Cherry Sauce.

$\mathcal{S}$emifreddo di Mascarpone con Salsa di Lampone

MASCARPONE SEMIFREDDO WITH RASPBERRY SAUCE

Serves 8

RASPBERRY SAUCE

2 10-ounce packages frozen raspberries in syrup, thawed

1 teaspoon cornstarch dissolved in 2 tablespoons water

1 teaspoon fresh lemon juice

3 large eggs, separated, at room temperature

1/3 cup sugar

8 ounces (1 cup) mascarpone, at room temperature

1 1/2 teaspoons vanilla extract

1/2 teaspoon grated lemon zest

2 ounces semisweet chocolate, finely grated

Fresh raspberries

continued

1. To make the sauce: In a food processor or blender, purée the raspberries. Force the purée through a fine sieve into a small saucepan. Bring the purée to a simmer. Stir in the cornstarch mixture and lemon juice. Bring to a boil and cook, stirring frequently, for 1 minute. Let cool. Cover and chill.

2. Line a 9- by 5- by 3-inch metal loaf pan with plastic wrap, leaving a 2-inch overhang on the ends. Chill the pan in the freezer.

3. In the large bowl of an electric mixer, beat together the egg yolks and sugar until the mixture is thick and pale. Beat in the mascarpone, vanilla, and zest until smooth.

4. In a large bowl, beat the egg whites until they just hold stiff peaks. Gently but thoroughly fold the whites into the yolk mixture.

5. Spoon half the mascarpone mixture into the chilled pan, and sprinkle the grated chocolate evenly over it. Spoon on the remaining mascarpone mixture, and smooth the surface. Cover with plastic wrap and freeze for at least 8 hours, or overnight.

6. Unmold the semifreddo onto a serving dish. Garnish with fresh raspberries and serve with the Raspberry Sauce.

Semifreddo allo Zabaglione con Pistacchi

ZABAGLIONE AND PISTACHIO SEMIFREDDO

Serves 8

5 large egg yolks

¾ cup sugar

3 tablespoons dry Marsala

3 large egg whites, at room temperature

¾ cup heavy cream

¾ cup chopped unsalted pistachio nuts

Fresh strawberries

1. Line a 9- by 5- by 3-inch metal loaf pan with plastic wrap, leaving a 2-inch overhang on the ends. Chill the pan in the freezer.

2. In the top of a double boiler or in a metal bowl, beat together the egg yolks, ¼ cup of the sugar, and the Marsala until well blended. Place over simmering water and beat until the mixture has quadrupled in volume. Remove from the heat. Place the pan or bowl into a larger bowl filled with ice water and let cool, stirring occasionally.

3. In a large bowl, beat the egg whites until they are frothy. Gradually beat in the remaining ½ cup sugar, and beat until the mixture just holds stiff peaks.

4. In a large chilled bowl, beat the cream until it just holds stiff peaks. Gently but thoroughly fold in the whites. Fold in the yolk mixture and then ½ cup of the pistachios. Scrape the mixture into the chilled pan. Cover with plastic wrap and freeze for at least 8 hours, or overnight.

5. Unmold the semifreddo onto a serving dish. Sprinkle with the remaining ¼ cup pistachios. Serve sliced, garnished with the strawberries.

Torta di Semifreddo

SEMIFREDDO TORTE

Serves 10 to 12

When I want to serve a fancy-looking dessert, I make this one. It consists of two meringue layers filled with a creamy frozen mousse. At first glance, it looks like a classic iced white cake. But I like it better because of the contrasting textures of the crispy meringue and creamy filling. There are any number of ways to vary it, by stirring chopped chocolate, crushed cookies, or nuts into the filling or by serving it with different sauces or fruits.

The recipe is based on one I tasted in Bologna, the semifreddo capital of Italy, at Trattoria da Silvio where it is served smothered in hot chocolate sauce.

The recipe seems long but it is only because I have given very detailed instructions for making the meringue layers, which can be prepared at least one day before the filling is added. Don't attempt to make meringues on a damp or rainy day, or they will not dry properly. The entire cake can be assembled and kept tightly wrapped in foil in the freezer for up to three days.

MERINGUE LAYERS

5 large egg whites (⅔ cup), at room temperature

2 tablespoons plus ⅔ cup granulated sugar

2 teaspoons vanilla extract

¾ cup confectioners' sugar

FILLING

1 cup granulated sugar

¼ cup water

2 egg whites, at room temperature

2 cups heavy cream

2 tablespoons orange or amaretto liqueur

1 pint blueberries

2 cups Strawberry Sauce (page 207)

1. To make the meringue layers: Line two large baking sheets with parchment paper. Using the *inside* of the rim of a 9-inch springform pan as a guide, trace three circles onto the paper.

2. Place one oven rack in the upper third of the oven and the second rack in the lower third. Preheat the oven to 225°F.

3. In the large bowl of an electric mixer, beat the egg whites on medium speed until foamy. Gradually add 2 tablespoons of the granulated sugar and continue beating until soft peaks form. Beating constantly, gradually add the remaining ⅔ cup granulated sugar in a steady stream. Add the vanilla, and beat 2 to 3 minutes longer, or until stiff peaks form when the beater is lifted and a small amount of the mixture rubbed between your fingers feels smooth and not grainy, indicating that the sugar is dissolved.

4. Place the confectioners' sugar in a sieve and sift it over the beaten egg whites. With a large rubber spatula, gently fold the confectioners' sugar into the egg whites just until it is incorporated. Do not overmix or the whites will lose their volume.

5. Divide the mixture evenly among the circles on the parchment paper. With a spatula, spread the egg whites out to just within the pencilled lines. (Stay within the lines so you will not have to trim the meringue disks after baking.)

6. Bake the layers for 60 to 75 minutes, rotating the pans halfway through the baking time. If the meringues begin to color, reduce the oven temperature slightly. The meringues are done when they feel firm when lightly pressed in the center. Turn off the oven, open the door completely, and let the meringues cool in the turned-off oven. When cool, slide a metal spatula under the disks and remove them from the paper. Wrap tightly in aluminum foil and store in a dry place.

7. To make the filling: In a small saucepan, combine the sugar and water and bring to a boil over medium heat. Swirl the pan occasionally until the sugar is dissolved, then boil the mixture until large bubbles form and the syrup is slightly thickened, about 2 minutes.

8. Meanwhile, in the large bowl of an electric mixer, beat the egg whites until just frothy.

9. With the mixer on medium speed, gradually add the boiling sugar syrup and beat until the whites are thick and hold stiff peaks. Then continue beating until cool, 8 to 10 minutes longer.

10. In a large chilled bowl, beat the heavy cream and liqueur until soft peaks form. Gently fold the cream into the cooled egg white mixture.

11. Set aside the best-looking of the three meringue layers. Place one of the remaining layers in the bottom of a 9-inch springform pan. If the meringue layers do not fit into the pan, carefully trim them with a knife. Scrape the cream mixture into the pan, and smooth the surface. Top with one reserved meringue layer, pressing it gently onto the filling. Cover tightly and freeze until firm, several hours or overnight.

12. To serve, chop the remaining meringue layer into small pieces. Run a metal spatula around the inside of the springform pan and remove the rim. Pat the crumbled meringue against the sides of the cake. Place on a serving platter. Serve with the blueberries and the Strawberry Sauce.

Salse Dolci

DESSERT SAUCES

A dessert sauce can make an ordinary dessert seem special and a special dessert seem extraordinary. In addition to the sauces in this chapter, there are a number of others throughout this book, paired with the recipes with which they are particularly compatible. This does not mean that they are inseparable, however, and you might enjoy mixing and matching them with other desserts.

These other sauces appear on the following pages:

Strawberry Sauce, page 207
Cherry Sauce, page 216
Hot Chocolate Sauce, page 208
Burnt Orange Sauce, page 213
Raspberry Sauce, page 217
Honey Mascarpone Cream, page 118
Warm Berry Sauce, page 112
Light Chocolate Sauce, page 146
Zabaglione and Variations, pages 140 to 144

Salsa di Caramella alla Panna

CARAMEL CREAM SAUCE

Makes about 1 cup

1 cup sugar

¼ cup water

½ cup heavy cream

1 tablespoon dark rum

1. In a heavy medium saucepan, combine the sugar and water. Cook over medium heat, swirling the pan occasionally, until the sugar caramelizes and turns an even light golden brown.

2. Remove the pan from the heat and swirl the caramel until the bubbles begin to subside. Slowly pour in the cream. The caramel will harden.

3. Place the pan back over medium heat and cook, stirring, until smooth. Remove from the heat, and let cool slightly. Stir in the rum. Serve warm or at room temperature. The sauce can be reheated over low heat.

Fior di Latte

Serves 4 as a dessert, 8 as a sauce

Fior di latte means "flower of the milk," and it is a name that has numerous applications. A variety of ice creams and cheeses are called fior di latte, implying that they are made from the best milk.

This recipe comes from Chef Andreas Hellrigl, owner of New York's spectacular Palio Restaurant. The chef is from the Alto Adige region, near Austria, where this delightful cream is used as a topping or filling or even as a dessert on its own. Try it with Buckwheat Cake (page 52) or as a filling for Cookie Cups (page 35).

¼ cup dark raisins

½ cup hot brewed tea

1 cup heavy cream

2 tablespoons sugar

1 tablespoon kirsch

¼ cup toasted pine nuts

¼ cup crushed vanilla wafers

1. Soak the raisins in the hot tea until the liquid is cool. Drain and pat the raisins dry.
2. In a large chilled bowl, using an electric mixer with chilled beaters, whip the cream with the sugar until stiff peaks form. Beat in the kirsch. Fold in the raisins and the remaining ingredients. Chill for 1 hour.

Crema di Mascarpone

MASCARPONE CUSTARD SAUCE

Makes 2½ cups

§ This sauce goes perfectly with Warm Apple Cake (page 50). Or serve it with toasted panettone. It can be made up to one day in advance and re-heats well.

1¾ cups milk

⅓ cup sugar

1 tablespoon all-purpose flour

1 large egg

½ cup (4 ounces) mascarpone

1 teaspoon vanilla extract

½ teaspoon grated lemon zest

1. In a small saucepan, heat the milk until small bubbles form around the edge. Remove from the heat.

2. In a small bowl, combine the sugar and flour. Beat in the egg. Whisk in the hot milk. Transfer the mixture to the saucepan. Cook over medium heat, stirring constantly, until the sauce comes to a simmer. Cook for 1 minute longer.

3. Pour the sauce into a bowl. Add the mascarpone, vanilla, and lemon zest, and whisk until smooth. Serve warm.

Salsa di Cioccolato al Latte

MILK CHOCOLATE SAUCE

Makes about 2 cups

❧ Serve this light chocolate sauce over ice cream or cake.

3 ounces semisweet chocolate, coarsely chopped
¼ cup sugar
½ hot milk
½ cup heavy cream

1. Place the chocolate and sugar in a heatproof bowl. Add the hot milk. Let stand for 1 minute to soften, then stir until smooth. Let cool to room temperature.
2. In a chilled bowl, using an electric mixer with chilled beaters, beat the cream until soft peaks form. Stir in the cooled chocolate mixture. Chill.

Salsa Mocha

MOCHA SAUCE

Makes about ¾ cup

4 ounces semisweet chocolate, coarsely chopped
½ cup brewed espresso
2 tablespoons unsalted butter
1 tablespoon Cognac, rum, or grappa

1. In a small saucepan, combine the chocolate, espresso, and butter. Heat over low heat until the chocolate is almost melted. Remove from heat and stir until completely smooth.
2. Stir in the Cognac. Serve warm.

Crema di Miele

HONEY CREAM SAUCE

Makes about 3 cups

A rich and sophisticated topping for fresh fruit or plain cakes.

2 *large egg yolks*

⅓ *cup honey*

2 *tablespoons Armagnac or Cognac*

1 *cup heavy cream*

1. In the top of a double boiler or in a medium heatproof bowl, whisk the yolks, honey, and Armagnac until blended. Place over simmering water and cook, stirring, until slightly thickened. Remove from the heat and let cool to room temperature.

2. In a large chilled bowl, using an electric mixer with chilled beaters, beat the cream until soft peaks form. Gently fold in the honey mixture. Serve immediately or refrigerate for up to 4 hours.

Salsa di Mascarpone

MASCARPONE SAUCE

Makes 1¼ cups

🌀 Since mascarpone differs in thickness from one manufacturer to the next, the amount of cream needed to make a smooth sauce will vary. This is lovely served over fresh berries, chocolate or other cake, fruit salads, crostate—in fact, just about any dessert. It keeps for several days.

4 ounces (½ cup) mascarpone

1 to 2 tablespoons confectioners' sugar, to taste

1 tablespoon dark rum

About ½ cup heavy cream

1. In a large bowl, beat the mascarpone with the confectioners' sugar and rum until blended.

2. With a wire whisk, slowly beat in enough cream to make a smooth, thick sauce. Serve immediately, or cover and refrigerate for up to 3 days.

Salsa di Fragole Caramellizata

CARAMEL STRAWBERRY SAUCE

Makes about 3½ cups

At the Locanda da Angelo in Sarzana, this sauce is made tableside and spooned warm over vanilla gelato. I like to serve it with Almond Semifreddo (page 208), though there are plenty of other uses. Any leftover sauce is good chilled.

1 cup sugar

½ cup water

2 pints strawberries, hulled and thickly sliced

2 tablespoons dark rum

1. In a large heavy saucepan, stir together the sugar and water. Bring to a boil over moderately high heat, stirring occasionally. Continue boiling until the syrup is a very light golden color and falls off the end of a spoon in a slow stream, about 10 minutes.

2. Add the strawberries, reduce the heat to moderate, and cook, stirring occasionally, until the strawberries are soft, about 3 minutes. Remove from the heat and stir in the rum. Serve warm, at room temperature, or chilled.

Salse alla Frutta Fresca
FRESH FRUIT SAUCES
Makes about 2 cups

Fruit sauces can be made from purées of many types of soft seasonal or frozen fruit, though it is best to avoid varieties that darken easily, such as bananas or pears, unless they will be used immediately.

The following is a basic recipe that can be adapted according to the fruit used. If you decide to combine fruits, do consider the color that will result, as well as their flavors. Serve with plain cakes, Yogurt Cream (page 152), or gelati.

2 cups fruit, such as whole berries or cut-up kiwis, peaches, nectarines, cantaloupe, or honeydew melon

1 to 2 teaspoons fresh lemon or lime juice to taste (optional)

1 to 3 tablespoons sugar, to taste (optional)

In a blender or food processor, purée the fruit until smooth. Add lemon or lime juice and sugar to taste. Thin to the desired consistency with a tablespoon or so of cool water. For a smoother sauce, pass the purée through a strainer.

Salsa Calda al Rhum

WARM RUM SAUCE

Makes 1½ cups

Yet another variation on zabaglione, this warm, foamy sauce is heavenly with chocolate or gianduja gelati.

> 1 cup heavy cream
>
> 2 large egg yolks
>
> ⅓ cup sugar
>
> 3 tablespoons dark rum, amaretto, or orange liqueur

In the top half of a double boiler or in a heatproof bowl, combine all the ingredients. Place over simmering water, and beat with a hand-held mixer or a wire whisk until thick and foamy, 10 to 20 minutes. Serve warm.

Formaggio

§§§§

CHEESE

Other than fruit, cheese is probably the most popular way for Italians to end a meal. Especially when a dinner is light on meat or other protein, one or two cheeses often are served either alone or with fruit. In addition, there are many desserts made with cheese.

Depending on the region of Italy, the cheese may be made from cow's, sheep's, or goat's milk. Though many Italian cheeses are imported here, some Italian-style cheeses are poor copies that give the real thing a bad name.

On the other hand, just because a cheese is made in Italy does not guarantee that it will be good. Cheese is perishable and if it is too old or has been mishandled, it can be disappointing. It is important to find a good source for cheese. Look for a market with a regular turnover so that the cheese will be fresh. A good store will allow you taste a cheese before buying it and will slice the cheese to your order, instead of selling it only in prewrapped pieces. If you are not satisfied with the look and taste of the cheese you are offered, try another variety.

Store cheese in the refrigerator, tightly wrapped in plastic. For best flavor and texture, remove cheese from the refrigerator at least an hour before serving so that it has a chance to come to room temperature.

Serve some crusty bread or breadsticks or fresh fruit with the cheese. The fruits can be served whole or cut up. Also good with cheese are dried fruits like dates, figs, or prunes and all kinds of toasted unsalted nuts. An artfully arranged platter of cheese with fresh and dried fruits and nuts makes an elegant and easy dessert.

Following are descriptions of some Italian cheeses and suggestions for serving them.

Asiago. From the area around Venice, Asiago is a semi-hard to hard cheese made from cow's milk. It has a natural brown rind and a creamy yellow interior with lots of tiny holes. When young, it has a rich flavor and creamy texture; as it ages it becomes firm and suitable for grating. Serve Asiago with apples or pears.

Bel Paese. Bel Paese is actually the brand name of a semi-soft, mild, and creamy cheese from Lombardy. The flavor is delicate and nutty. It is lovely with strawberries.

Caprino. This is more a category of cheese than a specific variety. The name is derived from the word *capra*, meaning "goat," and caprino is the name given to many different goat cheeses. They can be mild and fresh or aged and sharp. There are many good goat cheeses produced in this country that can be substituted for Italian varieties.

Fontina Val d'Aosta. One of the greatest cheeses of Italy, real Fontina has a rich, nutty flavor and semi-firm texture. Unfortunately, there are many disappointing imitations. Fontina Val d'Aosta has a natural rind—no colored wax or plastic coating. Serve Fontina Val d'Aosta with cherries and red wine or with coarse, whole-grain bread and pears.

Gorgonzola. Italy's best-known blue cheese, made from cow's milk, Gorgonzola can be *dolce* (sweet) or *piccante* (sharp). Either way, it is delicious, with a creamy, buttery texture. Make sure that the cheese looks fresh and not brown or dried out. If possible, smell it. If there is any trace of an ammonia smell, the cheese is too old. Gorgonzola goes beautifully with walnuts and most fruits. If you like a milder Gorgonzola flavor, look for *torta di Gorgonzola*, a layered terrine of Gorgonzola and mascarpone. It is heavenly with strawberries or pears.

Mascarpone. A fresh, soft, cow's milk cheese that tastes like a cross between cream cheese and whipped sweet butter. Super-rich mascarpone can be used in many dessert recipes, but it is also good as a spread or dip for fresh strawberries or dried figs. In fact, mixed with chopped dried fruits and nuts, it would make a delicious, if slightly unorthodox, dip to be served with wine or cocktails. Mascarpone is also good on toast or panettone.

Parmigiano-Reggiano. If I could choose only one cheese, it would be Parmigiano-Reggiano. Authentic Parmigiano is made only in a limited area around the cities of Parma and Reggio Emilia in Italy. Nothing else comes close to it for flavor. A nutty, firm cheese made from cow's milk, it is ideal for cooking and for eating. Always look at the rind of the cheese. The words *Parmigiano-Reggiano* should be stamped into the surface, along with the year in which the cheese was made. A young Parmigiano, about two years old, is best for eating. Older Parmigiano becomes drier, harder, and more piquant. Since it keeps well, I always have a large chunk of Parmigiano on hand. Parmigiano is delicious with dried figs or dates and many kinds of fresh fruit. One of the best combinations I can think of is Parmigiano with toasted walnuts, fresh pears, and red wine.

Pecorino. Like caprino, *pecorino* refers to an entire category of cheeses. *Pecora* is the word for "sheep," and pecorino sheep's milk cheese. There are many varieties of pecorino, mostly made in Central and Southern Italy. They range from the firm, sharp, and salty Pecorino Romano to the mild semi-firm and subtle Pecorino Toscano. Locatelli, a commonly seen cheese, is actually the brand name of a type of Pecorino Romano. For a dessert cheese, choose a mild, semi-firm pecorino. In Tuscany, it is often served drizzled with a fruity extra-virgin olive oil and a sprinkling of pepper. Pecorino is also good with a drizzle of flavorful honey. Serve pecorino with pears, apples, or grapes and nuts.

Ricotta. Sweet, soft ricotta is used in many Italian desserts. Some Italian markets make their own ricotta. Fresh ricotta really is a treat. Try ricotta with fruit or sprinkled with honey or sugar for a simple dessert. It is also good on breakfast toast topped with jam. Some of the best Sicilian pastry is made with sheep's-milk ricotta. Though ricotta is usually made from cow's milk, sheep's-milk ricotta has a lot more character and flavor. Unfortunately, it is hard to find here.

Robiola. From Piemonte, robiola may be made from cow's, sheep's, or goat's milk or a combination. There are many varieties of robiola. It is usually shaped in small, flat rounds and sold as a fresh cheese, though it can be aged until it is very sharp. Both fresh and aged robiola are good marinated with olive oil and pepper or served with a sweet and tart prune purée.

Taleggio. A flat, square cheese with a light orange crust and a creamy, soft interior, rich and savory taleggio is good with ripe pears.

Gorgonzola con Salsa di Fichi

GORGONZOLA WITH FIG SAUCE

Serves 4

Al Bersagliere in Goito near Verona is an elegant restaurant perched on the banks of a small river. We have enjoyed many meals there and always leave room for the cheese course. The restaurant has a splendid assortment of locally made cheeses that are difficult to find elsewhere. My husband especially looks forward to this dish, which is wonderful accompanied by vin santo or another rich dessert wine.

1 cup dried figs

1 cup water

¼ cup sugar

1 2-inch strip lemon zest

4 thin slices Gorgonzola piccante

1. Trim off the hard stems of the figs. Chop the figs fine.

2. In a small saucepan, combine the figs, water, sugar, and lemon zest. Bring to a simmer and cook, stirring occasionally, until the liquid is reduced and thickened, about 20 minutes. Let cool. Discard the lemon zest.

3. Place the Gorgonzola on serving plates. Serve the fig sauce on the side.

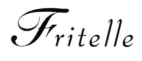

Fritelle

RICOTTA PUFFS

Serves 4 to 6

Crisp and brown on the outside and creamy on the inside, these tender little puffs are nice plain or with a fresh strawberry sauce.

½ cup all-purpose flour

1 teaspoon baking powder

½ teaspoon salt

2 large eggs, at room temperature

2 tablespoons sugar

1 cup whole-milk ricotta cheese

1 teaspoon vanilla extract

Vegetable oil, for deep frying

Confectioners' sugar

1. Combine the flour, baking powder, and salt.

2. In a large bowl, whisk the eggs and sugar until light. Stir in the ricotta and vanilla until blended. Stir in the flour mixture.

3. Fill a deep fryer with oil or pour 1 inch of oil into a deep heavy skillet and heat the oil to 375°F.

4. Drop the ricotta mixture by level tablespoons into the hot oil, and fry until browned on all sides, about 2 minutes. Drain on paper towels. Serve immediately, sprinkled with confectioners' sugar.

Digestivi, Vini da Dessert, e Liquori

§§§§

DIGESTIVES, DESSERT WINES, AND LIQUEURS

Whether it is a digestivo, liqueur, grappa, brandy, or a dessert wine, Italians frequently indulge in an after-dinner drink.

Dessert wines precede the coffee, but the other beverages named may follow it. The custom dates back to a time when elixirs made from distillates or alcohol infusions containing fruits, nuts, herbs, barks, berries or roots were brewed up by alchemists for various health purposes. Eventually, many of these brews were made at home to be shared with friends or family on special occasions. Others were made in monasteries by monks who dispensed them as medicine to their followers or sold them as a means of supporting themselves. Even today, an air of mystery and romance lingers about digestivi and liquori, and their complex formulas traditionally are divided up among two or three trusted custodians who keep the ingredients and proportions a closely guarded secret.

Each region has its own specialties and it has been estimated that there are over three hundred different kinds of after-dinner drinks made in Italy—not including the many kinds of dessert wines.

*D*igestivi

Life would not be as sweet without a touch of bitterness. Perhaps this is why Italians are so enamored of bitter drinks both before and after meals, though they say it is because these bitter drinks, called *amari*, stimulate the appetite and improve the digestion by virtue of their ability to get the gastric juices flowing. Most are lower in alcohol than liqueurs, brandy, and the like.

Some amari are only slightly bitter and make a pleasant, refreshing change from sweet liqueurs. Others are so bitter, harsh, and medicinal that they will leave you gasping, wondering why on earth anyone would voluntarily drink such a thing. But many Europeans enjoy amari, so obviously it is a taste that can be acquired.

The Milanese say that you must try bright red bitter Campari three times before you learn to like it. Campari is usually served as an apperitivo, that is, a drink taken before a meal, but the same advice can be applied to the digestivi taken after a meal.

Digestivi are normally served straight up in tall, narrow glasses, though some people like them with seltzer or mineral water and ice. If you have never tried a bitter digestivo before, this last preparation might be a good way to start. When a digestivo is served neat, a glass of water accompanies the drink so that you can alternate sips.

As a rule, digestivi are not served chilled. Sometimes in winter they are warmed, with a twist of orange or lemon peel. Some people like to pour a small amount of an amaro into their coffee.

Averna. Probably the most popular amaro, Averna comes from Sicily. It is milder than most other types, with a pleasantly bitter flavor that hints of coffee and chocolate. Averna was supposedly the favorite of the kings of Italy in the nineteenth century, so the coat of arms of the House of Savoy appears on the label.

Braulio. Created by Francesco Peloni, the son of a famous doctor and pharmacist in the Valtellina region, Braulio is made from a combination of herbs including yarrow, wormwood, gentian, and juniper that grow on Mount Braulio. Braulio is one of the more pleasant tasting amari.

Fernet Branca. Fernet, as it is commonly called, comes in two varieties, regular and mint. Both are extremely bitter and medicinal tasting, but the Italians swear by them as a cure for digestive problems. Once you have tried them, just the thought of it should be enough to frighten your stomach into submission. Fernet was developed by a Swedish doctor, then perfected by the Branca brothers in nineteenth-century Milan. Its secret formula includes spices and herbs that are cured in oak barrels.

Montenegro. One of the mildest of the digestivi, Montenegro, which comes from Bologna, has a pleasant light chocolate and cherry flavor. The great Italian poet Gabriel D'Annunzio called Montenegro "the liqueur of virtues."

Ramazotti. A mildly bitter amaro, Ramazotti has a flavor somewhere between Averna and Fernet. Among the many herbs and other flavorings in its secret formula is ginseng, an Oriental root that supposedly has aphrodisiac powers.

Unicum. In its cute round bottle, this is one of the more potent amari, a close relation to Fernet. Unicum is made in Solaro, Italy by a Swiss family named Zwack.

Vini da Dessert

Although there are many delicious dessert wines made all over Italy, some of the best come from Sicily, where the strong hot sun concentrates the flavor of the grapes and makes them sweet. Dessert wines go best with plain cakes, biscotti, and cheeses. Don't hesitate to dunk a piece of biscotti into the wine as the Italians do.

Abbazia di Rosazzo Ronco della Abbazia. From the Friuli-Venezia-Giulia region, this is a delicious sweet white wine that tastes of peaches. It is made from Picolit and Verduzzo grapes.

Moscato Passito di Pantelleria. A rich dessert wine produced from dried Muscat grapes grown on the volcanic island of Pantelleria just off the southwestern tip of Sicily. It has a delicious orange and apricot flavor. One of the best is made by De Bartoli and is called Bukkuram.

Caluso Passito. Made from Erbaluce grapes, Caluso has a delicately nutty flavor. It comes from Piedmont.

Malvasia delle Lipari. From the Lipari islands off the coast of Sicily, this rich, smooth, amber-colored wine has a flavor of apricots and honey. Hauner is a good producer.

Moscato d'Asti. A delightful low-alcohol dessert wine with a delicate flavor of orange blossoms, Moscato d'Asti is slightly sparkling. Some of the best is made by Cascinetta.

Asti Spumante. Similar to Moscato d'Asti, Asti Spumante is slightly sweeter and more intensely bubbly. It is delicious alone or with cheese, cookies, or panettone. Try adding a few drops of orange or raspberry liqueur to a glass of Asti Spumante. Good producers include Martini and Rossi, and Cinzano.

Marsala. From Sicily and made in many different styles, both sweet and dry. Dry Marsala is good for cooking or as an apperitivo, while sweet Marsala is best for sipping after a meal. Some of the best producers are De Bartoli, Pellegrino, Florio, and Rallo. Serve Marsala with Parmigiano and almonds.

Picolit. Produced in small quantities in Friuli, this very expensive wine is golden yellow with a delightful floral aroma. Two of the best producers are Ronco del Gnemiz and Livio Felluga.

Recioto di Valpolicella. A rich red wine that goes well with many aged cheeses, particularly Gorgonzola. Bertani is a good producer.

Vin Santo. Most vin santo comes from Tuscany, and it is the quintessential wine for dipping biscotti. It is made by crushing partially dried Malvasia and Trebbiano grapes, then fermenting the juice for three years in wood barrels. Vin santo has a golden amber color and a smooth, rich taste. Good producers include Lungarotti, Frescobaldi, and Castello di Ama.

Recioto di Soave. Made from partially dried grapes of the same varieties used to make soave, one of Italy's most popular white table wines, this wine is not too sweet. Good producers include Masi and Pieropan.

Liquori

Liquori, or liqueurs, are sometimes called cordials. The name *cordial* derives from the Latin word *cordialis*, meaning "of the heart," a reference to the time when these drinks were prescribed for health reasons or as love potions.

Italian cordials are quite sweet. They can be made from all kinds of fruits, nuts, seeds, herbs, and spices. At one time, these drinks were made at home simply by infusing alcohol with sugar and flavorings.

Liquori or cordials can be served straight or on the rocks. Many are good in mixed drinks or with seltzer or mineral water as well. Liquori are also important as flavorings in many desserts.

Ala (Antico Vino Amarascato). Ala is made from an ancient formula that dates back to the Greco-Roman period. The Duca di Salaparuta of Sicily supposedly discovered the recipe and had it recreated for his ballerina girlfriend, who liked to drink it with chocolate candy. It is made from red wine infused with sugar, wild cherry leaves, and almonds. Serve it straight or over ice with a twist of orange.

Amaretto. There are two kinds of amaretto. Most are made from apricot pits, which have a bitter almond flavor, but one company, Lazzaroni, makes theirs in part from the little almond cookies known as amaretti. Amaretto is sweet and mild with a pronounced almond flavor.

Anisette. Clear, licorice-flavored anisette is made from anise seed and is best known as an accompaniment to coffee. Anesone is similar to anisette but not as sweet. It has a higher alcohol content.

Frangelico. With its pronounced hazelnut flavor and bottle shaped like a monk, Frangelico is named for a seventeenth-century hermit. Use it sparingly in desserts, as the flavor tends to be overwhelming.

Galliano. A bright yellow liqueur made from a blend of herbs, berries, and spices. The flavor is a cross between vanilla and anise. Galliano, named for Major Giuseppe Galliano, a hero of the Ethiopian War, comes in a tall bottle featuring the figure of its namesake. It is good straight or in mixed drinks.

Maraschino. A clear, slightly bitter drink made from the marasca, a sour cherry that grows in Northern Italy and Yugoslavia. Maraschino, sold in a straw-covered square bottle, is traditionally used to flavor fruit compotes and many other desserts.

Nocello. A walnut-flavored liqueur in a walnut-shaped bottle, it was traditionally made at home to celebrate a daughter's wedding day.

Rosolio. At one time, every Italian household seemed to have a bottle or two of homemade rosolio tucked away to offer to guests on special occasions. Rosolio is made from alcoholic infusions of rose petals, orange blossoms, cinnamon, cloves, or jasmine flowers. The resulting liquid is clear and pastel-colored, with a mild perfumelike flavor. Today rosolio in a variety of flavors is produced by a number of big manufacturers.

Sambuca. Though it has an anise or licorice flavor, similar to anisette, sambuca actually is made from the berries of a small shrub. Like anisette, crystal-clear sambuca is often served with coffee. There is also a black sambuca, which is flavored with a hint of lemon. One popular way to serve sambuca is *con le mosche*, literally, "with flies." The flies in this case are actually coffee beans, which float in the glass of sambuca. Sometimes the sambuca is set aflame, the idea being that the flames will roast the coffee beans, adding a coffee flavor to the liqueur. I do not recommend trying this in your best crystal glasses. Whether they're been flamed or not, you are supposed to chew on the coffee beans while you sip the sambuca. Sambuca is also good in a cup of espresso.

Strega. Another bright yellow liqueur. The name means "witch." Strega comes from Benevento, near Naples, and is said to contain more than sixty herbs, fruits, barks, and spices. It has a mild, vanillalike flavor.

Tuaca. Said to date back to Renaissance times, Tuaca comes from Livorno on the coast of Tuscany and the label bears the coat of arms of the Medici family. It has a mild but complex flavor hinting of oranges, vanilla, almonds, and coconut.

$$\mathcal{SSSS}$$

Grappa. Grappa belongs in a separate category because it is actually a brandy. After the grapes have been pressed to make wine, the skins that remain are called *vernaccia*. This vernaccia is mixed with water and distilled to make grappa, a fiery drink that is clear when young, amber-colored when aged. At one time, grappa was a peasant drink, but nowadays it has become quite trendy and often is sold in gorgeous Venetian glass bottles. Some grappas are flavored with fruits, herbs, or roots. Good producers include Marolo Brothers, Nonino, and Ceretto.

Caffè

〰〰〰〰

COFFEE

Some part of most Italians' days are spent at the local coffee bar. Neighbors and co-workers meet to discuss current events, have breakfast or a snack, read a newspaper, or hang out—all this over un buon caffè, a good cup of coffee.

Of course, caffès offer more than just coffee. There is no differentiation made in Italy between places that can sell wine and liquor or soft drinks, so caffès, also called bars, usually offer a full range. Wines, liquor, apperitivi, digestivi, and cocktails are offered along with fruit juice, mineral water, sandwiches, sweet rolls, desserts, and snacks. More formal places, like cocktail lounges, are called "American bars."

Food or drink can be had standing at the counter, or seated at a table. The choice is up to you, but you will be charged extra for the use of a table. However, you can sit there all day long and no one will mind. Especially during the morning and afternoon rush, standing at the counter can be fun since you will be in the midst of the action, rubbing elbows with the locals.

Italian caffès offer many variations on the coffee theme. Basic coffee, called espresso or caffè normale, is brewed in an espresso machine from dark-roasted beans. The barman grinds the beans to a fine powder just before using them, and the coffee is brewed fresh a cup at a time for each customer.

The espresso machine is a handsome sight. Usually it is made of polished stainless steel, though you may occasionally encounter one of gleaming copper and brass. Glass tubing and pressure dials make it look very complicated and scientific, but it is really a simple device. Fresh water is pumped directly into the machine from a water line. The water is heated to a relatively low temperature (198°F. is optimal) and forced through the coffee grounds under high pressure. The result is a strong, concentrated coffee with a light layer of foam, called crema, on the surface. The coffee is deep, rich and concentrated, and almost syrupy. A little bit goes a long way, so just a few sips of coffee are served. The tiny cups, called demitasses (meaning half cups), are never filled more than one half full; one third full is most common.

A twist of lemon peel and maybe even a sugared cup rim have come to be associated in this country with good espresso service, but these are absolutely not done in Italy. A well-made cup of coffee does not need lemon, which would only disguise the flavor; and sugar should be added to taste. Most Italians seem to add quite a lot.

If you prefer your coffee a little less concentrated, you can request a caffè lungo, or long coffee, sometimes called caffè alto, or tall coffee. It is made with the same amount of coffee grounds but slightly more water is added. Stronger coffee, made with less water, is called caffè ristretto.

In the summer months, you can order caffè freddo, espresso that is sweetened and refrigerated (often stored in an old wine bottle). If you want your caffè freddo without sugar, you must specify it.

Milk is often added to espresso, though the milky cappuccino, named for the tan robes of the Capuchin monks, is only drunk at breakfast or mid-morning. Cappuccino is a larger serving of espresso topped with a foamy layer of hot steamed milk (not whipped cream). Italians consider it strange to drink cappuccino, which an Italian friend once described as "a big, milky drink," after a meal. The habit of sprinkling chocolate or cinnamon on a cappuccino depends on the bar where it is ordered and the taste of the customer.

Caffè macchiato is a regular espresso with just a macchia, or spot, of steamed milk added. Caffè latte, served at breakfast in a big cup, combines equal parts of coffee and hot milk.

Caffè corretto is espresso "corrected" with a splash of liquor or brandy. Once, when we were staying in Rome for a month, my husband and I got into the habit of stopping every morning at a local bar for breakfast. After a few days, he noticed that his coffee tasted different. The proprietor had slipped him a caffè corretto, fortified with a splash of grappa—quite an invigorating way to start the day.

Decaffeinated espresso goes by the name of caffè Hag, which is actually the name of a popular brand. All of the above coffee variations can be ordered decaffeinated.

American-style coffee is hard to come by in Italy. Since coffee beans there are roasted to a dark color, you are likely to get espresso with cold milk added, so the taste will not be the same.

Making Coffee

When I was growing up, dinner always ended with espresso. Though we would drink American coffee in the morning, espresso would always follow our evening meal, and I was generally assigned the task of making it, probably because I liked it so much. It was not until I became an adult that I learned to make "brown coffee," as we called the American variety.

You can buy an inexpensive stovetop espresso maker to make espresso. There are many variations, but the simplest, called a *machinetta,* has three parts, with a reservoir on the bottom for the water and a central basket for the coffee. When the water is heated, steam pressure forces it up through the coffee grounds and the brewed coffee fills the upper chamber.

Another type, called a *Napoletana*, is actually a drip pot. It also has three sections, but instead of letting the water rise up through the coffee, the pot is inverted. The water is heated in the bottom compartment, and the pot is turned upside down. The water drips through the grounds as opposed to being forced through by steam. The Napoletana is preferred in Southern Italy.

There are also a number of electric espresso makers for the home. Unfortunately, some of the less expensive models do not build up enough steam pressure to make good coffee and the result is insipid. The imported Italian espresso makers do a much better job, though they are also far more costly. But if you love good espresso, it may be worth the investment.

As important as the equipment is the kind of coffee used. Though I have always read that one should grind beans fresh, I find it difficult to grind them as fine as is necessary for my electric espresso maker. On a visit to Trieste, I tasted the most delicious coffee, not just in one coffee shop, but practically everywhere I went. It was made by the Illy company. When I returned home, I learned that Illy Caffè is imported here both as whole beans and ground to a fine powder in decaf and regular varieties. Now I buy the ground coffee by the case—it brews up into the most perfect cup of rich espresso this side of Italy, with a fine crema on top.

Once you have made your espresso, you might want to make it into cappuccino. There are all manner of ways to heat and steam the milk, but if you do not want to purchase the equipment, you can accomplish the same thing with a blender. Just heat the milk gently, then pour it into the blender. Blend on high speed for a minute or until foamy. Pour the espresso into a cup and top with the foamed milk and a dash of cinnamon.

Cioccolata Calda

HOT CHOCOLATE MILANESE STYLE

Serves 4

Winter in Northern Italy can be very cold and wet. We spent one New Year's holiday in Milan, where the gray skies constantly threatened snow, the streets were icy, and a damp wind blew. It was great weather for eating, though. Hearty dishes like polenta, risotto, and bollito misto never tasted so good. Between meals we warmed up with steaming cups of thick hot chocolate accompanied by warm custard-filled *bomboloni* (doughnuts) from our favorite coffee bar.

2 cups milk

6 ounces semisweet chocolate, coarsely chopped

¼ cup sugar

2 teaspoons cornstarch

½ teaspoon vanilla extract

Pinch of cinnamon

1. In a heavy saucepan, combine the milk and chocolate. In a small bowl, stir the sugar and cornstarch together to blend, and add to the saucepan.

2. Heat the mixture, stirring constantly with a whisk, until the chocolate melts and the mixture comes to a boil. Simmer for 1 minute, or until thick. Stir in the vanilla and cinnamon. Serve immediately.

Frullato

FRUIT AND MILK WHIP

Serves 2

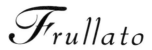 In Rome, frullati are often served as a mid-afternoon refresher or an afternoon snack. Some coffee bars specialize in frullati made with all kinds of fruits, ordinary and exotic, that they will mix up to your order. Kids and adults love them. You can make frullati with just one fruit or with an assortment. Sometimes liqueurs are added.

> 1 cup ripe fruits, such as berries, sliced bananas, or peaches, etc.
>
> ¾ cup milk
>
> 2 to 3 tablespoons sugar, to taste
>
> 2 to 4 ice cubes

In a blender, purée the fruit with the milk and sugar at high speed. Add ice cubes one at a time and blend until smooth. Serve in tall glasses.

$\mathcal{B}$arbajada

HOT COFFEE AND CHOCOLATE DRINK

Serves 2

Neither as sweet or rich as chocolate nor as strong as coffee, this hot chocolate-coffee drink is pleasantly in-between.

   2 teaspoons Dutch-process cocoa powder

   1 to 2 teaspoons sugar, to taste

1½ cups milk

   ½ cup brewed espresso or strong coffee

1. In a small saucepan, combine the cocoa and sugar to taste. Stirring constantly, add a tablespoon or so of the milk, just enough to make a smooth paste.

2. Gradually stir in the remaining milk and the coffee. Heat gently, stirring with a whisk until hot and foamy. Serve immediately.

Caffè dell'Amicizia

VAL D'AOSTA FRIENDSHIP CUP

Serves 4

🌀 This hearty coffee drink is a favorite in the mountainous Val d'Aosta in northwestern Italy. It is traditionally served in a *grolla,* a beautifully carved lidded wood bowl with four or more spouts that is passed around the table from guest to guest until everyone has drunk their fill.

Not everyone adds red wine to their caffè dell'amicizia, but the grappa is essential.

½ *cup brewed espresso*

¼ *cup red wine (optional)*

¼ *cup grappa*

1 *2-inch strip lemon zest*

2 *tablespoons sugar*

1. In a small saucepan, combine the espresso, wine, grappa, lemon zest, and sugar. Heat gently until steaming.

2. Keeping the pan away from your face, carefully light the mixture with a long match. Let simmer until the flames die down, then pour into a grolla or four cups. Serve immediately.

Cappuccino Freddo

ICED CAPPUCCINO

Serves 2

A nice summertime drink. I make the coffee in the morning and leave it at room temperature until I am ready to drink it.

½ cup hot brewed espresso

Sugar to taste

1 cup milk

2 to 4 ice cubes

Ground cinnamon

1. Sweeten the espresso with sugar to taste. Let cool.
2. In a blender, combine the milk and ice cubes. Blend until foamy.
3. Pour the espresso into two glasses. Top each with the foamy milk and a dash of cinnamon.

Tartufi di Cioccolata

CHOCOLATE GRAPPA TRUFFLES

Makes about 40

❦ This recipe did not quite fit into any of the other chapters in this book, so I include it here as these go so well with coffee.

> 8 ounces semisweet or bittersweet chocolate, coarsely chopped
> 4 tablespoons unsalted butter
> ¼ cup strong brewed espresso
> ¼ cup grappa
> About 1 cup Dutch-process cocoa powder

1. In a metal bowl set over a pan of barely simmering water, melt the chocolate with the butter, stirring occasionally until the mixture is smooth.

2. Remove the bowl from the heat and stir in the espresso and grappa. Let cool slightly, then cover and chill for at least 3 hours, or overnight.

3. Spread the cocoa powder on a plate. Scoop up a rounded teaspoon of the chocolate mixture and shape it into a ball. Roll the ball in the cocoa powder, coating it completely. Repeat with remaining chocolate and cocoa, placing the truffles as they are coated in paper candy cups or a wax paper–lined container. The truffles will keep in an airtight container in the refrigerator for 2 weeks.

Bibliography

Artusi, Pellegrino. *La Scienza in Cucina e l'Arte di Mangiar Bene*. Rome: Newton Compton, 1988.

Bastianich, Lidia. *La Cucina di Lidia*. New York: Doubleday, 1990.

Boni, Ada. *Il Talismano della Felicita*. Rome: Editore Colombo, 1972.

Della Salda, Anna Gosetti. *Le Ricette Regionali Italiane*. Milan: Solares, 1980.

Donati, Stella. *Il Grande Manuale della Cucina Regionale*. Milan: SugarCo Edizioni, S.r.l., 1982.

Field, Carol. *The Italian Baker*. New York: Harper & Row, 1985.

———. *Celebrating Italy*. New York: William Morrow & Company, Inc., 1990.

Giacomozzi, Mauro. *I Dolci in Casa*. La Spezia: Fratelli Melita Editori, 1989.

Gosetti, Fernanda. *Il Dolcissimo*. Milano: Fabbri Editori, 1984.

Hazan, Marcella. *The Classic Italian Cookbook*. New York: Knopf, 1976.

———. *More Classic Italian Cooking*. New York: Knopf, 1978.

Malgieri, Nick. *Great Italian Desserts*. Boston: Little, Brown & Company, 1990.

Palazzetti, Adalgisa. *Super Gelati*. Milano: Giovanni De Vecchi Editore, 1985.

Parenti, Giovanni Righi. *La Grande Cucina Toscana*. Vols. 1 and 2. Milan: SugarCo Edizioni S.r.l., 1986.

Piccinardi, Antonio, and James M. Johnson. *The Gourmet's Tour of Italy*. Boston: Little, Brown & Company, 1987.

Romano, Franca Colonna. *Il Sole ai Fornelli*. Milan: Rizzoli, 1982.

Serra, Piero, and Lya Ferretti. *Il Grande Libro della Pasticceria Napoletana*. Napoli: Franco di Mauro Editore, 1983.

Simeti, Mary Taylor. *Pomp and Sustenance*. New York: Knopf, 1989.

Index

G-4

PLEASE SHARE YOUR THOUGHTS
ON THIS BOOK:

COMMENTS:	COMMENTS:
Very good	
COMMENTS:	COMMENTS:
excellent	
COMMENTS:	COMMENTS:
A Real Treat ! Lemon Grita was Excellent	
COMMENTS:	COMMENTS:
COMMENTS:	COMMENTS:
COMMENTS:	COMMENTS: